Viva Practice for the FRCS(Urol) and Postgraduate Urology Examinations

Second Edition

Viva Practice for the FRCS(Urol) and Postgraduate Urology Examinations

Second Edition

Edited by

**Manit Arya, Iqbal S Shergill, Herman S Fernando,
Jas S Kalsi, Asif Muneer and Hashim U Ahmed**

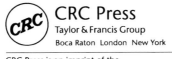

CRC Press
Taylor & Francis Group
Boca Raton London New York

CRC Press is an imprint of the
Taylor & Francis Group, an **informa** business

CRC Press
Taylor & Francis Group
6000 Broken Sound Parkway NW, Suite 300
Boca Raton, FL 33487-2742

© 2018 by Taylor & Francis Group, LLC
CRC Press is an imprint of Taylor & Francis Group, an Informa business

No claim to original U.S. Government works

Printed on acid-free paper

International Standard Book Number-13: 978-0-8153-6621-8 (Paperback)
978-0-8153-6731-4 (Hardback)

Visit the Taylor & Francis Web site at
http://www.taylorandfrancis.com

and the CRC Press Web site at
http://www.crcpress.com

To Maanvii and Krishan, who light up my life.

To Navroop, Mehtaab and Partap, for their support and motivation.

To my parents, Rani and Stanley, who have always stood by me, and my
wife, Deepa, and my daughter, Aditi, for their love and support.

To Harwinder, Serena, Sian and Hari, I thank you for enriching my
life and for all the love and support you give me every day.

To Iaisha, Adam and Jemima, for all your patience and support.

To all my family and friends, without whom nothing in my career would have been possible.

CONTENTS

PREFACE

The Fellowship of the Royal Colleges of Surgeons (FRCS) (Urol) examination is set to test the required standard of a recognised urology specialist in the United Kingdom, i.e. a day one National Health Service (NHS) UK/Ireland consultant. The examination is divided into two parts. The first part is devoted entirely to multiple choice questions (MCQs) and extended matching questions (EMQs) which aim to test the entire urology syllabus in depth.

The second part uses clinical scenarios to form the basis of the *viva voce* section of the examination. These vivas test the candidate on the domains of overall professional capability, knowledge and judgement, logical thought process, safe practice and communication skills.

The aim of this book is to provide a selection of common clinical scenarios together with a guide to answering these questions. Each chapter has been written by consultant urological surgeons or senior urology trainees who have already been successful in passing the examination. The book is intended primarily to be used as a revision tool in conjunction with a larger urology textbook supplemented by lectures and urology journals. In order to avoid an exhaustive list of references, only selected ones are included together under 'References' with some suggested 'Further Reading'. In several chapters a longer list of references has been included as this was deemed appropriate by the editors.

In addition to the FRCS(Urol) examination we hope that the scope of this book will extend to individuals sitting the Fellow of the European Board of Urology (FEBU) and equivalent postgraduate urological examinations in the United States, Australia and Asian countries. Established consultants may also find the text useful as a 'refresher' in areas outside their subspecialist interest.

This book is unique in that it is the first revision book to be published specifically for candidates sitting the FRCS(Urol) examination. This second edition has been published due to continual changes in practice and significant demand. Additionally, the chapters on urological cancers including prostate cancer, bladder cancer and renal cancer have seen important updates due to the emergence of new evidence and changes in National Institute for Health and Care Excellence (NICE), European Association of Urology (EAU) and American Urological Association (AUA) guidelines. Substantial revisions have also been made to other sections such as paediatric urology, female urology, urinary stone disease, benign prostatic hyperplasia and uro-technology to meet standards of current best practice. An extra chapter on the tumour, node and metastasis (TNM) classification of urological cancers has been added. We have made every effort to ensure the information in this book is as accurate as possible and we would like to apologize for any errors contained – please use this book in conjunction with other materials and texts.

The journey from the initial conception of the idea to the final publication involved hard work, frustration and significant time commitment but nonetheless was both exciting and challenging.

We would like to thank all the authors and contributors for their time and hard work.

To the candidates – 'Good luck!'

EDITORS

Manit Arya, FRCS, MD(Res), FRCS(Urol), is a consultant urological surgeon at Imperial College Healthcare NHS Trust, London, University College Hospital, London, and The Princess Alexandra Hospital, Harlow, United Kingdom. His research interests include investigating the molecular basis of prostate cancer – he has been awarded a MD Higher Research degree from the University of London in this field. He has published extensively throughout the urology literature particularly in the field of prostate cancer – he is an editor of 10 textbooks and has published approximately 150 articles in peer-reviewed journals. He is a principal investigator of several National Clinical Trials involving focal therapies (cryotherapy and high-intensity focused ultrasound [HIFU]) for prostate cancer.

Iqbal S Shergill, BSc(Hons), MRCS, FRCS(Urol), FEBU, is a consultant urological surgeon in Wrexham Maelor Hospital, Betsi Cadwaladr University Health Board, Wales. In addition, as recognition of his academic achievements, he is honorary senior lecturer in Manchester Medical School, The University of Manchester; honorary senior lecturer in Division of Biological Sciences, University of Chester; honorary senior lecturer in Division of Medical Sciences, Bangor University; and honorary clinical teacher in Cardiff University School of Medicine, Wales. He has an active interest in teaching, education and research. Currently, he is an assigned educational supervisor for urology trainees, lecturer on National Core Urology Course, panellist at National Selection for Urology Training and course director of Rapid Revision Course for FRCS(Urol). He is also on the Executive Committee for Academic Urology (BAUS) and clinical director at the North Wales and North West Urological Research Centre.

Herman S Fernando, MS, DNB, MRCSEd, MD, FRCS(Urol), FEBU, is a consultant urological surgeon at University Hospital of North Midlands NHS Trust and an honorary clinical lecturer at Keele University. He undertook a period of research in Cardiff University. He is actively involved in teaching, assessments, standard setting and examinations for various regional and national institutions (Royal College and GMC). His main clinical areas of interest are robotic/laparoscopic upper tract oncology and stone diseases.

Jas S Kalsi, BSc(Hons), MRCS(Eng), FRCS(Urol), is a consultant urological surgeon and andrologist at Imperial College in London and at Frimley Health in Surrey and Berkshire. He runs a regional andrology service based at Charing Cross Hospital and at Wexham Park. He is currently clinical lead and clinical governance lead at Wexham Park and Heatherwood hospitals. He is actively involved in education and is a national trainer for Holmium laser enucleation of the prostate (HoLEP) in the United Kingdom. He has been Foundation Training Programme director and educational supervisor for the Oxford Deanery. He is a member of the urology STC in North Thames. He is on the Trust patient safety and consent committee and has a commitment to patient safety and governance. His main clinical interests include andrology (Peyronie's disease, male factor infertility and severe erectile dysfunction) and the management of benign prostate hyperplasia, including the management of large and complex prostates using HoLEP surgery.

Asif Muneer, BSc(Hons), MB, MD, FRCSEd, FRCS(Urol), is a consultant urological surgeon and andrologist based at University College London (UCL) Hospital, United Kingdom. Having completed his higher degree (MD) at UCL he went on to higher surgical training in Oxford. He has published widely on all aspects of urology with main interest in andrology and has also edited *Textbook of Penile Cancer, Atlas of Male Genitourethral Surgery* and *Prosthetic Surgery in Urology*. He has lectured both nationally and internationally and is the president of the British Society for Sexual Medicine and the chair of the BAUS Section of Andrology.

Professor Hashim U Ahmed, FRCS(Urol), PhD, BM, BCh, MA, is chair of urology at Imperial College London. He is an internationally renowned expert in prostate cancer diagnosis, imaging and biopsy as well as minimally invasive therapies for prostate cancer. He has taught dozens of surgeons in these techniques in the United Kingdom and around the world and given numerous invited international lectures in this area as well as has been visiting professor in a number of institutions. He majors in methodological research in imaging and surgical methods and has an extensive research portfolio with about £6M in grant income as a principal applicant and co-applicant to a research programme of approximately £14M. He has published over 150 peer-reviewed papers in areas that have led to key changes in the way we diagnose and treat men with localised prostate cancer.

CONTRIBUTORS

Aruna Abhyankar
Children's Hospital for Wales
Cardiff, United Kingdom

Jim Adshead
Lister Hospital
East and North Hertfordshire NHS Trust
Stevenage, United Kingdom

Jane Boddy
Royal Wolverhampton NHS Trust
Wolverhampton, United Kingdom

Emma Bromwich
Bournemouth and Christchurch NHS
    Foundation Trust
Bournemouth, United Kingdom

John A Bycroft
Lister Hospital
East and North Hertfordshire
    NHS Trust
Stevenage, United Kingdom

Daniel Cohen
Lister Hospital
East and North Hertfordshire NHS Trust
Stevenage, United Kingdom

Ananda K Dhanasekaran
Sandwell General Hospital
Birmingham, United Kingdom

Alan Doherty
Department of Urology
University Hospitals Birmingham NHS
    Foundation Trust
Birmingham, United Kingdom

Gidon Ellis
Whipps Cross University Hospital
London, United Kingdom

Lyndon Gommersall
University Hospital of North Midlands
    NHS Trust
Stoke-on-Trent, United Kingdom

Rizwan Hamid
National Hospital for Neurology and
    Neurosurgery
University College Hospitals
London, United Kingdom

Dominic Hodgson
Solent Department of Urology
Portsmouth Hospital NHS Trust
Portsmouth, United Kingdom

Basharat Jameel
Wrexham Maelor Hospital
Wrexham, United Kingdom

Thomas Johnston
Addenbrookes NHS Foundation Trust
Cambridge, United Kingdom

Vinay Kalsi
Frimley Park Hospital
Camberley, United Kingdom

Farooq A Khan
Luton and Dunstable University Hospital
Luton, United Kingdom

Muhammad Jamal Khan
Frimley Health Foundation Trust
Berkshire, United Kingdom

Ciaran Lynch
Royal Liverpool University Hospital
Liverpool, United Kingdom

David Mak
University Hospital of North Midlands
    NHS Trust
Stoke-on-Trent, United Kingdom

William J McAllister
Broomfield Hospital
Chelmsford, United Kingdom

Suks Minhas
University College London Hospitals
    NHS Trust
London, United Kingdom

Vibhash Mishra
Royal Free Hampstead NHS Trust
London, United Kingdom

Christian Nayar
Wye Valley NHS Trust
Hereford, United Kingdom

Ahmed Qteishat
The Princess Alexandra Hospital NHS Trust
Harlow, United Kingdom

Tina Rashid
Imperial College Healthcare NHS Trust
London, United Kingdom

Mark Rochester
Norfolk and Norwich University Hospital
Norwich, United Kingdom

Julian Shah
National Hospital for Neurology and
    Neurosurgery
University College Hospitals
London, United Kingdom

Davendra M Sharma
St Georges's Hospital
London, United Kingdom

Arash K Taghizadeh
Evelina London Children's Hospital
Guys and St Thomas' NHS Trust
London, United Kingdom

Oliver Wiseman
Addenbrookes NHS Foundation Trust
Cambridge, United Kingdom

CHAPTER 1
PROSTATE CANCER

Hashim U Ahmed, Jane Boddy, Alan Doherty,
Lyndon Gommersall and Manit Arya

Contents

PROSTATE-SPECIFIC ANTIGEN (PSA) AND PROSTATE CANCER DETECTION

Q. A 66-year-old man with a PSA of 5.3 is referred to you. Testing was performed during a routine health check with his GP. He has mild lower urinary tract symptoms but is otherwise fit and well. Examination revealed a small benign feeling prostate. How would you assess this man?

A. A full urological history should be taken with an emphasis on lower urinary tract symptoms (LUTS), age, race, family history and history of urinary infections. If advanced disease is suspected then a history of bone pain, leg swelling, anorexia, weight loss, coagulopathy and new onset peripheral neurology is important. A general urology examination should be performed along with a digital rectal examination. If there is high-quality multiparametric MRI (mpMRI) available in my unit, then I would offer an mpMRI prior to biopsy. I would then offer a transrectal ultrasound (TRUS) guided systematic prostate biopsy with targeting of any suspicious areas, quoting a 1%–2% risk of severe sepsis. Almost all patients experience some bleeding (rectal bleeding/haematuria/haematospermia) following this procedure which then resolves. Treatment is dependent on the grade and stage of the tumour as well as any co-morbidity.

Q. What is PSA?

A. PSA is a 34 kD serine protease. This glycoprotein was first discovered in 1970. Also known as human kallikrein 3 (HK3) it has 261 amino acids. HK2 and HK1 also exist. It is encoded by a gene on chromosome 19. It is secreted uniquely by prostatic ductal epithelial cells and its biological effect is to liquefy the seminal coagulum within the ejaculate. It is synthesised as pre-pro-PSA which is converted to pro-PSA and then PSA. PSA exists in three forms in serum:

1. Free – Unbound with a half-life of between 2 and 3 hours.
2. Bound to alpha-1 antichymotripsin (ACT – a serine protease inhibitor or serpin), this form has some epitopes exposed which affects free to total PSA measurement. It has a half-life of 4–5 days.
3. Bound to alpha-2 macroglobulin (AMG – all five PSA epitopes are covered making this more difficult to quantitate) with a half-life of 4–5 days.

Overall PSA has a half-life of between 2 and 3 days. Total PSA therefore equates to:

$$\text{Total PSA} = \text{Free PSA} + \text{Complexed PSA}$$
(i.e. ACT bound PSA but not including AMG bound PSA)

The measurement of PSA is now automated using a monoclonal antibody assay technique and commercially produced antibodies.

Q. What is a normal PSA?

A. There is no PSA cut-off that completely predicts the absence of prostate cancer. However in clinical practice a normal PSA can be defined as either being lower than an absolute figure (generally considered as 3 or 4 ng/mL) or as a range of values related to the patient's age. Oesterling described the most commonly used age-specific reference ranges for PSA [1]. This is reproduced in Table 1.1. More recently Sun et al. have reported on 12,078 patients who have been retrospectively reviewed following prostate biopsy [2]. In this study receiver operative characteristics (ROC) analysis of the PSA results demonstrated a normal PSA cut-off as 2.3 ng/mL. An analysis of the Swedish Cancer Registry data showed that a very low PSA at the age of 50 years (usually less than 1.2 ng/mL) confers a very low (about 1%) probability of cancer-specific mortality over 15 years.

PSA is prostate specific but not prostate cancer specific. It is also elevated in benign prostatic hyperplasia, prostatitis, catheterisation and other non-malignant conditions.

Note: *The threshold of 4 ng/mL was defined from the use of ROC analysis, a technique used in radar detection of enemy aircraft during the Second World War. From the 1970s this approach was applied to medical testing in general. For a range of values this technique delineated when a given signal is more likely to be enemy aircraft than radar artefact. When applied to PSA readings it showed that PSA can distinguish between benign disease or malignancy at a certain threshold.*

The original clinical work on PSA was performed by Catalona et al. in the early 1990s [3]. This study investigated men invited to attend for a PSA blood test. They were stratified into three groups according to their PSA. The first group had a PSA between 0 and 4 ng/mL, the second between 4 and 10 and the third over 10. Each patient with a PSA greater than 4 ng/mL was offered a prostate biopsy. Prostate cancer was detected in 26% of the patients with a PSA between 4 and 10 ng/mL and in 53% of patients with a PSA of greater than 10 ng/mL. More recently the prostate cancer prevention trial (PCPT) gives further insight into the percentage of positive biopsies for a 'normal' PSA [4]. These data are reproduced in Table 1.2. This landmark study reveals the high proportion of patients with prostate cancer with low PSA readings. A criticism of the PCPT is the overdiagnosis of prostate cancer, i.e. a man's lifetime risk of developing prostate cancer is approximately 16% but in the PCPT trial, prostate cancer was detected in 24.4% of patients analysed.

Table 1.1 Oesterling's age-specific reference ranges

Age	PSA (ng/mL)
40–50	2.5
50–60	3.5
60–70	4.5
70–80	6.5

Source: Adapted from Oesterling JE et al. *JAMA* 1993; 270: 860–864.

Table 1.2 Prevalence of prostate cancer among men with a prostate-specific antigen level less than 4 ng/mL

PSA range (ng/mL)	Prevalence of prostate cancer (%)
<0.5	6.6
0.6–1.0	10.1
1.1–2.0	17.0
2.1–3.0	23.9
3.1–4.0	26.9

Source: Adapted from Thompson IM et al. *N Engl J Med* 2004; 350: 2239–2246.

Gerstenbluth et al. reported on the positive predictive value of PSA. A PSA of greater than 20 ng/mL relates to an 87% chance of prostate cancer being detected on biopsy. Table 1.3 reports the positive predictive value for PSA ranges from this same paper [5].

Table 1.3 Positive predictive value for various PSA ranges

PSA range (ng/mL)	Positive predictive value (PPV) (%)
PSA 20–29	74
PSA 30–39	90
PSA 50–99	100
PSA >20	87

Source: Adapted from Gerstenbluth RE et al. *J Urol* 2002; 168: 1990–1993.

Q. What do you know about PSA velocity (PSAV)?

A. PSA is not a specific test. To improve the accuracy of detection of prostate cancer many adaptations of PSA have been described (Table 1.4). PSAV is defined as the rise in PSA per year in ng/mL/y. A rise in PSA of greater than 0.75 ng/mL/y is associated with an increased risk of prostate cancer [6]. Sun et al. use a PSAV cut-off of 0.6 ng/mL/y [2]. Ideally at least three PSAs are required to produce a PSAV reading due to the variability of the test. This is calculated with the following equation:

$$PSAV = 0.5 \times (PSA2 - PSA1/time\ 1\ in\ years + PSA3 - PSA2/time\ 2\ in\ years)$$

Table 1.4 PSA derivatives and normal values

PSA derivative	Normal
PSA velocity	<0.6–0.75 ng/mL/year
PSA doubling time	More than 3 years
PSA density	<0.15 ng/mL/mL
PSA transitional zone density	<0.35 ng/mL/mL
Free to total PSA	>20%
Supersensitive PSA	<0.01 ng/mL

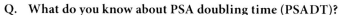

Q. What do you know about PSA doubling time (PSADT)?

A. PSADT is defined as the length of time that a patient's PSA takes to double in months or years. PSADT is useful in patients under surveillance for high PSA readings and negative biopsies, active surveillance for low-risk disease or patients with a rising PSA following radical treatment. It is calculated using regression analysis of the PSA tests recorded. The Marsden experience with active surveillance uses a PSADT of less than 2 years. The data on active monitoring provide useful information on how to follow patients with a high PSA who have negative biopsies. Following radical prostatectomy biochemical progression can be due to local recurrence, lymph node positive disease or metastatic disease. Calculation of the PSA doubling time can elucidate between these two scenarios. In one study a PSADT <4.3 months suggested metastatic disease and a PSADT of >11.7 months suggested local recurrence [7]. This is important in deciding whether adjuvant local treatment is appropriate. Similar data exist for post radiotherapy biochemical progression.

Q. What do you know about PSA density (PSAD)?

A. PSAD is defined by the serum PSA per millilitre of prostate tissue. Prostate volume can be measured using the ellipsoid volume formula:

$$\text{Prostate volume} = \text{Height} \times \text{Width} \times \text{Length} \times 0.52$$

A PSAD of >0.15 ng/mL/mL of prostate tissue is more likely to lead to a diagnosis of prostate cancer [8]. Other authors have not proven the utility of PSAD. This may relate to the inability to accurately measure prostate volume and the considerable variability of PSA production from benign prostate epithelium. PSAD when applied to equivocal mpMRI findings of the prostate was much more useful in reducing the false-negative rate of mpMRI.

The PSA transitional zone density (PSATZD) can also be quantified. This is defined as the amount of PSA per millilitre of transitional zone tissue. Djavan et al. described a normal value of 0.35 ng/mL and published a PPV of 74% for PSA levels less than 10 ng/mL [9]. This result has not been replicated.

Q. What do you know about free to total PSA (f/T PSA)?

A. f/T PSA is defined as the percentage free PSA compared to the total PSA in serum. PSA exists in serum as either free PSA or bound to ACT and AMG. Prostate cancer has a significantly lower f/T PSA value compared with BPH in the PSA range 4–10 ng/mL [10]. A cut-off of greater than 25% suggests benign disease. Despite several early meta-analyses which showed the clinical utility of f/T PSA had not been clearly defined, recent studies in developing nomograms have shown that it can be predictive.

Q. What do you know about supersensitive PSA (sPSA)?

A. sPSA enables PSA to be detected to a threshold of 0.003 ng/mL. Following radical prostatectomy 10%–40% of patients will develop biochemical relapse. An undetectable PSA is defined as <0.01 ng/mL. In a study of 200 patients following radical prostatectomy if the PSA nadir was <0.01 then biochemical progression occurred in only 3% of patients compared to 75% if this level was not attained [11]. This assay therefore allows the early detection of biochemical relapse after radical prostatectomy and can expedite the use of secondary interventions.

Q. Does digital rectal examination (DRE) change the PSA results?

A. Many factors alter the serum PSA level. In a series of 202 patients the DRE significantly changed the PSA by only 0.26 ng/mL. It was concluded that PSA elevation due to DRE was clinically insignificant [12].

Q. What is uPM3 or PCA3?

A. The uPM3 test detects prostate cancer antigen 3 (PCA3), a non-coding segment of mRNA. It is a gene specifically produced by prostate epithelial cells 60–100 times more in prostate cancer than benign prostatic disease [13]. A uPM3 or PCA3 test is performed by collecting the first 20–30 mL of urine voided following vigorous prostatic massage. The ratio of PCA3 to PSA mRNA can then be calculated. The test claims to have a specificity of 70%. It is sometimes used in men with a negative TRUS biopsy prior to further biopsy in the event of persistently elevated serum PSA.

Q. Is screening for prostate cancer justified?

A. Prostate cancer screening has a considerable evidence base but there is controversy about offering it within healthcare systems. Therefore it is not currently undertaken in the United Kingdom or Europe as a whole. In the United States, the U.S. Preventative Services Taskforce issued guidelines in 2012 advocating against wholesale PSA screening. Recently, in 2017, these guidelines were changed to advocate discussing PSA testing with men between the ages of 55 and 69 years with appropriate informed decision making with the patient. In the United Kingdom a policy of early detection through case finding is recommended via the prostate cancer risk management programme (www.cancerscreening.nhs.uk/prostate). This aims to ensure concerned individuals receive clear and balanced information about the advantages and disadvantages of the PSA blood test and treatment of prostate cancer before receiving the test.

Prostate cancer screening is controversial and does not fulfil all the Wilson and Junger's (World Health Organisation [WHO]) criteria for a good screening programme (Table 1.5). Prostate cancer is an important health problem with a 16% lifetime risk of developing it and a 3% risk of dying from prostate cancer. In the United Kingdom in 2014 the incidence was over 46,000 cases (Office of National Statistics data). The disease has a long latent period often allowing the patient to die of other causes rather than prostate cancer. PSA is an acceptable screening test for patients but lacks sensitivity and specificity. Digital rectal examination, TRUS and prostate biopsy are invasive which would be required by a large group of men in a screened population.

The European Screening trial and the prostate, lung, colorectal and ovarian (PLCO) trial from the United States have differed in their conclusions on the benefit of screening reducing mortality with the European Screening study showing a survival benefit using screening and the PLCO study showing no survival benefit. It is now accepted that the PLCO had significant contamination in that many men in the control arm had PSA testing anyway. Estimates put this at well over 50% and possibly even 70%–90%.

Although localised prostate cancer can be treated with surgery, radiation or more novel techniques, some recent randomised controlled trial (RCT) data have drawn light on the small benefit on reduction in metastases and mortality using treatment compared to active monitoring or watchful waiting.

However, one of the first groups to report was the Scandinavian Prostate Cancer Group – this study has reported a number of published papers on the success of radical prostatectomy versus watchful waiting. The group has reported that radical prostatectomy significantly improved local progression, metastasis and prostate cancer death (both prostate cancer specific mortality and importantly overall mortality) at a median follow-up of just over 8 years [14]. The latest article in the series published the results at approximately 13 years median follow-up and demonstrated that the significant overall survival benefit was more notable in men less than 65 years of age and also that radical prostatectomy reduces metastatic disease burden, androgen deprivation therapy and palliative treatments across all age groups as compared with watchful waiting [15].

In contrast in 2012, Wilt et al. showed that in men randomised between radical prostatectomy and watchful waiting diagnosed early in the PSA screening era of the United States, there was no overall survival or cancer-specific survival difference between the two arms. Subgroup analyses showed that there was a benefit in treating high-risk disease and probably in intermediate-risk disease but not in low-risk disease [16].

In 2017, Hamdy et al. reported on the ProtecT (prostate testing for cancer and treatment) trial which randomised men between radiotherapy, surgery and active monitoring [17]. They showed no survival difference at 10 years between these three arms which recruited from men diagnosed in the screening arm of the UK screening study called CaP. There were no differences in subgroups in this study. They showed a slight reduction in metastases in favour of treatment but there is criticism that ProtecT did not carry out modern active surveillance which might have not even showed this difference.

Radical treatment can obviously also have side effects with surgical and radiotherapy series reporting significant problems with erectile dysfunction (ED), incontinence, voiding LUTS and rectal toxicity [18]. The multidisciplinary team framework and recent National Institute for Health and Care Excellence (NICE) guidelines solidify the indication for treatment at all stages of prostate cancer. Without definitive evidence that prostate cancer screening decreases prostate cancer-specific mortality the cost per year of life saved is difficult to quantify. Overall it seems unlikely that such a programme will exist in the near future.

Table 1.5 Wilson and Junger criteria for a screening programme

1. The condition sought should be an important health problem for the individual and community.
2. There should be an accepted treatment or useful intervention for patients with the disease.
3. The natural history of the disease should be adequately understood.
4. There should be a latent or early symptomatic stage.
5. There should be a suitable and acceptable screening test or examination.
6. Facilities for diagnosis and treatment should be available.
7. There should be an agreed policy on whom to treat as patients.
8. Treatment started at an early stage should be of more benefit than treatment started later.
9. The cost should be economically balanced in relation to possible expenditure on medical care as a whole.
10. Case finding should be a continuing process and not a once and for all project.

Source: Adapted from Wilson JMG and Junger G. *J R Coll Gen Pract* 1968; 16: 318 [49].

In terms of the evidence for prostate cancer screening, several studies are now quoted:

1. *The Quebec study* – In the Quebec study patients were randomised to screened and non-screened populations. Initial reports showed a 70% decrease in prostate cancer death rates in the screened population. However this trial has been widely criticised due to cross-contamination of the patient groups. Further analysis on an intention to screen basis has shown no difference in mortality.
2. *The Tyrol study* – The Tyrol study is a natural experiment comparing two areas of Austria. In the Tyrol free PSA testing was introduced and a 70% uptake achieved. This resulted in a 44% decrease in prostate cancer mortality in 2000. However this effect was too rapid to explain this outcome. To elucidate the efficacy of localised disease treatment would take a far longer period of time and therefore these results probably represent aggressive treatment of locally advanced and metastatic disease.
3. *The Seattle and Connecticut study* – Seattle and Connecticut have very disparate socioeconomic populations. Seattle is prosperous and has more PSA screening and aggressive treatment of prostate cancer than in Connecticut. However no difference in prostate cancer mortality was demonstrated in these two populations.
4. *European Randomised Study of Screening for Prostate Cancer (ERSPC)* – This was conducted in several countries and has reported several times. The most recent was after 13 years of median follow-up and showed that one prostate cancer death was averted per 781 men invited for screening and that 27 screened men would have to be treated to prevent 1 death.

5. *The U.S. Prostate, Lung, Colon and Ovary (PLCO) trial* – This showed no mortality difference between systematic PSA testing and opportunistic PSA testing although recent data show that PSA testing in the control arm was likely to be as high as 90%.

Q. What do you know about the Prostate Cancer Prevention Trial (PCPT)?

A. The PCPT reported on 18,882 men randomised to receive prostate cancer chemoprevention with finasteride 5 mg od or placebo for 7 years [19]. The entry criterion was simply a PSA of less than 3 ng/mL. Prostate biopsies were performed if an abnormal DRE or PSA >4 ng/mL was found. All patients were offered an end-of-study biopsy. The study closed 15 months early due to significant results being achieved. It was then published in the *New England Journal of Medicine* in 2003. The study found a relative risk reduction in prostate cancer of 24.8% in the finasteride group. However a higher incidence of high-grade cancer (Gleason score 7, 8, 9 or 10) was detected in the finasteride arm (6.4%) compared to the placebo arm (5.1%). This worrying effect has been discussed at length in the urological literature. The main issues are first that cancer was detected in four times the number of patients than expected, and second that cancers were low or intermediate grade. The possible explanations of these findings have been discussed by Grover et al. among others [20]. They concluded that

- Finasteride may induce histological changes that mimic those seen in high-grade cancer.
- High-grade tumours are resistant to androgen deprivation and are unaffected by finasteride.
- Treatment created an environment that promotes the growth of high-grade tumours.
- These results may be an artefact due to increased detection (finasteride reduces prostate volume).

The REDUCE (Reduction by Dutasteride of Prostate Cancer Events) trial was an international, multicentre, double-blind, placebo-controlled chemoprevention study using the dual inhibitor of 5 alpha reductase subtypes I and II, dutasteride. In this trial patients were enrolled with a negative prostate biopsy within 6 months of entry and a PSA of between 2.5–10 ng/mL (50–60 years) and 3–10 ng/mL (>60 years). Repeat biopsy was performed at 2 and 4 years. The trial showed a relative risk reduction in detected cancer on biopsy with dutasteride of 22.8% over the 4-year study period [21]. However, once again there were some concerns in the numbers of higher-grade cancers detected in the dutasteride group in years 3–4 of the study.

MANAGEMENT OF THE PATIENT WITH AN ELEVATED PSA

Q. A 62-year-old man is referred urgently from his GP with a raised PSA of 6.4 ng/mL. He had the PSA blood test performed due to deterioration in his urinary symptoms. A midstream specimen of urine (MSU) was negative and he is otherwise well. He is concerned and is anxious about further assessment. How would you assess this patient in clinic?

A. A full urological history should be taken including his age, race, LUTS, urinary tract infection, bone pain and family history of prostate cancer. A general examination would precede examination of his external genitalia and a DRE. If advanced disease is suspected one should also look for leg swelling, anorexia, weight loss, bone tenderness and neurological defects suggesting spinal cord compression. This relatively young patient has an abnormal PSA reading and therefore he should be counselled about further tests, either upfront TRUS prostate biopsy with an explanation that we are concerned about a diagnosis of a prostate cancer or, as is becoming more common, *pre-biopsy* multiparametric MRI of the prostate, if I have access to a high-quality service for this locally. I will explain the pros and cons of biopsy to him including the risks of severe bleeding (1%), severe infection (1%–2%), pain and urinary retention. Many men will experience haematospermia, rectal or urethral bleeding or both following this procedure. If his upfront biopsy results are negative, one would continue to follow him up with a further PSA blood test in 6 months' time. If another biopsy is indicated, then I would consider an initial mpMRI or a transperineal template biopsy. If his biopsy is positive then he should be counselled regarding the available treatment options. He may need further investigation of his lower urinary tract symptoms prior to treatment.

Q. How do you perform a prostate biopsy?

A. Transrectal prostate biopsy is performed with a 7.5 MHz transrectal ultrasound probe. Many are now bidirectional allowing multiplanar views. Antibiotic prophylaxis is required. Regimes vary between hospitals but commonly intravenous gentamicin, rectal metronidazole and three doses of a quinolone are prescribed. After informed consent, including the risks of bleeding, infection, pain and acute urinary retention, a digital rectal examination is first performed assessing the prostate for size and consistency. The ultrasound probe is then inserted into the rectum. The prostate is then scanned to detect any capsular breach or hypoechoic areas within the periphery of the prostate. Using the ellipsoid volume formula (height × breadth × width) × 0.52 the prostate volume can be calculated. The PSAD can then be calculated. Local anaesthetic peri-prostatic injections have been shown to reduce the pain of prostate biopsy in a RCT [22]. A total of 12 biopsy cores are now considered standard and is an acceptable compromise between increased cancer detection and the morbidity from the procedure. Targeting of the periphery of the prostate is essential due to the higher proportion of prostate cancers diagnosed in this anatomical location (approximately 85% of prostate cancers are found in the peripheral zone of the prostate and 15% in the transition zone).

Q. What are the chances of finding prostate cancer in further biopsies?

A. Djavan et al. looked at prostate biopsies in a series of 1051 men with a normal DRE and PSA between 4 and 10 ng/mL. This study reported that the chance of finding a prostate cancer on the first, second, third and fourth biopsy were 22%, 10%, 5% and 4%, respectively [23]. The more biopsies that are taken, the lower the Gleason score of the cancer is when it is detected. Therefore a second biopsy is often considered in many patients with serial abnormal PSAs, but the more biopsies that are taken the more confident the clinician can be that the disease will be insignificant.

Q. Is there a role for pre-biopsy MRI in men with an elevated PSA?

A. There have been a number of studies, such as the UK PROMIS study [24], which have shown multiparametric MRI of the prostate can detect higher-risk disease with better sensitivity than TRUS biopsy. The important point about MRI of the prostate is that it has to be multiparametric (including T2-weighting, diffusion weighting, dynamic contrast enhancement), with a high-quality 1.5 Tesla or 3 Tesla scanner and reported by an expert uro-radiologist. There is still controversy about how to manage men with a negative or non-suspicious mpMRI of the prostate as the false-negative rate can vary between 5% and up to 25%. This is often because of difference in expertise and experience between and within centres, different ways of comparing the mpMRI to histology and different definitions of what is high-risk cancer. Most urologists would still biopsy the prostate if the mpMRI is negative because of concern about missing some Gleason 7 tumours and concern about the inter-observer variability of reporters. In this case of a non-suspicious MRI, I would discuss with my patient the false-negative rate of mpMRI and TRUS biopsy, the risks and benefits of biopsy and the problems of missing important cancer if we do not biopsy and overall advise he undergo a systematic biopsy.

Q. The multiparametric MRI is as shown in Figure 1.1. What can you see?

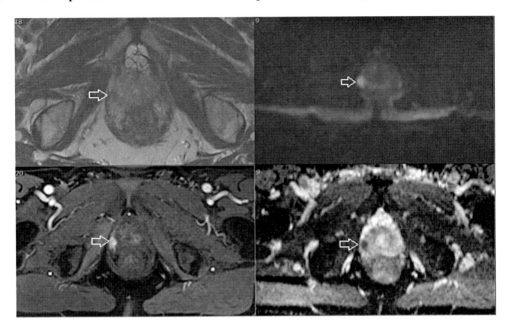

Figure 1.1

A. I would want to see the full series of scans (T2, diffusion weighted and dynamic contrast-enhanced images) using a dedicated DICOM software viewer or a PACS system. I would want this reported by a dedicated uro-radiologist.

However, I can see the following on these images provided:

- *Top left* – This is an axial T2-weighted MRI scan of the prostate delineating the peripheral zone and the transition clearly. In the right peripheral zone I can see a *hypo*intense/low signal area that is potentially suspicious.
- *Top right and bottom right* – These are diffusion weighted images (DWIs).
  - *Top right* – This is the long b DWI image that shows restricted diffusion with high signal intensity in the area of concern in the right peripheral zone.
  - *Bottom right* – This is the ADC (apparent diffusion coefficient) map in which the lesion is seen as an area of low signal intensity.
- *Bottom left* – This is a contrast-enhanced image (contrast used in mpMRI is gadolinium) in which the corresponding area is shown to have early intense contrast enhancement (tumours have early contrast enhancement and also demonstrate early washout of contrast).

In summary the lesion enhances early with contrast and has a diffusion signal so this lesion would be scored highly suspicious on the MRI and would need to be targeted with biopsies (in addition to taking systematic biopsies of the prostate).

Q. What is the PIRADS score on MRI?

A. PIRADS, Prostate Imaging Reporting and Data System, is a standardised way of reporting the level of suspicion that a radiologist has for there being clinically significant prostate cancer on a multiparametric MRI. There is an alternative scale called Likert that is similar. The scale means the following:

1 = Highly unlikely for the presence of clinically significant prostate cancer
2 = Unlikely for the presence of clinically significant prostate cancer

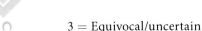

3 = Equivocal/uncertain

4 = Likely for the presence of clinically significant prostate cancer

5 = Highly likely for the presence of clinically significant prostate cancer

The higher the score, the greater is the chance of finding high-risk prostate cancer.

Q. The highly suspicious lesion on mpMRI of the prostate in the previous questions is scored 5 on the Likert scale. What are the different ways you might target this?

A. The broad approach to targeting is whether one does this using a cognitive (or otherwise known as visually estimated) approach or using software and devices to help guide the needle. Most of the studies so far have shown no significant difference between cognitive and image-fusion targeting in expert hands. Fusion can be done using rigid or elastic methods, with elastic fusion taking into account the deformation that occurs when a TRUS probe is used. There is no definite evidence that this makes a difference in fusion. Targeting can also be done inside the MRI scanner although this can be expensive and take a significantly longer time. Targeting can be done using a transrectal approach or a transperineal approach with most of the transperineal cases being done under general anaesthetic. Recently, some groups have used local anaesthetic and sedation to do transperineal biopsies.

Q. How would you manage a patient with high-grade prostatic intraepithelial neoplasia (HGPIN) on biopsy?

A. HGPIN has been proposed as a precursor to prostate cancer but this remains unproven. If HGPIN is found in one core then the patient has a 20% chance of prostate cancer on further biopsies. If more than one core identifies HGPIN then the next biopsy can be positive for prostate cancer in up to 70%. In 82% of radical prostate specimens HGPIN is shown, but only 40% of BPH specimens show HGPIN after transurethral resection of the prostate (TURP). HGPIN does not secrete PSA. With an overall positive biopsy rate of 24% on second biopsy, this is similar to the detection of prostate cancer in the PCPT trial. Clinically the European Association of Urology (EAU) guidelines recommend repeat biopsy if HGPIN is found in three or more prostate biopsies but the interval is unclear.

Q. How would you manage a patient with atypical small acinar proliferation (ASAP) on biopsy?

A. ASAP has a 40% detection of prostate cancer on repeat biopsy compared to 24% with HGPIN. The EAU guidelines recommend repeat biopsy but the interval is unclear. Due to the higher detection of prostate cancer on subsequent biopsy with ASAP a more aggressive approach to repeat biopsy is often undertaken. Recent studies in which MRI-targeted biopsies have found ASAP, the rate of Gleason 7 or more cancer on repeat biopsies is very low so men evaluated in this manner could just undergo PSA surveillance.

Q. What do you know about epidemiology, diet and chemoprevention in prostate cancer?

A. Prostate cancer affects 100 in 100,000 men in the Western world. Post-mortem series suggest that the prevalence is very high with 30% of 50-year-olds having the disease, increasing to 80% at 80 years. However, only a small proportion of these patients develop clinically significant, life-threatening cancer. In the United Kingdom in 2014, over 46,000 men developed prostate cancer making the disease a significant health problem.

Dietary factors have been shown to affect the risk of prostate cancer. The factors that increase the risk of prostate cancer include obesity (relative risk 1.1), meat (not much data) and dairy products (higher risk). A reduced risk of prostate cancer has been publicised for many components of a man's diet with limited evidence. These include fruit and vegetables (no benefit), beta-carotene 50 mg (no benefit), lycopene (possible benefit), vitamin D (no benefit), vitamin E and selenium (both no benefit – in fact results from the Selenium and Vitamin E Cancer Prevention Trial, SELECT, demonstrated that men should avoid selenium or vitamin E supplementation at doses that exceed recommended dietary intakes as this resulted in an increased risk of being diagnosed with prostate cancer including high-risk cancers). In addition, the PCPT trial has shown the possible chemoprevention benefit of finasteride compared to placebo in decreasing the incidence of prostate cancer, although this may be at the expense of an increase in higher-grade cancers (see previous discussion).

Q. **What do you know about hereditary prostate cancer?**

A. Familial prostate cancer represents about 9% of prostate cancer patients and relates to a clustering of prostate cancer cases within a family. Hereditary prostate cancer by definition must have three generations affected with three first-degree relatives or three relatives under the age of 55 years. In addition, prostate cancer in a family infers an increased risk of prostate cancer. If one relative is affected then a 2–3× risk is transferred, if two relatives are affected then a 5× risk is transferred and for three relatives an 11× risk is transferred. Familial breast cancer confers a greater risk of prostate cancer within a particular family. The BRCA 2 gene particularly has been implicated in this relationship.

LOCALISED PROSTATE CANCER

Q. **A 65-year-old man is referred to your clinic with an elevated PSA of 11.1 ng/mL, found on a routine medical check. How would you assess this patient in your clinic?**

A. Take a focused history and perform a clinical examination, including a DRE to assess the prostate gland.

Q. **What features in the clinical history would you be interested in and why?**

A. The important factors are discussed in Table 1.6.

Table 1.6 Important factors in the history of patients with suspected prostate cancer

Age	The risk of prostate cancer increases with age.
Race	Afro-Caribbean patients are at higher risk of prostate cancer than Caucasian patients [25] who are at higher risk than Asian patients.
Previous urological history	A history of inflammation (i.e. prostatitis) or infection (i.e. UTI) may account for an artificially elevated PSA. Previous surgery (i.e. TURP) may affect potential treatment options (e.g. brachytherapy).
Family history	The risk of familial prostate cancer increases with the number of first degree relatives affected.
	Hereditary prostate cancer accounts for approximately 9% of cases and may be related to a single gene defect on Chr1q24-25 (HPC-1).
Past medical history	The presence of co-morbidities is important to help determine life expectancy and therefore the most appropriate management and treatment options.
Drug history	Identifying whether the patient is on warfarin or clopidogrel is important if requesting a TRUS biopsy.

Q. **He has no preceding urinary symptoms and is otherwise fit and well. DRE reveals a 40 g prostate with a firm irregular left lobe. You organise a TRUS prostate biopsy. What does the histology slide in Figure 1.2 show?**

A. Figure 1.2 is a histological slide of a prostate biopsy demonstrating prostatic acinar and stromal tissue. (Thanks to Dr Rupali Arora, Consultant Histopathologist, University College Hospitals, London, UK, for providing this image.)

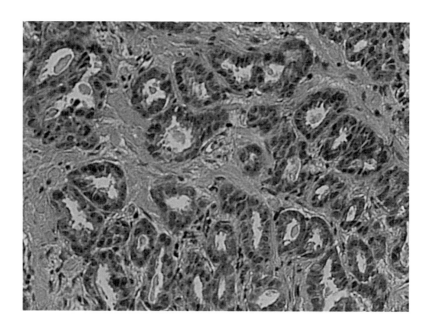

Figure 1.2

Q. Can you determine the Gleason score in Figure 1.2?

A. The glands demonstrate an irregular shape with irregular spacing in-between and loss of the basal cell layer, consistent with a Gleason grade 3. As there is only one predominant pattern the Gleason score is 3 + 3.

Note: *The Gleason scoring system was described by Donald Gleason in 1974 [26] after he compared tumour architecture with clinical outcome. The Gleason score is derived by assigning a score to the most common and also the second most common tumour pattern within a specimen. The tumour pattern is assessed by examining the glandular architecture at low magnification. The glandular features which determine the Gleason grade are shown in Table 1.7.*

Table 1.7 Gleason's grading system for prostate cancer

Grade 1	Well-demarcated nodule (the whole periphery must be seen)
Grade 2	Irregular spacing between glands and irregular outline (cannot be diagnosed on biopsy)
Grade 3	Variability in gland shape and spacing
Grade 4	Gland fusion
Grade 5	Diffuse solid sheet of undifferentiated cells

Source: Adapted from Pareek G et al. *J Urol* 2001; 166: 894–897.

Q. What is the clinical stage of this tumour using the 2017 TNM classification?

A. The clinical stage is T2bNxMx. T2b as the whole of the left lobe is involved and Nx Mx as investigations have not been performed to assess for lymph node involvement or metastases.

The prefix 'c' is used to describe clinical staging, while the prefix 'p' is used to describe pathological stage following radical prostatectomy. The TNM scoring system for prostate cancer is reproduced in Table 1.8.

Table 1.8 The 2017 TNM classification of prostate cancer (8th edition)

T	Primary tumour
Tx	Primary tumour cannot be assessed
T0	No evidence of primary tumour
T1	Clinically inapparent tumour not palpable or visible by imaging
T1a	Tumour incidental histological finding in 5% or less of tissue resected
T1b	Tumour incidental histological finding in more than 5% of tissue resected
T1c	Tumour identified by needle biopsy following elevated PSA (neither palpable nor visible)
T2	Tumour confined within the prostate
T2a	Tumour involves one-half of one lobe or less
T2b	Tumour involves more than half of one lobe, but not both lobes
T2c	Tumour involves both lobes
T3	Tumour extends through the prostatic capsule
T3a	Extracapsular extension (unilateral or bilateral)
T3b	Tumour invades seminal vesicle(s)
T4	Tumour is fixed or invades adjacent structures other than seminal vesicles: bladder neck, external sphincter, rectum, levator muscles, or pelvic wall
N	Regional lymph nodes
Nx	Regional lymph nodes cannot be assessed
N0	No regional lymph node metastasis
N1	Regional lymph node metastasis
M	Distant metastasis
Mx	Distant metastasis cannot be assessed
M0	No distant metastasis
M1	Distant metastasis
M1a	Non-regional lymph node(s)
M1b	Bone(s)
M1c	Other site(s)

Q. **Are you aware of a risk stratification system for prostate cancer? What is its role?**

A. The NICE guidelines 2008 describe a stratification system which enables patients to be divided into three groups according to their risk of having metastatic disease: low-, intermediate- and high-risk groups (Table 1.9). The patients are assigned a group based upon their PSA level, Gleason score and clinical stage. This is similar to D'Amico and the National Comprehensive Cancer Network (NCCN) risk groups. Establishing which risk group a patient is in enables you to determine the most appropriate staging investigations and treatment for that individual.

Table 1.9 Risk stratification system reproduced from the NICE guidelines 2008

Risk group	PSA	Gleason score	Clinical stage
Low	<10	≤6	T1-T2a
Intermediate	10–20	7	T2b-T2c
High	>20	8–10	T3-T4

Q. What is this patient's risk group?

A. His PSA is 11.1, his Gleason score is 6 and his clinical tumour stage is T2b putting him in the intermediate-risk group.

Q. What should happen next in the management of this patient?

A. This is a newly diagnosed cancer and therefore it should be discussed at the local and specialist multidisciplinary team (MDT/SMDT) meeting with the aim of confirming the histology, determining the need for staging investigation and identifying the most appropriate treatment options.

Q. What factors need to be considered when discussing a case at the MDT meeting?

A. The factors which influence the need for staging investigations and treatment options include the following:

1. Disease profile (risk group):
   a. Baseline PSA
   b. Clinical 2017 TNM stage
   c. Gleason score
2. Patient profile:
   a. Age
   b. Co-morbidities
   c. Life expectancy
   d. QoL
   e. Associated urinary symptoms/urological pathology

Q. What is a nomogram?

A. A nomogram is a statistically derived tool or two-dimensional diagram which can be used to help predict risk.

Q. What are Partin's tables and what is their role?

A. Partin's tables are a group of nomograms, based upon the outcomes of several thousand radical prostatectomies, which were designed to help predict the post-operative pathological T and N stages [27]. Four clinical risks can be assessed: organ confined disease, capsular penetration, seminal vesicle involvement and positive lymph nodes. These tables use three clinical variables: PSA level (pre-operative), Gleason score (on biopsy) and clinical T stage.

It is important to acknowledge that nomograms are only as strong as the variables used to calculate them. For example, Partin's tables are based on radical prostatectomies where only a limited lymph node dissection (obturator fossa and external iliac vein) was performed. It has been shown that prostate cancer can metastasise outside of this area and hence the risk of having positive lymph nodes may in fact be higher than that calculated using Partin's tables.

Q. What staging investigations would you perform in this case and why?

A. This is a 65-year-old man who is otherwise fit and well and therefore curative treatment is an option. If curative treatment is being considered then the need for staging investigations must be addressed including an MRI scan, if the patient has not had one for diagnostic purposes before biopsy. The 2014 published NICE Prostate Cancer guidelines suggest that multiparametric MRI (or computed tomography [CT] if MRI is contraindicated) should be considered for men with histologically proven prostate cancer if knowledge of the T or N stage could affect management.

In this particular patient the PSA is below 20 ng/mL and he has clinical stage T2b, Gleason 6 disease; therefore, he is intermediate risk and my local guidelines suggest that a mpMRI should be performed if one has not already been performed pre-biopsy (in our region almost all men have a pre-biopsy MRI). In addition the risk of having bone metastases is less than 2% (0.5% if the PSA is less than 10 ng/mL [28]) and therefore I would not perform a bone scan (again refer also to local guidelines). In high-risk cases the presence or absence of extracapsular spread seen on mpMRI will determine whether a radical prostatectomy is a viable treatment option or whether radical radiotherapy may be more appropriate.

Determining lymph node status is important when planning radiotherapy for potentially curative treatment of high-risk cases. However, according to Partin's tables in those patients with stage T2 disease or less, PSA <20 ng/mL and a Gleason score ≤6 the risk of lymph node involvement is less than 10% but most local guidelines in the United Kingdom would recommend mpMRI prior to radiotherapy treatment. MRI or CT can be used to identify suspicious nodes defined as those over 1 cm in diameter. CT of the pelvis, abdomen and chest is helpful in planning treatment in those cases with locally advanced tumours where there is a possibility of non-regional lymph node metastasis.

Q. **Look at Figure 1.3. A prostate MRI has been performed in this patient. What does Figure 1.3 show?**

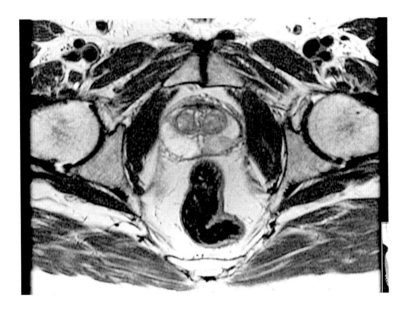

Figure 1.3

A. This is the T2-weighted sequence of a prostate MRI and demonstrates a low signal/ hypoechoic lesion in the peripheral zone of the left lobe causing a bulge to the capsule but no obvious capsular breach. I would like to see the other sequences including DWI and if performed also the contrast-enhanced images.

Note that a period of at least 6–8 weeks should be allowed before performing an MRI post-biopsy as haemorrhage can mimic a prostate tumour. (Some suggest that an mpMRI should not be performed ideally for at least 4 months after prostate biopsy as there is evidence to suggest that it takes this long for the intraprostatic haemorrhage to completely resolve.)

Q. **Your mpMRI confirms an apparently localised tumour to the left lobe. What treatment options are available for this man with intermediate-risk disease?**

A. The NICE guidelines 2008 and updated in 2014 recommendations for the preferred treatment of intermediate-risk disease include radical prostatectomy and conformal radiotherapy

(Table 1.10). Other options include watchful waiting (WW) and active surveillance. Brachytherapy may also be considered if the required criteria for prostate size are met. Cryotherapy and high-intensity focused ultrasound (HIFU) are currently only recommended as part of a clinical trial or part of a national NICE-approved registry under special arrangements at each hospital (Table 1.10).

Table 1.10 Treatment options as recommended by the NICE guidelines according to the risk stratification group

	Low risk	Intermediate risk	High risk
Watchful waiting	Option	Option	Option
Active surveillance	Preferred	Option	Not recommended
Prostatectomy	Option	Preferred	Preferred[a]
Brachytherapy	Option	Option	Not recommended
Conformal deep x-ray therapy (DXT)	Option	Preferred	Preferred[a]
Cryotherapy	Not recommended[b]	Not recommended[b]	Not recommended[b]
HIFU	Not recommended[b]	Not recommended[b]	Not recommended[b]

Note: Conformal DXT should be given at min dose of 74 Gy (max 2 Gy per fraction).
[a] Offer if there is a realistic prospect of long-term disease control.
[b] Unless part of clinical trial.

Q.   What is watchful waiting (WW) and why is it offered?
A.   WW is the conscious decision to avoid treatment in a patient until it is required usually when symptoms of progressive disease develop or the PSA rises above an arbitrary cut-off point. WW is offered to men with well or moderately differentiated tumours who have a life expectancy of less than 10–15 years as it has been shown that the majority of these men will die from other causes due to competing co-morbidities [29].

The indications for WW include

- Life expectancy less than 10–15 years
- Low-grade cancer
- Low-stage cancer
- Significant co-morbidities

Q.   What is active surveillance?
A.   Active surveillance is a management option for men who have potentially curable prostate cancer but who wish to avoid the complications associated with intervention (Table 1.11). However, the patient should be suitable for radical treatment if there is evidence of disease progression. The aim is to avoid treatment in those men with indolent cancers, by only treating those whose cancers show signs of progression. It requires regular reassessment of their risk category. It is reported that this management option may avoid radical intervention in up to 60%–80% of patients.

Table 1.11 Summary of the differences between WW and active surveillance

	Watchful waiting	Active surveillance
Aim	Avoid treatment	Treat only if necessary
Protocol	Occasional PSA	Frequent PSA
	No biopsies	Frequent biopsies
Treatment indication	Symptoms	PSA increase (PSADT)
		Upgrading of Gleason score
Treatment timing	Late	Early
Treatment intent	Palliative	Radical (curative)

Q. What criteria are needed for active surveillance to be considered?

A. In order for active surveillance to be offered the patient should be suitable for radical treatment if he shows signs of disease progression. Therefore, the patient needs to be medically fit for radical intervention with a life expectancy of over 10–15 years. He also needs to have localised disease which is low to moderately differentiated.

The Royal Marsden criteria for active surveillance include [30]

- Age 50–80 years
- Fit for radical treatment
- PSA <15 ng/mL
- Stage T1-2
- Gleason ≤3 + 4
- <50% positive cores

The NICE guidelines recommend active surveillance to all men at low risk who are considered suitable for radical treatment, particularly those with features matching Epstein 1994 criteria for 'insignificant' disease: T1c, Gleason 6, PSAD <0.15 ng/mL, less than three cores positive, no core more than 50% positive or >10 mm [31]. There is some concern about young men with a long life expectancy being on active surveillance as they may miss the opportunity of curative intervention. Active surveillance might also be advised for men with intermediate-risk disease where the mpMRI is reassuring and there is a small amount of Gleason 3 + 4 disease in older men but it is not recommended for those at high risk. All men considering this option should have had an initial minimum of a 12 core prostate biopsy protocol and recent NICE guidelines also ask that they have an mpMRI of the prostate at enrolment of active surveillance if this has not previously been performed.

Q. How would you follow up a patient on active surveillance?

A. Different regimens are described. NICE guidance recommends that an mpMRI of the prostate should be performed at enrolment of active surveillance if this has not previously been performed. NICE then suggests that PSA is measured every 3–4 months for the first year and every 6 months thereafter until surveillance ends. (PSA doubling time and velocity should be monitored.) A DRE is performed every 6–12 months until the end of year 4 and annually thereafter. A prostate biopsy is performed 12 months after commencing surveillance but not routinely thereafter unless there are clinical changes or concerns as regards PSA at which point an mpMRI and/or repeat biopsy are performed.

Interestingly, some alternative protocols now follow up this group of patients with regular PSAs and regular mpMRIs (one to two yearly). Prostate biopsy is not offered unless the PSA velocity or doubling time is worrying or unless the mpMRI shows changes. There is ongoing research looking into the role of mpMRI as a surveillance tool. One of the dilemmas in offering active surveillance is the lack of consensus about the ideal follow-up regime and when to intervene.

Q. What are the indicators for disease progression on active surveillance?

A. PSADT and grade progression on repeat biopsy are the primary factors used to assess disease progression. A PSADT of less than 2 years and a re-biopsy primary Gleason grade 4 or above or more than 50% positive cores are the main indicators for initiating treatment although 10%–20% of men sometimes choose treatment despite no clinical progression because of anxiety.

Q. Can you quote any outcomes for active surveillance?

A. Klotz has published an update of the original Canadian active surveillance series in 2005 [32]. At 8 years follow-up the overall survival was 85% and the disease-specific survival was 99% with only two patients succumbing to prostate cancer. This is a series of favorable risk prostate cancer patients (stage pT1b to pT2b N0 M0, Gleason Score 7 or less and PSA of

15 ng/mL or less). Of the total cohort 34% of patients came off active surveillance for rapid biochemical progression (15%), clinical progression (3%), histological progression (4%) and patient preference (12%).

Q. **The patient asks you if there is any evidence about which treatment option is best. How will you answer this?**

A. There are three RCTs assessing the role of primary therapy in prostate cancer – there has been initial discussion about these trials earlier in this chapter. The first compared radical prostatectomy (RP) with WW. This study was published by the Scandinavian study group, SPCG-4, initially by Holmberg in 2002 [33], updated by Bill-Axelson in 2005 [14] and then again in 2014 [15]. It included 695 men (348 RP, 347 WW) with a mean age of 65 years with localised (T2 or less), well or moderately differentiated cancer. Patients were followed up for a median of just over 13 years. The primary endpoint was death due to prostate cancer while secondary endpoints included death from any cause, metastasis and disease progression. In the surgery group 63 deaths occurred, and 99 in the watchful-waiting group were due to prostate cancer; the relative risk was 0.56 (p = 0.001), and the absolute difference was 11.0%. Men under the age of 65 years benefited more from treatment as they had longer life expectancy.

There are a number of limitations with this study which should be acknowledged. First only 12% of patients had T1c tumours (PSA detected) while 75% were T2 tumours in contrast to current day practice where only 15% of cases are T2 and additionally the median PSA was high at 13 indicating most men were clinically diagnosed on DRE and not based on PSA screening. The criteria for local progression, which included DRE and bladder outflow symptoms requiring TURP, could have resulted from BPH. In addition there was limited pathological data such that it is unknown how many were up-staged secondary to positive margins and there were only a small number of deaths. Finally the cancer-specific survival was only improved in men less than 65 years of age.

PIVOT (Prostate cancer Intervention Versus Observation Trial) is an American study comparing watchful waiting versus surgery [16]. In 2012, Wilt et al. showed that in men randomised between radical prostatectomy and watchful waiting diagnosed early in the PSA screening era of the United States, there was no overall survival or cancer-specific survival difference between the two arms. Subgroup analyses showed that there was a benefit in treating high-risk disease and probably in intermediate-risk disease but not in low-risk disease. Criticisms of this study are that it recruited from the Veterans Health Administration system in the United States and therefore the socioeconomic background and general health of these men was much worse than the general population as indicated by a rather high overall mortality in all arms from all causes. There was also poor compliance to WW with some men undergoing radical therapy.

In 2017, Hamdy et al. reported on the ProtecT trial which randomised men between radiotherapy, surgery and active monitoring. They showed no survival difference at 10 years between these three arms which recruited from men diagnosed in the screening arm of the UK screening study called CaP [17]. There were no differences in subgroups in this study. They showed a slight reduction in metastases in favour of treatment but there is criticism that ProtecT did not carry out modern active surveillance which might have not even showed this difference and also that the follow-up period is too short when treating screen detected prostate cancer.

Q. **The patient would like to know what complications may occur if he undergoes a radical prostatectomy.**

A. The complications which may occur as listed on the British Association of Urological Surgeons (BAUS) consent form are reproduced in Table 1.12.

Table 1.12 Complications of radical prostatectomy reproduced from the BAUS consent form

Mortality	0%–1.5%
Infection	5%–10%
Bleeding	5%–10%
Rectal injury	5%
Impotence (and no ejaculation)	40%–60%
Incontinence	50% early (5%–10% long term)
Anastomotic stricture, stenosis	10%
Anaesthetic (chest infection, deep vein thrombosis and pulmonary embolism, myocardial infarction, death)	5%–10%

Note: Complications have been shown to be less common when performed in high-volume departments.

Q. The patient is particularly concerned about urinary incontinence and if there is any treatment for this?

A. All patients should be taught to perform pelvic floor exercises before surgery. Despite this, up to 50% of patients get mild urinary incontinence which tends to improve over 12–18 months. Approximately 5%–10% will have severe, long-term incontinence requiring the use of more than one pad per day. If after 12 months severe incontinence persists then invasive intervention can be considered. Options include urethral bulking agents, the bulbourethral sling and the artificial urinary sphincter (AUS). The AUS, which has an 80% success rate, is currently the only option recommended by NICE.

Bladder neck stenosis and detrusor overactivity may also present with incontinence and therefore must be excluded with a flow rate, post-micturition residual and uro-dynamics prior to intervention.

Q. The patient, who has an active sex life, is also concerned about the risk of impotence and asks if this risk can be reduced.

A. This patient has palpable disease on one side and hence is eligible for a unilateral nerve-sparing (NS) RP. He does need to be aware that there is no guarantee that the right neurovascular bundle can be preserved and sometimes it does have to be sacrificed to enable a curative operation to be performed. His risk of impotence with a unilateral NS procedure is approximately 50% (over 60% if bilateral). I would advise that this patient starts a PDE5I (PDE5 inhibitor) at his first post-operative visit at 6 weeks, although there is some evidence to suggest that treatment is more beneficial if started pre-operatively. Post-operative alternatives to PDE5I include intraurethral and intracavernosal prostaglandin E1. The vacuum pump can also be considered and recently it has been reported that its use may prevent post-operative shrinkage of the penis while awaiting the return of normal erectile function. Following surgery all patients should have access to a specialist clinic for follow-up of their ED.

Contraindications to a NS-RP include palpable disease (although the contralateral side can be spared if unilateral), apical tumour extension and high-risk Gleason 8 or more. An mpMRI in expert hands is used by some surgeons to decide on nerve preservation. Some centres are also evaluating the NeuroSAFE technique, which involves fresh frozen sections at the time of the operation to guide decisions about nerve preservation.

Q. The patient is interested in hearing your thoughts about whether using open or laparoscopic or the robot is better for radical prostatectomy?

A. I would explain that the evidence shows a laparoscopic or robotic approach seems to be better for length of stay, transfusion rates and post-operative pain. The technical advantages of a laparoscopic/robotic RP include field magnification ×10–15 allowing for potentially better nerve sparing and a more precise anastomosis. However, there is no proven benefit that using a laparoscopic or robotic approach improves long-term incontinence or ED. The laparoscopic, robotic and open techniques for radical prostatectomy have similar oncological outcomes. The EAU guidelines suggest that all approaches, open/laparoscopic/robotic are acceptable because none has clearly shown superiority in terms of functional or oncological results.

There is very good evidence that the experience of the surgeon is very important and that high-volume surgeons and centres seem to have better results. The disadvantage of laparoscopic RP is a longer learning curve. It is important that if I am doing this operation, I explain what approach I will take and explain my own experience and results/outcomes.

Q. **The patient undergoes a successful RP. Histology confirms that the capsule is not breached by the tumour and that the resection margins are negative. How will you follow this patient up?**

A. Following discharge I will arrange for the patient to attend for a trial without catheter 7–14 days following surgery. Assuming no complications I will then review the patient in the outpatient department (OPD) at 6 weeks. This visit is primarily to assess the patient's recovery, exclude early complications and discuss the histology. At this visit it is also important to ensure that the patient is performing pelvic floor exercises. A PDE5I can also be offered to begin rehabilitation of erectile function. The second review occurs at 3 months post-operatively and it is at this point that the PSA level is checked to ensure that it is un-recordable. At this visit it is also important to review the degree of incontinence and impotence to provide appropriate ongoing specialist care and follow-up. Assuming the PSA is un-recordable and the patient has made a good recovery, follow-up is then on a six-monthly basis with a PSA check at each visit.

Q. **The patient attends his 3-month visit and asks you about his chances of survival. Can you briefly outline the 10-year survival figures for a RP?**

A. The 10-year survival figures following a radical prostatectomy are

- PSA free survival: 65%–75%
- Metastasis free: 85%–90%
- Overall survival: >95%

The 10-year PSA progression rate following RP is approximately 30%. Of these 80% will fail within 3 years of their RP. Without additional treatment, the time to development of clinical disease after PSA progression averages 8 years [34].

Q. **Is there any role for neoadjuvant hormone treatment prior to RP for localised disease?**

A. Neoadjuvant hormone treatment, which is defined as the administration of hormone treatment prior to definitive local curative treatment, has been shown to reduce the prostate volume and positive surgical margin rate. However, there is no evidence that it improves overall survival or disease-free survival compared to RP alone. Currently it is not recommended outside of a clinical trial.

Q. **A 73-year-old man is found to have a PSA of 15 ng/mL. His past medical history includes hypertension, atrial fibrillation and a previous TURP. His DRE reveals a 30 g suspicious feeling prostate. An mpMRI suggests bilateral disease which is organ confined. He undergoes a targeted and systematic transrectal prostate biopsy which confirms bilateral adenocarcinoma Gleason 4 + 4 with MCCL of 9 mm. His bone scan is negative for metastatic disease.**

What treatment options would you advise for this patient?

A. This patient has high-risk disease with a Gleason score of 8. The treatment options therefore include radical radiotherapy, radical prostatectomy (if there is a realistic prospect of long-term disease control) or hormone treatment. Active surveillance and brachytherapy are not recommended for high-risk disease while HIFU and cryotherapy should not be offered.

Q. What is radiotherapy and how does it work?

A. Radiotherapy is the use of ionizing radiation to achieve fatal damage to neoplastic cells. When x-rays are passed through proliferating tissue a proportion of the energy is absorbed and results in DNA damage. Radiotherapy utilises high-energy photons produced by linear accelerators which have excellent tissue penetration. The interaction of photons (packets of energy) and outer atoms leads to formation of free radicals (e.g. OH^-). These result in DNA damage and double-strand breakage which are irreparable. The optimisation and effects of radiation can be summarised as follows:

1. *Repair* – DNA repair occurs following the delivery of radiotherapy. Cells are more radiosensitive in the G2 or S phase of cell division. Fractionation results in more cells entering the sensitive phases of the cell cycle as well as arresting the repair process.
2. *Reoxygenation* – Oxygen is important for free radical formation. As cells die then more oxygen becomes available for free radical formation.
3. *Reassortment* – Cells are more sensitive to radiotherapy in the G2 and S phase of the cell cycle. Damage that occurs may not be appreciable until cell division has occurred.
4. *Repopulation* – Further cell division results in tumour growth which compromises efficacy.

Q. What types of radiation can be used for prostate cancer?

A. The types of radiation therapy used in prostate cancer treatment include external beam radiation therapy and brachytherapy:

- External beam radiation therapy (EBRT) uses a linear accelerator to produce high-energy x-rays which are directed in a beam towards the prostate. In the 1990s conformal radiotherapy was introduced and more recently intensity modulated radiotherapy (IMRT). IMRT utilises computer-controlled linear accelerators to deliver precise radiation to a specified area. Like conformal radiotherapy it shapes the beam to fit the target area, but unlike conformal radiotherapy it can alter the dose depending upon the shape of the prostate. This enables the dose administered to be increased to 80 Gy within the target volume, while reducing bladder and rectal toxicity. NICE guidance states a minimum dose of 74 Gy to the prostate at no more than 2 Gy per fraction should be given. The CHHiP trial in 2016 [35] showed that hypofractionated radiotherapy using 60 Gy in 20 fractions is non-inferior to conventional fractionation using 74 Gy in 37 fractions.
- Low dose rate (LDR) brachytherapy involves the placement of small 'seeds' containing radioactive material (such as iodine-125 or palladium-103) with multiple needles through the perineum directly into the prostate. The seeds, which eventually become inert, emit lower-energy radiation capable of travelling only short distances and thereby limiting damage to the bladder and rectum. Brachytherapy can be used as monotherapy in low-risk and low-volume intermediate-risk disease or as combination therapy with external beam radiation for high-risk cases.
- High dose rate (HDR) brachytherapy is the delivery of radiation from a source that is inserted through thin plastic tubes placed under general anaesthetic. Once delivered, no implants or radioactive sources remain in the prostate. The radioactive source often used is Iridium-192.

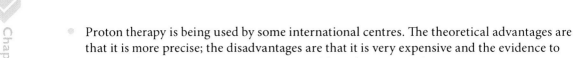

- Proton therapy is being used by some international centres. The theoretical advantages are that it is more precise; the disadvantages are that it is very expensive and the evidence to date has shown no toxicity or cancer control benefits compared to IMRT.

Q. What are the complications of EBRT to the prostate?

A. The complications of radiotherapy are reproduced in Table 1.13.

Table 1.13 Complications of radiotherapy to prostate

Cystitis	20%
Haematuria	18%
Proctitis	30% (severe long term in 3%)
Urethral stricture	4%–8%
Urinary incontinence	1% severe long term
Leg oedema	6%
ED	25%–60% (occurs over several years)
Second cancer	1 in 300 (1 in 70 in long-term survivors)

Q. Are you aware of any contraindications to EBRT to the prostate?

A. There are a number of contraindications to radiotherapy including severe lower urinary tract symptoms, inflammatory bowel disease and previous pelvic irradiation.

Q. What is the role of neoadjuvant and adjuvant hormone treatment with EBRT in a patient with high-risk localised disease?

A. There has been a large EORTC RCT by Bolla et al. [36] which clearly demonstrated a benefit to *adjuvant* hormone treatment (3 years) in terms of disease-free survival and overall survival in those with high-risk localised and locally advanced disease (see below).

The NICE guidelines 2014 advise that *neoadjuvant* hormones should be given for 3–6 months to all patients with intermediate- to high-risk localised and locally advanced disease receiving radiotherapy. *Adjuvant* hormones are recommended for up to 3 years after radiotherapy in high-risk localised prostate cancer or locally advanced disease.

The EORTC 22863 study by Bolla et al. [36] addressed the role of adjuvant hormone treatment in conjunction with EBRT. The study included 415 patients with T1-2 high-grade disease or stage T3-4 N0-N1 M0 over a median follow-up period of 4.5 years. Patients were randomised to 3 years of hormone ablation with EBRT (195 patients) versus EBRT alone (190 patients). The disease-free survival (DFS) figures for those with and without adjuvant treatment were 74% and 40%, respectively, while the overall survival (OS) figures were 78% and 62%, respectively. This demonstrated that an luteinizing hormone-releasing hormone (LHRH) analogue given during and for 3 years after EBRT improves both DFS and OS.

Q. The patient undergoes radiotherapy without any significant complications. How will you monitor this patient in clinic and how do you define treatment failure?

A. After the initial follow-up has been completed I would see the patient in the outpatient department every 4–6 months to assess his symptoms and monitor his PSA level. There are two main definitions for PSA recurrence following radiotherapy. The American Society of Therapeutic Radiation Oncologists 1996 (ASTRO) [37] definition is three consecutive PSA increases measured 4 months apart. Time to recurrence is midway through the three PSA measurements. More recently, the Radiation Therapy Oncology Group (RTOG)-ASTRO consensus conference [38] created a new definition, with failure being a PSA rise of 2 ng/mL above the post-treatment PSA-nadir (lowest value).

Q. What treatment options are available if the patient does develop disease recurrence post radiation therapy?

A. Hormone therapy is the mainstay of treatment. These confer systemic side effects such as weight gain, lethargy, hot flushes, breast tenderness/enlargement, osteoporosis and metabolic syndrome. Hormones offer no further chance of cure and the time to castrate resistance is a median of 18–24 months. Local salvage therapy is an option in the absence of metastatic disease and can help with a further chance at cure, delay time to hormones and time to castrate resistance. However, the patient must understand the significant additional complications associated with salvage RP which is also technically very demanding. Whole-gland or focal salvage therapy using cryotherapy or HIFU seem to have fewer complications and side effects, encouraging medium biochemical control but have less long-term data. They should only be offered in approved centres.

Local failure after radiation therapy is confirmed by mpMRI and a positive prostate biopsy. Each centre uses different staging imaging studies which can include various combinations of isotope bone scan, cross-sectional CT, positron emission tomography (PET) imaging or whole-body MRI. However, such a workup is only necessary if local salvage therapy (salvage cryotherapy, salvage HIFU or salvage prostatectomy) is being considered.

Q. A 76-year-old man who underwent radiotherapy for Gleason 4 + 3, T2/3 disease has developed PSA recurrence 2 years after completing his 3 years of adjuvant hormone treatment. His PSA is currently 2.7 ng/mL, PSADT 2.5 years. The patient has read about cryotherapy in the newspaper and asks if this is a treatment option for him.

A. Cryotherapy has been shown to have a role in salvage therapy for organ-confined prostate cancer. In this case the time to PSA recurrence and the PSADT suggest localised disease and assuming this is confirmed on re-staging scans, cryotherapy is an option for this patient.

Cryotherapy is one of two minimally invasive treatment options, the other being HIFU. Both have a potential role in salvage therapy for organ-confined recurrent disease following radical radiotherapy (both techniques have been proposed as treatment options also for localised primary prostate cancer but current NICE guidelines only recommend their use in this group as part of a clinical controlled trial).

Q. What does the technique of cryotherapy involve?

A. Cryotherapy involves the insertion of trans-perineal ultrasound guided cryoprobes which are used to deliver argon or liquid nitrogen to achieve a sustained temperature ideally at least as low as −40°C. Freezing is alternated with thawing (helium gas is used in the thawing process). Two cycles of freeze-thaw are administered, resulting in cellular necrosis. The diameter of the ice ball is generally monitored on ultrasound. A urethral warming catheter and thermosensors are used during the procedure to protect the urethra, external sphincter and rectal wall.

Q. What is the mechanism of cell death during cryotherapy?

A. The two freeze-thaw cycles result in

- Cellular dehydration and protein denaturation
- Direct rupture of cellular membranes by ice crystal formation
- Endothelial damage resulting in vascular stasis and microthrombi resulting in ischaemia and coagulative necrosis

The complications of cryotherapy include erectile dysfunction, incontinence, urinary symptoms/urethral sloughing/retention, pelvic pain, transient perineal numbness and recto-urethral fistula. All of these complications are more common in the salvage setting.

Q. A 70-year-old man with a PSA of 13 ng/mL is diagnosed with adenocarcinoma of the prostate, Gleason score 4 + 5. He has undergone a previous TURP and suffers with chronic obstructive pulmonary disease (COPD). Staging MRI confirms localised disease. The patient has a friend who had brachytherapy and he would like to know if it is an option for him?

A. Brachytherapy is *not* an option for this patient due to his previous TURP and high-risk disease. The contraindications to brachytherapy include

- Life expectancy less than 5 years
- Coagulation disorder
- Previous pelvic radiation
- Gleason grade 5 disease
- Previous TURP (high risk of incontinence)
- Large prostate >50 cc or large median lobe (difficult seed implantation) (LHRH agonists can be used to decrease prostate volume)
- Moderate to severe LUTS (risk of retention and worsening LUTS)

Q. Which patients would be suitable for brachytherapy?

A. The NICE guidelines advise that brachytherapy is an option for patients with low- and intermediate-risk disease:

- Stage: T2c or less
- Gleason score: 7 or less
- PSA: 20 ng/mL or less

However, local guidelines vary and many brachytherapists only treat patients with PSA up to 10 and Gleason 3 + 4 with additional criteria and limitations on percent core involvement and percent of cores positive.

Q. If the patient had been a suitable candidate for brachytherapy, what are the complications that the patient needs to be warned about?

A. The complications associated with brachytherapy include

- Development of irritative voiding symptoms
- Urinary incontinence (particularly if the patient requires TURP following brachytherapy for urine retention)
- Acute urinary retention
- Erectile dysfunction (in 50% over several years)
- Perineal haematoma
- Proctitis

Q. What do you understand by the term PSA 'bounce'?

A. PSA 'bounce' refers to the benign rise in the PSA level that occurs after its initial fall following radiotherapy (can occur with either EBRT or brachytherapy). The level should, however, remain less than 1.5 ng/mL. The mean time to a PSA bounce is approximately 9 months. It can be seen in up to 30% of patients after brachytherapy and tends to occur later following this treatment, often in the second year post therapy.

Q. The patient asks about HIFU. He would like to know if this treatment is available.

A. NICE interventional guidance only recommends HIFU as a treatment option for localised prostate cancer as part of a clinical trial or a prospective national registry in centres under special arrangements. HIFU treatment uses focused ultrasound waves emitted from a rectal transducer. These focused ultrasound waves are used to cause coagulative necrosis through both mechanical and thermal effects. HIFU requires a general anaesthesia. There is a lot of recent interest in focal therapy using HIFU (or cryotherapy). Studies are ongoing on this concept which involves treating only the areas of cancer or the main (index) cancer and monitoring the rest of the prostate. It is controversial as the disease is multifocal, mpMRI and biopsy can miss cancers, the untreated tissue might develop new cancers and there is no long-term or RCTs assessing its cancer control compared to radiotherapy or surgery. Studies have shown that one-fifth of men need to have the treatment again over 5 years because of residual or recurrent cancer. Its potential advantages are that incontinence (any pad usage) is about 1%–2%, impotence 5%–15% and recto-urethral fistula 0.1% [39].

LOCALLY ADVANCED PROSTATE CANCER

Q. **A fit and well 68-year-old man is referred to your clinic with an elevated PSA of 14.3 ng/mL. Examination reveals a nodule in the left lobe of the prostate. A pre-biopsy mpMRI scan raises the possibility of a lesion on the left and likely capsular breach. A targeted trans-perineal biopsy with systematic cores is performed under sedation and local anaesthetic. It confirms Gleason 3 + 4, 15 mm maximum cancer core length involvement on the left. Three of five targeted cores were positive; one systematic core from the right showed 2 mm of Gleason 6. What are the treatment options available for this patient?**

A. This patient is an intermediate-risk patient with possible high-risk disease given the potential capsular extension on mpMRI. Depending on life expectancy and co-morbidities, the preferred treatment options are EBRT and RP. In this otherwise fit and well patient RP is an option but the risk of residual disease must be carefully explained. Recent evidence suggests a multimodal approach (surgery followed by radiotherapy) may be advantageous in terms of biochemical control although side effects are higher and there is no current convincing evidence that survival is improved. Alternative non-curative options include WW and hormone treatment if the patient cannot accept the associated side effects with curative treatment.

Q. **The patient elects to undergo an RP despite the potential risk of residual disease. Histology confirms a capsular breach on the left with a positive resection margin but negative lymph nodes. You see the patient in the OPD at 6 weeks and explain the histology result. He wants to know what his risk is of developing tumour recurrence.**

A. Studies have shown between 30% and 60% of patients with T3 disease will develop biochemical progression at 5 years.

Q. **The patient is concerned about the possible risk of residual cancer and asks if there is any further treatment that can be given.**

A. The adjuvant treatment options available to him following RP include adjuvant radiotherapy and adjuvant hormone treatment. Adjuvant hormone therapy following an RP for localised disease has not been shown to be of additional benefit [40]. The role of adjuvant radiotherapy is less clear, in particular it is not known whether immediate radiotherapy is more beneficial than delayed radiotherapy when PSA relapse occurs. Currently I would follow the NICE guidelines and advise close PSA surveillance every 3 months, offering radiotherapy if the PSA relapses, ideally before it reaches 1 ng/mL.

 The only RCT conducted and which has subsequently reported results to assess the role of immediate post-operative radiotherapy in positive surgical margins and T3 disease is the EORTC 22911 study by Bolla et al. [41]. This assessed immediate post-operative EBRT (502 patients) compared to delayed EBRT at the time of biochemical progression (503 patients) in those with pT3N0M0 disease but with one or more risk factors suggests stage T3. The study found that immediate EBRT was well tolerated and that it improves biological free survival at 5 years from 51.8% to 72.2%. However, there was no evidence that it improves overall survival and therefore its role remains controversial.

The EAU guidelines advise that those patients with stage T2/T3 disease with positive margins or capsular breach can be offered immediate EBRT or clinical monitoring and salvage EBRT when the PSA is >0.5 ng/mL but <1 ng/mL. In contrast the 2008 NICE guidelines do not recommend immediate radiotherapy for margin positive disease after RP, favouring PSA surveillance and salvage radiotherapy on relapse. The role of adjuvant radiotherapy may be clarified when the results of the RADICALS (Radiotherapy and Androgen Deprivation In Combination After Local Surgery) study are available. This RCT assesses adjuvant versus salvage EBRT after RP with or without adjuvant short- and long-term hormones [42].

Adjuvant androgen deprivation therapy (ADT) has been assessed in the early prostate cancer (EPC) studies by McLeod et al. [43]. The EPC program comprises three RCTs involving 23 countries and 8113 patients. The studies evaluate the efficacy and tolerability of high-dose bicalutamide (150 mg/day) versus placebo given in addition to standard care (RP, EBRT, AS). For localised disease there was no benefit to progression-free survival (PFS) by adding bicalutamide to standard care although there was a trend towards decreased survival in patients otherwise undergoing WW. In those with locally advanced disease there was a significantly improved PFS for those given EBRT, a trend for those treated with WW (p = 0.06) but it was not significant for those who underwent an RP.

Q. **The patient was reviewed in the OPD at 3 months and his PSA was <0.1 ng/mL. He was kept under regular surveillance over the next 3 years and his PSA remained <0.1 ng/mL. When he attends your OPD you find that his latest PSA has increased to 0.3 ng/mL. What do you tell the patient and how would you manage this?**

A. This PSA level indicates biochemical recurrence. There are a number of definitions for biochemical recurrence following an RP but a widely accepted definition is a PSA above 0.2 ng/mL. I would therefore explain to the patient that this is likely to indicate residual *local* disease following which I would discuss potential treatment options. If the patient wishes to try and cure the cancer then salvage radiotherapy is an option assuming there are no contraindications. If the patient wishes to avoid the complications of radical treatment then ADT can be given. ADT is best given early in the presence of systemic relapse as it has been shown to decrease the frequency of clinical metastases [44]. With localised recurrence, delaying ADT until the development of clinically evident metastatic disease is more appropriate as the median time for the development of metastasis is 8 years and median time from metastasis to death another 5 years [34]. There is no role for ablative cryotherapy or HIFU in this setting.

Q. **A fit and well 71-year-old man is referred to your clinic with an elevated PSA of 19.1 ng/mL and an abnormal DRE. An MRI reveals capsular breach bilaterally and invasion of the left seminal vesicle. TRUS systematic and targeted biopsies confirm maximum Gleason 4 + 4 and overall Gleason 4 + 3 disease. What treatment options are available for this patient?**

A. This man has locally advanced high-risk disease. Curative treatment can be attempted with the use of conformal EBRT but RP is not routinely recommended in the presence of seminal vesicle invasion. Alternative options include hormone treatment and WW. There is some evidence that a multimodal approach with surgery followed by radiotherapy might be beneficial in terms of biochemical control but there is no convincing evidence that survival is improved. Side effects are higher with multimodal treatment.

Q. **A 70-year-old man who had radiotherapy for G3pT1 bladder cancer 2 years ago was found to have an elevated PSA of 24 ng/mL and clinically T3 prostate cancer. The biopsy confirms Gleason 3 + 4 disease and his MRI scan demonstrates capsular penetration and seminal vesicle invasion bilaterally. His bone scan is negative. What treatment options are available to him?**

A. This man has locally advanced disease, which is not curable with RP. Conformal radiotherapy is also not an option given his previous pelvic irradiation. Treatment options therefore include hormone treatment or WW. Some centres might consider cysto-prostatectomy but there is no evidence to guide this approach.

Q. A 70-year-old man is diagnosed with Gleason 3 + 4 disease (PSA 12 ng/mL). His bone scan is negative and the MRI suggests possible capsular breach on the left. The patient elects to undergo an RP. The histology report shows a positive margin in the left lobe with one positive obturator lymph node. What management options are available for this patient?

A. This patient has lymph node positive disease and therefore the treatment options include early hormone therapy or delayed hormone therapy when the patient develops clinically symptomatic disease.

Messing et al. assessed the use of immediate hormonal therapy compared with observation after radical prostatectomy in 98 men with node-positive prostate cancer [45]. Men were randomly assigned to receive immediate ADT, with either goserelin or bilateral orchidectomy, or to be followed until disease progression. After a median of 7.1 years of follow-up, 7 of 47 men who received immediate ADT had died, as compared with 18 of 51 men in the observation group. The cause of death was prostate cancer in 3 men in the immediate-treatment group and in 16 men in the observation group. At the time of the last follow-up, 36 men in the immediate-treatment group (77%) and 9 men in the observation group (18%) were alive and had no evidence of recurrent disease. They concluded that immediate ADT after radical prostatectomy with positive lymph node disease improves survival and reduces the risk of recurrence in patients with node-positive prostate cancer. With the use of supersensitive PSA an argument could be made for observation followed by introduction of delayed ADT when progression occurs to limit side effects from treatment.

METASTATIC AND HORMONE REFRACTORY PROSTATE CANCER

Q. What is ADT and how does it work?

A. ADT refers to any treatment that lowers androgen activity. Prostate cells are physiologically dependent on androgens to function, stimulate growth and proliferate. Testosterone, although not tumourigenic, is essential for the growth and perpetuation of tumour cells. When androgen deprivation occurs, androgen-sensitive prostate cancer cells undergo apoptosis.

Q. Can you briefly outline the physiology behind androgen secretion?

A. Approximately 90%–95% of androgens are produced by the Leydig cells of the testes, with only 5%–10% being derived from the adrenal cortex. Testosterone secretion is regulated by the hypothalamic-pituitary-gonadal axis as shown in Figure 1.4.

The hypothalamic gonadotropin-releasing hormone (GnRH) stimulates the anterior pituitary gland to release luteinizing hormone (LH) and follicle-stimulating hormone (FSH). LH stimulates the Leydig cells of the testes to secrete testosterone. Within prostate cells, testosterone is converted by the enzyme 5-alpha reductase into dihydrotestosterone (DHT), which is approximately 10 times more active biologically. Once bound to the androgen receptor in the cytoplasm the androgen-receptor complex enters the nucleus where it interacts with DNA to influence cell growth and division. Peripheral aromatisation of testosterone into oestrogens, together with circulating androgens, exerts negative feedback control on hypothalamic LH secretion.

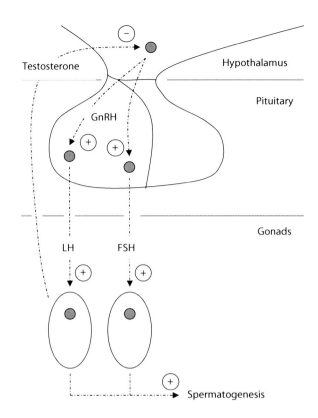

Figure 1.4 Hypothalamic-pituitary-gonadal axis.

Q. What are the different mechanisms used to induce androgen deprivation and what hormone treatment options are available for each?

A. Androgen deprivation can be induced by suppressing the secretion of testicular androgens, either medically or surgically, or by inhibiting their action at the androgen receptor using anti-androgens. Some, including oestrogen and steroidal anti-androgens have more than one mechanism of action. These actions are summarised in Table 1.14.

Both surgical and medical forms of castration have equivalent efficacy.

Table 1.14 The actions of hormonal manipulation in prostate cancer

Reduced androgen production	
Surgical castration	Removes Leydig cells
Medical castration	Reduces LH production
• LHRH agonists	Down-regulates pituitary GnRH receptors
• LHRH antagonists	Inhibits GnRH receptor
Blocks androgen effect	
Non-steroidal anti-androgens (e.g. bicalutamide, flutamide)	Blocks androgen at receptor level
Combined effect	
Oestrogen	Down-regulates LHRH secretion
	Inactivates androgen
	Suppresses Leydig cells
Steroidal anti-androgens (e.g. cyproterone acetate)	Down-regulates LHRH secretion
	Blocks androgen at receptor level

Q. **What are LHRH agonists and how do they work?**

A. LHRH agonists are long-acting synthetic analogues of GnRH. Chronic exposure to LHRH agonists eventually results in down-regulation of GnRH receptors with subsequent suppression of pituitary LH and FSH secretion and testosterone production. The level of testosterone decreases to castrate levels usually within 2 to 4 weeks. The two main types are goserelin and leuprorelin. They are delivered as depot injections on a 1 or 3 monthly basis.

Over 70%–80% of patients will respond to ADT. However, the development of androgen independence is inevitable with a mean time to disease progression of 14–36 months after commencement of treatment.

Q. **What are the side effects of LHRH agonists?**

A. Typical side effects of LHRH agonists include

- Flushing (vasomotor) 80%
- Erectile dysfunction
- Osteoporosis
- Hyperlipidaemia
- Gynaecomastia
- Cognitive decline
- Diabetes
- Anaemia
- Loss of muscle mass
- Reduced quality of life

Q. **What are the two types of anti-androgens and how do they differ?**

A. The two classes of anti-androgens are steroidal (cyproterone acetate) and non-steroidal (bicalutamide, flutamide). Non-steroidal anti-androgens act purely as competitors of androgens at the receptor level, enabling the testosterone level to be maintained or increased. Steroidal anti-androgens also compete at the receptor level but have additional progesterogenic activity which causes central inhibition of pituitary gland LH secretion and hence a reduced testosterone level.

Q. **The patient denies any urinary symptoms and has a good quality of life. He asks you if there are any benefits to starting the hormone treatment early.**

A. Hormone treatment tends to be reserved for patients with symptomatic metastatic disease. One argument against early hormones is their associated side effects, particularly in patients who are clearly asymptomatic from their disease. However, studies have suggested that in locally advanced and metastatic disease, early hormone treatment results in slower disease progression and reduced disease morbidity. These issues therefore need to be discussed with the patient and the risk-benefit ratio assessed for each individual.

Q. **The patient enjoys an active sex life and asks if there is any treatment that can be given which does not affect this.**

A. In those men wishing to avoid ED and reduced libido, bicalutamide 150 mg od, has been shown to be an alternative to LHRH agonists although its equivalence has not been proven [43].

Q. **The patient is commenced on bicalutamide treatment and his PSA falls to less than 0.1 ng/mL. He returns to your clinic 6 months later distressed about the painful breast swellings that he has developed. He would like to know if anything can be done for this.**

A. Approximately 75%–80% of patients develop gynaecomastia when taking non-steroidal anti-androgens and 50% develop pain. It occurs due to the peripheral aromatisation of testosterone to oestradiol. Prevention of gynaecomastia can be achieved with radiotherapy (8–10 Gy to each breast) but it does not prevent pain or tenderness. An alternative is tamoxifen 20 mg od particularly if there is no response to RT. However, once gynaecomastia has already developed or in the presence of severe pain the most effective treatment is a bilateral mastectomy.

Q. **The patient has a successful bilateral mastectomy. When he returns to your clinic 18 months later his PSA has increased on several occasions and is now 1.2 ng/mL. What do you do now?**

A. The patient has developed androgen-independent disease. Having been on anti-androgens alone I would commence an LHRH agonist and reduce his bicalutamide to 50 mg daily.

Q. **What is the aim of maximum androgen blockade (MAB)?**

A. MAB aims to prevent all androgen stimulation by blocking both the production of androgens by the testis and inhibiting the androgens produced by the adrenals at the receptor level.

Q. **What is the role of intermittent hormone treatment?**

A. Intermittent ADT is becoming an increasingly popular way of treating patients with localised disease, particularly in those patients who wish to limit the side effects of treatment.

The primary aim of intermittent ADT is to delay the development of an androgen-independent state. Androgen independence may begin early after the initiation of hormonal treatment, due to the arrest of androgen-induced differentiation of the prostatic epithelium. If ADT is stopped prior to the progression of androgen-independent cells, any subsequent tumour growth may remain androgen dependent, which potentially will be susceptible once again to androgen withdrawal. Although superiority has not been proven over continuous ADT it does have three clinical benefits including reduced side effects during the off-therapy periods, decreased bone loss and reduced cost. Side effects may, however, be slow to resolve after stopping treatment as the serum testosterone level can take up to 9 months to recover.

Q. **A 75-year-old man is referred to your clinic with an elevated PSA of 62 ng/mL and an abnormal DRE. TRUS biopsy confirms Gleason 4 + 4 disease. Figure 1.5 is an investigation this patient went on to have. What does Figure 1.5 show and what is it demonstrating?**

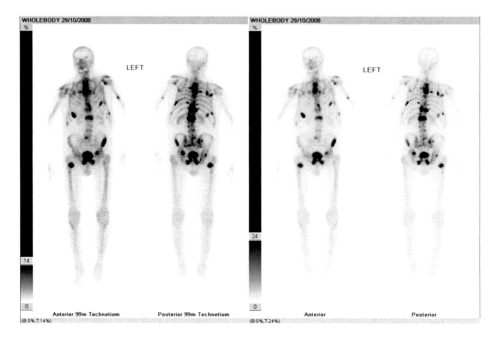

Figure 1.5

A. Figure 1.5 is a radionuclide whole-body isotope bone scan. It demonstrates several scattered hot spots within the ribs, thoracic spine, iliac bone and proximal long bones which given the history are consistent with bone metastases.

Q. The patient asks what treatment options are available.

A. The mainstay of treatment for metastatic prostate cancer is ADT, i.e. medical castration (with anti-androgens or LHRH analogues) or surgical castration (orchidectomy). In advanced disease this is best given at the time of diagnosis rather than at the time of symptomatic progression as it has been shown to reduce both disease progression and its complications [44]. Clinical disease progression after androgen deprivation will tend to occur after a median interval of about 12–18 months. Recent randomised trials have evaluated the role of upfront docetaxel chemotherapy and most, such as STAMPEDE [46] have shown a survival benefit for using upfront chemotherapy in such men, if they accept the side effects and can tolerate the regimen.

Q. What is tumour flare and how do you prevent it?

A. When first given, LHRH agonists stimulate the pituitary LHRH receptors, resulting in a transient rise in LH and FSH release. Consequently testosterone levels are temporarily increased, which is referred to as a testosterone 'surge' or 'flare'. The flare occurs within 2 or 3 days after the first injection and continues for approximately 1 week. This flare can have severe consequences such as spinal cord compression. To prevent this flare anti-androgens are given for 1 week before and 2 weeks after the first dose of the LHRH agonist.

Q. Who is at risk of tumour flare and what are its consequences?

A. The patients at risk of clinical flare are those with high-volume, symptomatic, bony disease, which accounts for only 4%–10% of metastatic patients. The typical consequences include spinal cord compression, fatal cardiovascular events due to hypercoagulation, ureteric obstruction, acute bladder outlet obstruction and increased bone pain.

Q. How can tumour flare be prevented?

A. Concomitant therapy with an anti-androgen, commencing on the same day or preferably a week before the first depot injection of LHRH agonist and continued for 2 weeks following it, can prevent tumour flare by blocking the androgen receptor. An alternative option in patients at high risk is to use LHRH *antagonists*, although this has been associated with significant side effects from histamine release. Surgical castration (subcapsular orchidectomy) has the benefit that no concomitant therapy is required (i.e. there is no tumour flare with surgical castration) and it is extremely effective in rapidly reducing circulating testosterone levels, which is useful in emergency situations.

Q. The patient would like to know what his prognosis is.

A. With asymptomatic disease the average survival is 2–3 years, which reduces to 12 months with symptomatic disease. The overall 5-year survival rate for a patient with metastatic disease is approximately 25%. These figures are historical and with contemporary interventions patients are clearly living longer.

Q. The patient responds to ADT initially but 22 months later his PSA starts to increase. His latest PSA is 54 ng/mL and he is now complaining of severe pain in his ribs. What options are available for the management of bone pain secondary to metastases?

A. In addition to analgesia, alternative options include

- Radiotherapy, which is particularly useful when the pain is localised
- Radioisotopes (i.e. strontium-89), which is useful for widespread disease

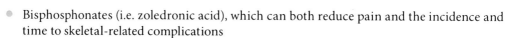

- Bisphosphonates (i.e. zoledronic acid), which can both reduce pain and the incidence and time to skeletal-related complications
- Oestrogens/steroids

Bisphosphonates act by inhibiting osteoclast mediated bone resorption. Saad et al. studied the role of bisphosphonates in 643 men with hormone-resistant prostate cancer and bone metastases [47]. Men were randomised to receive either zoledronic acid for 15 consecutive months or placebo. At 15 months and 24 months follow-up, there was a significant reduction in skeletal-related events in the zoledronic acid treated group compared to the placebo group (33% versus 44%) and the frequency of pathological fractures (13.1% versus 22.1%). Furthermore, zoledronic acid significantly prolonged the time to first skeletal-related event.

Q. What are the complications associated with metastatic prostate cancer?

A. The complications include

- Spinal cord compression
- Ureteric obstruction/renal failure
- Sepsis
- Hypercalcaemia
- Anaemia
- Hepatotoxicity
- Skeletal fractures
- Urinary retention

Q. An 82-year-old man is admitted as an emergency complaining of increasing lethargy and difficulty passing urine. Abdominal examination confirms an enlarged palpable bladder. DRE reveals a non-tender, malignant feeling prostate, cT3/4. What is your diagnosis?

A. This patient has chronic urinary retention, likely to be due to prostate cancer. His history of lethargy in association with this would raise concerns about associated renal failure.

Q. After completing a basic assessment, you insert a catheter and 1.5 L of urine is drained. His renal function results are as follows: urea of 18.1 mmol/L, creatinine of 364 μmol/L, potassium 5.2 mmol/L. Six months ago his renal function was normal. What is the diagnosis and how will you manage this patient now?

A. This patient has acute renal failure which may be secondary to high pressure chronic urinary retention or ureteric obstruction. Given his large residual and renal impairment he is at risk of a post-obstructive diuresis and therefore I would monitor his urine output every hour, and perform 4 hourly observations including blood pressure measurements to assess for postural hypotension. I would also check his weight and renal function on a daily basis. An ultrasound study of his renal tract will confirm the presence of hydronephrosis and exclude any other renal pathology. In order to confirm the diagnosis of prostate cancer he needs to have his PSA repeated (it may be artificially elevated secondary to retention) and a biopsy performed. If the PSA is very high (>100 ng/nL) then a biopsy may not be necessary and a bone scan can be requested instead.

If his renal function does not return to normal and the hydronephrosis persists despite catheter insertion then ureteric obstruction must be considered and percutaneous nephrostomy tubes inserted.

Q. A 78-year-old man on ADT for metastatic prostate cancer who has been complaining of back pain for the last 2 months is admitted to the accident and emergency department with a sudden exacerbation of his pain, 'off legs' and difficulty in passing urine? What is the likely diagnosis? How will you confirm this?

A. The likely diagnosis is spinal cord compression. A thorough history and clinical examination needs to be performed to assess for signs of cord compression and determine its level. The diagnosis is confirmed with an urgent MRI.

Q. **What does Figure 1.6 demonstrate?**

A. Figure 1.6 is an MRI of the spine. It demonstrates compression of the spinal cord at the level of L5. In fact, spinal cord compression occurs most commonly in the thoracic or upper lumbar regions of the spine. It is due to either vertebral collapse secondary to tumour invasion or from extradural tumour growth. Symptoms include radicular pain and peripheral neurological symptoms such as motor or sensory loss or both, including urinary retention.

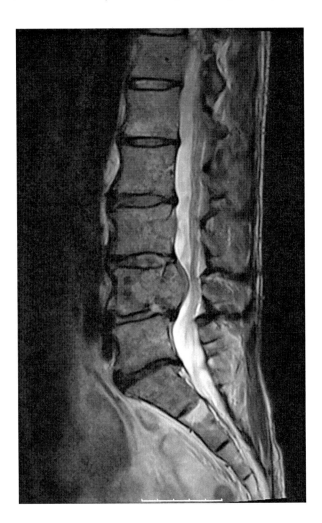

Figure 1.6

Q. **How do you manage spinal cord compression?**

A. Spinal cord compression is an acute surgical emergency. Steroid treatment should be administered immediately followed by definitive treatment with either radiotherapy or surgical decompression depending upon the patient and nature of cord compression. ADT should also be started on an urgent basis with anti-androgen cover to prevent tumour flare.

Q. What is the role of chemotherapy in androgen-independent prostate cancer?

A. Systemic chemotherapy is indicated in men with androgen-independent prostate cancer with proven metastatic disease. It is contraindicated in patients with significant renal, haematological or bone disease and poor performance status. Docetaxel-based regimens have been shown to give a 10 months median survival advantage if used upfront but only 2–3 months if used at time of castrate resistance [48].

Q. What is castrate resistance or hormone-relapsed prostate cancer?

A. Castrate-resistant prostate cancer (CRPC) or hormone-relapsed prostate cancer (HRPC) is defined by disease progression despite androgen-deprivation therapy and may present as one or any combination of a continuous rise in serum levels of PSA, progression of pre-existing disease, or appearance of new metastases. There are numerous agents which might be used in this setting such as abiraterone, enzalutamide, docetaxel or cabazitaxel chemotherapy and immunotherapies. Some are approved by NICE but many are under active investigation within randomised clinical trials. These cases are best managed under the care of a multidisciplinary team of urologists, medical oncologists and/or clinical oncologists.

REFERENCES

1. Oesterling JE et al. Serum prostate-specific antigen in a community-based population of healthy men. Establishment of age-specific reference ranges. *JAMA* 1993; 270: 860–864.
2. Sun L et al. Prostate-specific antigen (PSA) and PSA velocity for prostate cancer detection in men aged <50 years. *BJU Int* 2007; 99: 753–757.
3. Catalona WJ et al. Comparison of digital rectal examination and serum prostate specific antigen in the early detection of prostate cancer: Results of a multicenter clinical trial of 6,630 men. *J Urol* 1994; 151: 1283–1290.
4. Thompson IM et al. Prevalence of prostate cancer among men with a prostate-specific antigen level < or = 4.0 ng per milliliter. *N Engl J Med* 2004; 350: 2239–2246.
5. Gerstenbluth RE et al. The accuracy of the increased prostate specific antigen level (greater than or equal to 20 ng/mL) in predicting prostate cancer: Is biopsy always required? *J Urol* 2002; 168: 1990–1993.
6. Carter HB et al. Longitudinal evaluation of prostate-specific antigen levels in men with and without prostate disease. *JAMA* 1992; 267: 2215–2220.
7. Trapasso JG et al. The incidence and significance of detectable levels of serum prostate specific antigen after radical prostatectomy. *J Urol* 1994; 152: 1821–1825.
8. Benson MC et al. Prostate specific antigen density: A means of distinguishing benign prostatic hypertrophy and prostate cancer. *J Urol* 1992; 147: 815–816.
9. Djavan B et al. Prostate specific antigen density of the transition zone for early detection of prostate cancer. *J Urol* 1998; 160: 411–418.
10. Lee R et al. A meta-analysis of the performance characteristics of the free prostate-specific antigen test. *Urology* 2006; 67: 762–768.
11. Doherty AP et al. Undetectable ultrasensitive PSA after radical prostatectomy for prostate cancer predicts relapse-free survival. *Br J Cancer* 2000; 83: 1432–1436.
12. The Internal Medicine Clinic Research Consortium. Effect of digital rectal examination on serum prostate-specific antigen in a primary care setting. *Arch Intern Med* 1995; 155: 389–392.
13. Hessels D et al. DD3(PCA3)-based molecular urine analysis for the diagnosis of prostate cancer. *Eur Urol* 2003; 44: 8–15.
14. Bill-Axelson A et al. Radical prostatectomy versus watchful waiting in early prostate cancer. *N Engl J Med* 2005; 352: 1977–1984.

15. Bill-Axelson A et al. Radical prostatectomy or watchful waiting in early prostate cancer. *N Engl J Med* 2014; 370: 932–942.

16. Wilt TJ et al. Radical prostatectomy versus observation for localized prostate cancer. *N Engl J Med* 2012; 367: 203–213.

17. Hamdy FC et al. 10-year outcomes after monitoring, surgery, or radiotherapy for localized prostate cancer. *N Engl J Med* 2016; 375: 1415–1424.

18. Stanford JL et al. Urinary and sexual function after radical prostatectomy for clinically localized prostate cancer: The Prostate Cancer Outcomes Study. *JAMA* 2000; 283: 354–360.

19. Thompson IM et al. The influence of finasteride on the development of prostate cancer. *N Engl J Med* 2003; 349: 215–224.

20. Grover S et al. Do the benefits of finasteride outweigh the risks in the prostate cancer prevention trial? *J Urol* 2006; 175: 934–938.

21. Andriole GL et al. Effect of dutasteride on the risk of prostate cancer. *N Engl J Med* 2010; 362: 1192–1202.

22. Pareek G et al. Periprostatic nerve blockade for transrectal ultrasound guided biopsy of the prostate: A randomized, double-blind, placebo controlled study. *J Urol* 2001; 166: 894–897.

23. Djavan B et al. Prospective evaluation of prostate cancer detected on biopsies 1, 2, 3 and 4: When should we stop? *J Urol* 2001; 166: 1679–1683.

24. Ahmed HU et al. Diagnostic accuracy of multi-parametric MRI and TRUS biopsy in prostate cancer (PROMIS): A paired validating confirmatory study. *Lancet* 2017; 389: 815–822.

25. Ben Shlomo Y et al. The risk of prostate cancer amongst black men in the United Kingdom: The PROCESS cohort study. *Eur Urol* 2008; 53: 99–105.

26. Gleason DF et al. Prediction of prognosis for prostatic adenocarcinoma by combined histological grading and clinical staging. *J Urol* 1974; 111: 58–64.

27. Partin AW et al. Combination of prostate-specific antigen, clinical stage, and Gleason score to predict pathological stage of localized prostate cancer. A multi-institutional update. *JAMA* 1997; 277: 1445–1451.

28. Oesterling JE et al. The use of prostate-specific antigen in staging patients with newly diagnosed prostate cancer. *JAMA* 1993; 269: 57–60.

29. Albertsen PC et al. Competing risk analysis of men aged 55 to 74 years at diagnosis managed conservatively for clinically localized prostate cancer. *JAMA* 1998; 280: 975–980.

30. van As NJ et al. Active surveillance with selective radical treatment for localized prostate cancer. *Cancer J* 2007; 13: 289–294.

31. Epstein JI et al. Pathologic and clinical findings to predict tumor extent of nonpalpable (stage T1c) prostate cancer. *JAMA* 1994; 271: 368–374.

32. Klotz L. Active surveillance with selective delayed intervention is the way to manage 'good-risk' prostate cancer. *Nat Clin Pract Urol* 2005; 2: 136–142.

33. Holmberg L et al. A randomized trial comparing radical prostatectomy with watchful waiting in early prostate cancer. *N Engl J Med* 2002; 347: 781–789.

34. Pound CR et al. Natural history of progression after PSA elevation following radical prostatectomy. *JAMA* 1999; 281: 1591–1597.

35. Dearnaley D et al. Conventional versus hypofractionated high-dose intensity-modulated radiotherapy for prostate cancer: 5-year outcomes of the randomised, non-inferiority, phase 3 CHHiP trial. *Lancet Oncol* 2016; 17: 1047–1060.

36. Bolla M et al. Long-term results with immediate androgen suppression and external irradiation in patients with locally advanced prostate cancer (an EORTC study): A phase III randomised trial. *Lancet* 2002; 360: 103–106.

37. Shipley WU. PSA following irradiation for prostate cancer: The upcoming ASTRO symposium. *Int J Radiat Oncol Biol Phys* 1996; 35: 1115.

38. Roach M, III et al. Defining biochemical failure following radiotherapy with or without hormonal therapy in men with clinically localized prostate cancer: Recommendations of the RTOG-ASTRO Phoenix Consensus Conference. *Int J Radiat Oncol Biol Phys* 2006; 65: 965–974.

39. Donaldson IA et al. Focal therapy: Patients, interventions, and outcomes – A report from a consensus meeting. *Eur Urol* 2015; 67: 771–777.

40. Sternberg CN. Apples and oranges. Re: 7.4-year update of the ongoing bicalutamide Early Prostate Cancer (EPC) trial programme. *BJU Int* 2006; 97: 435–438.

41. Bolla M et al. Postoperative radiotherapy after radical prostatectomy: A randomised controlled trial (EORTC trial 22911). *Lancet* 2005; 366: 572–578.

42. Parker C et al. Radiotherapy and androgen deprivation in combination after local surgery (RADICALS): A new Medical Research Council/National Cancer Institute of Canada phase III trial of adjuvant treatment after radical prostatectomy. *BJU Int* 2007; 99: 1376–1379.

43. McLeod DG et al. Bicalutamide 150 mg plus standard care vs standard care alone for early prostate cancer. *BJU Int* 2006; 97: 247–254.

44. The Medical Research Council Prostate Cancer Working Party Investigators Group. Immediate versus deferred treatment for advanced prostatic cancer: Initial results of the Medical Research Council Trial. *Br J Urol* 1997; 79: 235–246.

45. Messing EM et al. Immediate hormonal therapy compared with observation after radical prostatectomy and pelvic lymphadenectomy in men with node-positive prostate cancer. *N Engl J Med* 1999; 341: 1781–1788.

46. James ND et al. Addition of docetaxel, zoledronic acid, or both to first-line long-term hormone therapy in prostate cancer (STAMPEDE): Survival results from an adaptive, multiarm, multistage, platform randomised controlled trial. *Lancet* 2016; 387: 1163–1177.

47. Saad F et al. Long-term efficacy of zoledronic acid for the prevention of skeletal complications in patients with metastatic hormone-refractory prostate cancer. *J Natl Cancer Inst* 2004; 96: 879–882.

48. Tannock IF et al. Docetaxel plus prednisone or mitoxantrone plus prednisone for advanced prostate cancer. *N Engl J Med* 2004; 351: 1502–1512.

49. Wilson JMG and Junger G. Principles and practice of screening for disease. *J R Coll Gen Pract* 1968; 16: 318.

CHAPTER 2
TESTICULAR CANCER

Farooq A Khan and Jas S Kalsi

Contents

CLINICAL ASSESSMENT OF TESTICULAR SWELLINGS, IMAGING AND STAGING

Q. A 26-year-old previously healthy man is referred to the urology clinic on the 2-week wait proforma with a right-sided testicular mass. How will you assess the patient in clinic?

A. I would take a pertinent history and perform a physical examination with specific reference to the following sections.

History

Related to the mass

- Length of symptoms
- Painful or painless mass
- Change in size of mass
- Any previous history of surgery on the genitalia
- Sexual history – Recent sexual contact or penile discharge
- Associated urinary symptoms
- Trauma – Does not cause testicular cancer but may be the cause of the testicular swelling in 10%–15%

Previous relevant history and risk factors

History of cryptorchidism (either side) – This increases the risk of testicular cancer between 4 and 13 times in the undescended testicle [1] with 7%–10% of testicular tumours arising in an undescended testis [2]. There still remains a 5%–10% risk of developing testicular cancer in the contralateral testis with those with a history of cryptorchidism [3,4].

Family history of testicular cancer – Especially in fathers and brothers – increases risk by six and eight times, respectively, with 1.35% providing a positive family history [5,6].

Race – Testicular cancer is three times more common in Caucasians and in Northern Europeans with the highest incidence in Scandinavia, 11 per 100,000 men (Norway and Denmark). In the United Kingdom the incidence is 7.1 per 100,000 men.

Maternal oestrogen exposure – Foetal exposure of diethylstilboestrol increases the risk of testicular cancer in the male offspring (relative risk 2.8%–5.3%). This is a difficult history to elicit [4].

History of subfertility and poor semen analysis parameters increases the risk of testicular cancer in some studies by 1.6 times and from the SEER (Surveillance, Epidemiology and End Results) database by 20 times.

Contralateral history of testicular tumour – There remains a 5%–10% risk of testis cancer in the remaining testicle.

HIV – Increased risk of seminoma – Cause unknown.

Q. What features are you particularly interested in on physical examination?

A. I would perform a general examination to include palpation of the supraclavicular nodes, chest examination and an abdominal examination to palpate for a retroperitoneal nodal mass and ensure there are no inguinal scars from childhood orchidopexy that the patient has failed to mention. I would complete my examination by examining the testicle for the mass, its size and whether it is painful or painless. I would also examine the contralateral testicle.

The presence of pain does not confidently discriminate infection from a neoplastic process as 10% of men presenting with a painful testicle, clinically resembling epididymo-orchitis, have a testicular tumour and up to 20% can present with testicular pain as their first symptom [1].

Q. His right testicle has a hard, irregular and painless mass arising from the upper pole. What would you do?

A. I would arrange an urgent scrotal ultrasound scan and in our department we would walk the patient round to the radiology department for this the same day (using a minimum of a 7.5 MHz transducer).

Q. The ultrasound shows the image presented in Figure 2.1. What do you see and how would you describe this?

A. Figure 2.1 shows a heterogenous, irregular mass in the upper pole of the right testis. Clinically this is a testicular tumour.

Q. Any other investigations you would like to do in clinic?

A. I would take tumour markers, namely, serum α-fetoprotein (AFP – half-life 5–7 days), β-human chorionic gonadotrophin (βhCG – half-life 24–36 hours) and lactate dehydrogenase (LDH) and arrange a contrast CT chest, abdomen and pelvis particularly if widespread metastases are suspected (the presence of widespread testicular metastases on imaging is an oncological emergency and the patient must be referred urgently to

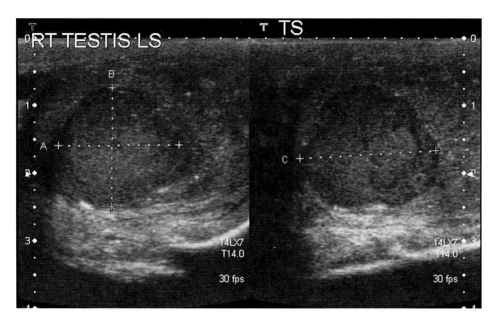

Figure 2.1

an oncologist – immediate chemotherapy may be necessary prior to radical inguinal orchidectomy in these cases).

Note: *Historically one would obtain a pre-operative CXR from clinic to elucidate the presence of widespread metastases but with the recent ease of access to CT scans pre-operative CXRs are performed less often.*

Q. Do all patients have raised tumour markers at presentation?

A. No. Across the board for all testicular tumours, 51% will have raised tumour markers. This varies for the type of tumour present. For germ cell tumours, 5%–10% of pure seminomas will have a raised βhCG (produced by syncytiotrophoblast elements). Pure seminomas do not secrete AFP.

For non-seminomatous germ cell tumours (NSGCTs) elevated tumour markers can be found in up to 90% of cases, with 50%–70% having raised AFP (produced by yolk sac elements) and ~40% having a raised βhCG. Elevated βhCG is found in 100% of choriocarcinoma and 40%–60% of embryonal carcinoma cases.

Q. What is the role of tumour markers in this case?

A. They are both diagnostic and prognostic. Measurement of tumour markers following orchidectomy and their half-life decline are useful in assessing the likelihood of retroperitoneal and metastatic disease. Given the half-life of the markers we would expect the βhCG to halve every 36 hours and the AFP every 5 days.

The presence of normal markers prior to orchidectomy does not exclude metastatic disease and equally normalisation of markers post-orchidectomy does not mean the absence of distant disease.

Q. What is the significance of measuring the LDH?

A. This is useful in determining tumour burden and is a surrogate marker for tumour volume and cell necrosis. This is usually helpful for seminomas and to the oncologist as a measure of tumour response. It is raised in approximately 10% of seminomas.

Q. Are there any other conditions in which the above tumour markers may be raised other than in testicular cancer?

A. Yes. Other malignancies can raise the βhCG such as pancreatic, liver, stomach, lung, breast, kidney and bladder and strangely in marijuana smokers. AFP can be raised with liver, pancreas, stomach and lung malignancies and with benign liver dysfunction.

In addition raised levels of luteinizing hormone in hypo-gonadotrophic patients may cross-react with some radio-immunoassay techniques for βhCG resulting in spuriously high results.

Q. Is there any other pre-operative imaging you might wish to undertake other than a scrotal ultrasound scan?

A. Ideally a contrast CT scan of the chest, abdomen and pelvis should be performed pre-operatively for staging purposes. However, surgery should be undertaken at the earliest opportunity and should not be delayed if CT scan cannot be performed in a timely manner in which case the CT can be performed *after* inguinal orchidectomy. Importantly, as mentioned earlier, in the scenario where widespread metastases are suspected on presentation pre-operative contrast CT of the chest, abdomen and pelvis (or CXR if CT not easily accessible) is mandatory.

There is no role for the routine use of pre-operative magnetic resonance imaging (MRI) or positron emission tomography (PET), as these do not alter the initial treatment plan. They may have a role in select cases in assessing the retroperitoneal nodes – in the case of MRI in patients with a contrast allergy preventing the use of CT, or in the case of PET in assessing whether a residual retroperitoneal mass after chemotherapy (in seminomas) can be safely watched or needs active treatment.

Q. What would you do with this young man?

A. I would arrange for an urgent radical inguinal orchidectomy (<1 week) and consideration for contralateral testis biopsy in high-risk cases.

Q. How do you perform a radical inguinal orchidectomy?

A. Through an inguinal incision, the tumour-bearing testicle is removed along with the epididymis and spermatic coverings and cord. *Prior* to manipulation of the testis the cord is isolated and clamped to allow control of the draining lymphatics to minimise tumour spill and metastatic release into the lymphatics towards the landing retroperitoneal nodes. The tumour-bearing testicle is resected to the deep inguinal ring and is transected and secured with one heavy tie (0 or 1 Vicryl) and a transfixation suture. Some suggest that a Prolene suture be used at the cut end of the cord to act as a marker for possible future nodal dissection. (We do not do this during our orchidectomies.)

I would warn him of the common complications of bleeding, infection and specifically loss of sensation on the inner thigh and ipsilateral scrotal wall or chronic groin pain as a consequence of damage to the ilio-inguinal nerve. It is also important to warn of possible reduced hormonal and fertility potential.

Q. Is there anything you would offer him or consider prior to inguinal orchidectomy?

A. I would offer him the opportunity to sperm-bank and consider insertion of a prosthesis. The EAU recommends that sperm-banking take place prior to orchidectomy although for adequate specimens to be banked practically means that this happens after orchidectomy in most units. If there is a history of sub-fertility or a small contralateral testicle and fertility is an issue for the patient then sperm-banking prior to orchidectomy is highly advisable. I would offer him a prosthesis at the same sitting but caution should be advised in those who are likely to need early post-operative chemotherapy (pulmonary metastases, markedly raised markers) because prosthesis-related infection (0.6%–2%) [7] may delay this. Some oncologists would therefore prefer not to offer this in this setting but at a later date.

Q. **How does a patient bank sperm? Are there any issues the patient needs to be aware of?**

A. The patient is asked to attend the local designated fertility clinic to provide three semen samples with a 2–3 day period of abstinence. A brief assessment of sperm quality is undertaken microscopically and then the sample is frozen in liquid nitrogen at −196°C. Patients should be aware of the following as part of the consent process for sperm-banking:

- Quality of sperm is not guaranteed if and when it is thawed.
- Illness prior to or at the time of sperm-banking may affect the quality of sperm. If chemotherapy is planned sperm-banking can still be done in the first week or so following its initiation as sperm produced prior to the start of chemotherapy will still be healthy and usable.
- There is some evidence that the quality of semen in men with germ cell tumours is poor in comparison to similarly matched healthy males and assisted conception techniques may be required [8].
- Maximum storage is for 10 years (until the age of 55 in the United Kingdom).
- The Human Fertilisation and Embryology Authority (HFEA) require all men banking sperm to be screened for HIV and hepatitis B and C prior to its transfer to a long-term storage facility. Men with HIV/hepatitis can bank sperm in separate storage vessels.
- At present the cost of initial consultations, blood tests and storage for the first year are met by the National Health Service (NHS). Most centres charge £200 per year of storage after the first year which at present is met by the patient.
- The patient may need to travel some distance to the nearest facility to be able to sperm-bank.

Q. **The patient decides he wishes to have a prosthesis. What complications would you warn the patient regarding prosthesis insertion?**

A. The complications based on a review of 2,500 prostheses for a variety of indications [7] include

- Extrusion from the scrotum – 3%–8%
- Scrotal contraction and migration – 3%–5%
- Chronic pain – 1%–3%
- Haematoma – 0.3%–3%
- Infection – 0.6%–2%

Q. **You mentioned a little earlier that you would consider a contralateral testis biopsy? How will you decide this for individual patients?**

A. The purpose of a contralateral biopsy is to identify the presence of carcinoma *in situ* or intratubular germ cell neoplasia (ITGCN) the risk of which is ~5%–9% of patients with testicular cancer. The EAU recommends that men under the age of 40 with a contralateral testis volume of <12 mL (relative risk for developing ITGCN is 3.78) have a 34% risk of ITGCN on biopsy [9]. Contralateral testicular biopsy should also be considered in men with a history of undescended testis (normal volume testis) and subfertility/poor spermatogenesis as these are associated with ITGCN [9,10].

Q. How would you biopsy the contralateral side?

A. Through a scrotal incision the tunica vaginalis is opened and the testicle is delivered. Small incisions of the tunica albuginea at each pole (5 mm) are made with a scalpel allowing extrusion of the seminiferous tubules. These are then cut with a pair of scissors or taken flush to the albuginea with a scalpel and placed into Bouin's solution (and not formalin). Using a double biopsy open technique (biopsies from each pole) it can be anticipated that 99% of ITGCN will be identified [11].

There is evidence that using a biopsy gun and Tru-Cut needle (with the testis delivered through a scrotal incision) provides the same quality of biopsy and detection rate for a diagnosis of ITGCN as does an open technique.

Q. Are there any occasions where an immediate orchidectomy is not undertaken?

A. Yes. In rare cases patients may present with extensive life-threatening metastatic disease (respiratory compromise from widespread metastases, severe back pain from retroperitoneal disease). In such cases an immediate orchidectomy is not required but urgent chemotherapy is under the care of an oncologist. A later orchidectomy may be required that may reveal the original tumour or often a residual scar in the testis.

In men with no obvious testicular tumour, but who have widespread disease of unknown origin, the diagnosis of a germ cell tumour should be considered and raised tumour markers can be diagnostic. Given that results of marker estimation will take some time before they are available, a urine pregnancy test can be considered to confirm the presence of urinary βhCG, which would be an indication that the widespread metastatic disease is in fact a germ cell tumour. Initial chemotherapy can then be given without delay.

Q. You perform the radical inguinal orchidectomy and your patient goes home the same day. What information do you want your pathologist to tell you about the orchidectomy specimen?

A. Macroscopically we want to know the size of the testicle and tumour and any macroscopic invasion of the epididymis, tunica vaginalis and cord structures.

Microscopically we would want to know the following:

- Histological type of tumour – Germ cell tumour, sex cord tumours
- Size
- Multiplicity
- Rete testis involvement
- Pathological stage
- Presence of ITGCN
- Presence of microvascular invasion
- If seminoma – Are there any non-seminomatous elements which would then dictate how the patient is managed in the long term?

Specifically for seminoma tumour size greater than 4 cm and rete testis invasion have been shown to be important prognosticators for relapse for stage I disease.

For NSGCT the presence of vascular and lymphatic invasion, the percentage of embryonal carcinoma (>50%) and the proliferation rate (>70%) predict for metastatic disease.

Note should be made of the pathological classification of testicular tumours which separates tumours into those of germ-cell origin (subdivided into those with one histological type and those with more than one histological type) and the less common sex cord and paratesticular tumours (see Table 2.1).

Table 2.1 Pathological classification of testicular tumours and comparison of the World Health Organisation (WHO) and British Testicular Tumour Panel and Registry (BTTP&R) pathological classifications of testicular germ cell tumours

WHO	BTTP&R
Germ cell tumours	Germ cell tumours
Seminoma	Seminoma
Spermatocytic seminoma	Spermatocytic seminoma

Non-seminomatous germ cell tumour
  1. Mature teratoma
  2. Embryonal carcinoma with teratoma (teratocarcinoma)
  3. Embryonal carcinoma
  4. Yolk sac tumour
  5. Choriocarcinoma
	Teratoma
	  1. Malignant teratoma differentiated (MTD)
	  2. Malignant teratoma intermediate (MTI)
	  3. Malignant teratoma undifferentiated (MTU)
	  4. Yolk sac tumour
	  5. Malignant teratoma trophoblastic (MTT)

Sex cord stromal tumours	
Leydig cell tumour	
Sertoli cell tumour	
Granulosa cell tumour	
Mixed	
Unclassified	
Mixed germ cell/sex cord stromal tumours	
Other tumours	
Adenocarcinoma of rete testis	
Lymphoma	
Metastatic	

Q. **Microscopically the specimen looks like this – Figure 2.2 – can you describe the likely histological diagnosis?**

A. Figure 2.2: There are islands and sheets of large cells with clear cytoplasm with densely staining nuclei of varying sizes with prominent nucleoli in keeping with the appearances of a seminoma. There are also fibrous glands traversing the tumour and an associated lymphocytic infiltrate which are also characteristic of a seminoma.

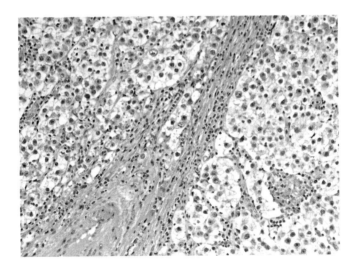

Figure 2.2

Q. **The pathologist agrees with you and reports the specimen as being a seminoma. What would you do now?**

A. I would complete the staging of the patient by way of a contrast abdominal and chest CT. In our department all patients with seminoma undergo this along with NSGCTs.

In addition, if there had been any elevated tumour markers pre-operatively I would repeat these and document the post-operative tumour marker kinetics.

SUMMARY AND KEY FACTS

- When asked 'How would you assess a patient?' always start with a history and examination and specifically tell them what things you want to know in the history, i.e. risk factors for testicular cancer.
- Ultrasound study in essence has almost 100% sensitivity for testicular tumour detection. MRI is just as good but expensive and therefore not cost effective.
- Overall 51% of new testicular tumours have raised markers.
- AFP is made by yolk sac elements and not raised with seminoma.
- βhCG is raised in all choriocarcinomas and only ~10% of seminomas. It is produced by the giant syncytiotrophoblastic cells.
- AFP half-life is 3–5 days. βhCG half-life is 36 hours.
- EAU guidelines recommend staging CT of abdomen/pelvis and chest for germ cell tumours.
- Always offer sperm-banking to a patient prior to orchidectomy, especially if there is a history of subfertility or small contralateral testis with patient desire to maintain fertility.
- EAU guidelines for a contralateral testis biopsy are as follows:
  - <40 years of age
  - Testicular volume <12 mL
  - Considered in men with history of undescended testis and subfertility
- The contralateral biopsy technique – open two-pole technique – will pick up 99% of ITGCN.
- Pathological prognostic factors for relapsing disease are as follows:

Seminoma:	Rete testis invasion
	Tumour size >4 cm
NSGCTs:	Microvascular/lymphatic invasion
	Embryonal cancer content >50%
	Proliferation rate >70%

INTRATUBULAR GERM CELL NEOPLASIA (ITGCN) AND MICROLITHIASIS

Q. **What do you understand by the term _testicular intraepithelial neoplasia_ (TIN) or intratubular germ cell neoplasia (ITGCN)?**

A. Intratubular germ cell neoplasia (ITGCN) is a malignant pre-invasive testicular germ cell lesion also known as carcinoma _in situ_. It is believed to be the precursor for all germ cell tumours except spermatocytic seminoma.

Q. **Why is ITGCN important?**

A. Its presence denotes that there is a 50% chance of progression to germ cell tumours over a 5-year period and a cumulative probability of 70% of developing cancer at 7 years [12].

Q. Pathologically how would you describe ITGCN? (Figure 2.3)

A. Histologically ITGCN is characterised by malignant germ cells lining seminiferous tubules containing Sertoli cells in a single row with nuclear pleomorphism with an intact basement membrane. The tubules are usually of smaller diameter than normal, with thickened walls, and show decreased or absent spermatogenesis. The atypical cells are usually aligned along the basement membrane and are similar in appearance to seminoma tumour cells – clear cytoplasm and large nuclei, round or irregular, with prominent nucleoli.

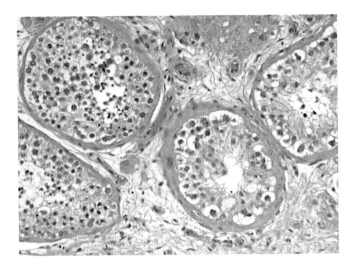

Figure 2.3 Intratubular germ cell neoplasia (ITGCN).

Q. How often do we see ITGCN in testicular tumours? Are there any other conditions associated with this condition?

A. It is present in the contralateral testis in about 5%–9% of patients; this number rises to 34% in those less than 40 years of age and with testicular volumes less than 12 mL, hence the recommended criteria for contralateral testis biopsy in this group of patients [9]. The presence of ITGCN in the tumour-bearing testicle has no bearing on overall prognosis. In the general population the overall incidence is ~0.8%.

Other risk factors for the development of ITGCN are as follows:

- Cryptorchidism (3%)
- Extra-gonadal germ cell tumour (40%)
- 45XO karyotype
- Subfertility (0.4%–1.1%)

Q. Does ITGCN raise tumour markers?

A. No.

Q. What would you tell the patient who has had an orchidectomy with ITGCN in the contralateral testis?

A. I would tell him that there is a risk of progression to invasive germ cell tumour over the following 5 years equating to 50%.

Q. The patient asks you what are you going to do about it?

A. This poses a difficult problem. The options for the patient are surveillance, treatment by way of radiotherapy or orchidectomy rendering the patient anorchic and reliant on testosterone replacement.

The case should be discussed with the patient. For those men who have not completed their family it is entirely reasonable to encourage them to do so naturally or by assisted conception techniques, if they wish, with a close surveillance programme. This will require regular self physical examinations and an annual ultrasound of the testis.

Radiation treatment is by way of a total dose of 20 Gy delivered at single 2 Gy doses over 5 days per week. This dose seems to be adequate to eliminate all foci of ITGCN but possibly at the loss of Leydig cell function necessitating the need for regular follow-up testosterone measurement. There is evidence that a smaller dose of 16 Gy is not adequate to completely eradicate ITGCN [13].

Undertaking an orchidectomy requires testosterone replacement therapy and loss of fertility.

Q. Is there any role for chemotherapy with ITGCN?

A. The answer to the question 'Will chemotherapy eradicate ITGCN in some patients?' is yes; but we would not use it routinely unless otherwise indicated.

Two-thirds of patients with ITGCN who need post-orchidectomy chemotherapy will have their ITGCN eradicated on follow-up biopsy. Any follow-up biopsy should be timed no earlier than 2 years after the completion of chemotherapy to minimise the risk of missing the ITGCN soon after chemotherapy. If the biopsies show persistent ITGCN then the above options can still be used although the likelihood of a low testosterone status is increased with radiation therapy at this stage.

Q. A young patient is referred by the GP with a testicular ultrasound showing widespread testicular microlithiasis. What is microlithiasis?

A. Microlithiasis is the presence of widespread calcifications present throughout the testicular parenchyma. Strictly the definition is the presence of more than five calcifications per image field on ultrasound with each calcification being less than 2 mm with no change in testicular shape or volume [14]. Its incidence in the population is 2%–6%.

Q. Is microlithiasis important? What would you tell the patient?

A. We now believe that microlithiasis is not as important as it once was thought to be. Originally, because of the finding of microlithiasis in association with testicular tumours, in some cases up to 74% of testicular cancer, it was believed that this may be a premalignant marker lesion and in some way aetiological in the development of testicular cancer. It is now clear that the rate of testicular cancer in with those with microlithiasis on long-term follow-up is no different to the rate of developing testicular cancer in the population as a whole [15], and for this reason we would not follow-up such patients in the urology clinic. Advice is given about self-examination and early referral on any palpable abnormality rather than annual testicular ultrasound that used to be the norm in many departments until recently.

Q. Is this advice true across the board for all patients?

A. Yes, although there is a suggestion that the risk of testicular cancer be stratified according to risk factors that the patient may have and the initial reason for the ultrasound.

Q. How would you stratify this risk?

A. For those without any risk factors for testicular cancer, advice on self-examination by the patient is given without urology follow-up. For those with risk factors an annual ultrasound is reasonable along with self-examination and possibly review with a urologist [16].

Q. What do you do in your department with a patient with microlithiasis?

A. We advise and educate patients to self-examine and do not undertake regular follow-up but will provide ultrasound testing to those patients who seek the additional reassurance this may provide, especially those who in the past may have been given advice that regular follow-up was recommended.

STAGING AND TREATMENT: CLINICAL STAGE I, II AND ADVANCED SEMINOMA

Q. **What do you understand by the term *staging* and why is it important in testicular cancer? What imaging modalities do we commonly use to stage testicular cancer?**

A. Staging is a process by which clinically, radiologically and pathologically the extent of the disease is defined to prognosticate for relapse and survival for the patient, and the need for additional treatments.

The mainstay of radiological staging is abdominal CT to assess retro-peritoneal nodes and chest CT to assess the lungs and mediastinum. The EAU recommends a chest CT for both seminomas and NSGCTs. Occasionally there can be a role in special select cases for MRI in those with a contrast allergy for whom a CT cannot be used and PET scanning in re-staging residual masses following chemotherapy, specifically in seminoma. CT scans of the head for brain metastases and liver imaging are used where clinically indicated.

Q. **What staging systems do you know for testis cancer?**

A. There are clinical and pathological staging systems. We use primarily the American Joint Committee on Cancer (AJCC) staging classification of TNM and serum markers (Table 2.2).

The AJCC TNM stage groupings of testicular germ cell tumours (Table 2.3) are similar to the Royal Marsden Staging System (Table 2.4). Stage I disease is that confined to the testis, stage II has varying degrees of retroperitoneal nodal involvement depending on size (stage IIA, B and C) and stage III indicates supra-diaphragmatic and visceral metastatic disease with varying degrees of raised tumour markers. The use of tumour markers in the TNM staging is unique to testis cancer.

Other staging systems include the Boden/Gibbs classification and the previously mentioned Royal Marsden system (Table 2.4), which are similar to the AJCC TNM stage grouping classification (Table 2.3).

Table 2.2 TNM classification of testicular cancer

pT	Primary tumour
pTX	Primary tumour cannot be assessed (T-Primary Tumour)
pT0	No evidence of primary tumour (e.g. histological scar in testis)
pTis	Intratubular germ cell neoplasia (carcinoma *in situ*)
pT1	Tumour limited to testis and epididymis without vascular/lymphatic invasion: tumour may invade the tunica albuginea but not tunica vaginalis
pT2	Tumour limited to testis and epididymis with vascular/lymphatic invasion, or tumour extending through tunica albuginea with involvement of tunica vaginalis
pT3	Tumour invades spermatic cord with or without vascular/lymphatic invasion
pT4	Tumour invades scrotum with or without vascular/lymphatic invasion
N	Regional lymph nodes clinical
NX	Regional lymph nodes cannot be assessed
N0	No regional lymph node metastasis
N1	Metastasis in a lymph node mass 2 cm or less in greatest dimension or multiple lymph nodes, none more than 2 cm in greatest dimension
N2	Metastasis in a lymph node mass more than 2 cm but not more than 5 cm in greatest dimension or multiple lymph nodes, any one mass more than 2 cm but not more than 5 cm in greatest dimension
N3	Metastasis in a lymph node mass more than 5 cm in greatest dimension

(Continued)

Table 2.2 (*Continued*) TNM classification of testicular cancer

pN	Pathological
pNX	Regional lymph nodes cannot be assessed
pN0	No regional lymph node metastasis
pN1	Metastasis in a lymph node mass 2 cm or less in greatest dimension and five or fewer positive nodes, none more than 2 cm in greatest dimension
pN2	Metastasis in a lymph node mass more than 2 cm but not more than 5 cm in greatest dimension and five or fewer positive nodes, none more than 2 cm in greatest dimension
pN3	Metastasis in a lymph node mass more than 5 cm in greatest dimension
M	**Distant metastasis**
MX	Distant metastasis cannot be assessed
M0	No distant metastasis
M1	Distant metastasis
M1a	Non-regional lymph node(s) or lung
M1b	Other sites
S	**Serum tumour markers**
SX	Serum tumour markers not available or not performed
S0	Serum marker study levels within normal limits

LDH (U/l)	hCG (mLU/mL)	AFP (ng/mL)
S1 <1.5 × N and	<5000 and	<1000
S2 <1.5–10 × N or	5000–50,000 or	1000–10,000
S3 >10 × N or	>50,000 or	>10,000

Note: N indicates the upper limit of normal for the LDH assay. LDH – lactate dehydrogenase; hCG – human chorionic gonadotropin; AFP – alpha-fetoprotein.

Table 2.3 AJCC stage groupings for testicular tumours

Stage	TNM classification
Stage I	pT1–4, N0, M0, SX
Stage II	Any pT/Tx, N1–3, M0, SX
IIA	Any pT/Tx, N1, M0, SX Any pT/Tx, N1, M0, S1
IIB	Any pT/Tx, N2, M0, S0 Any pT/Tx, N2, M0, S1
IIC	Any pT/Tx, N3, M0, S0 Any pT/Tx, N3, M0, S1
Stage III	Any pT/Tx, any N, M1, SX
IIIA	Any pT/Tx, any N1, M1a, S0 Any pT/Tx, any N1, M1a, S1
IIIB	Any pT/Tx, N1–3, M1a, S0 Any pT/Tx, any N, M1a, S2
IIIC	Any pT/Tx, N1–3, M0, S3 Any pT/Tx, any N, M1a, S3 Any pT/Tx, any N, M1b, any S

Table 2.4 Comparison of several staging systems for testicular cancer

Royal Marsden system	TNM system	Description
I	Tx, N0, M0	Disease confined to testis and peri-testicular tissue
II A <2 cm B 2–5 cm C >5–10 cm D >10 cm	Tx, N1 or N2a, M0	Fewer than six positive lymph nodes without extension into retroperitoneal fat; no node >2 cm (infradiaphragmatic)
	Tx, N2b, M0	Six or more positive lymph nodes, well-encapsulated and/or retroperitoneal fat extension; any node >2 cm
	Tx, N3, M0	Any node >5 cm
III	Tx, Nx, M1	Supradiaphragmatic and infradiaphragmatic lymphadenopathy (no extralymphatic metastasis)
IV		Disseminated disease (lungs, liver, bone)

Q. A patient has an orchidectomy and histologically this is a seminoma that is confined to the testicle. His staging CT of chest, abdomen and pelvis is normal and he has normal tumour markers. What stage disease does he have?

A. This is clinical stage I disease. Stage I is disease confined to the testicle and surrounding structures without nodal spread or metastatic deposits (T1-4, N0, M0).

Stage I disease can be broken down further into IA where the T stage is T1 (confined to testis with no involvement of tunica vaginalis and no vascular invasion, stage IB where the tumour stage is T2-T4 but normal markers and stage IS where any T stage is accompanied by elevated serum tumour markers.

Q. Does this man need follow-up and if so by whom? What would you do with this man with clinical stage I seminoma?

A. Such patients are normally followed up by the oncologist. The purpose of follow-up is to detect distant disease relapse especially in the retroperitoneum and initiate early treatment.

For clinical stage I seminoma, about 15%–20% of men have subclinical metastatic disease usually in the retroperitoneum and will subsequently relapse after orchidectomy alone [17]. To minimise this rate of relapse an informed discussion with patients about the need for adjuvant treatment is undertaken that reduces this risk balanced with the risks of treatment.

Q. What options does this young man have for clinical stage I seminoma following radical inguinal orchidectomy?

A. The options are surveillance, single-dose adjuvant chemotherapy (carboplatin) following orchidectomy or adjuvant radiotherapy to the retroperitoneum.

Q. This man is interested in surveillance given that you have indicated to him an approximately 80%–85% chance of being cured by orchidectomy alone. What would you tell him in light of the above information about surveillance?

A. I would tell him that patients who choose surveillance have an 80%–85% cure rate with orchidectomy alone but will need close regular follow-up with which they must be compliant to look for relapse. If relapse were to occur it can be treated with adjuvant treatment resulting in an overall cancer-specific survival of 97%–100%. Given that ~16% will relapse [18] over a 5-year period of follow-up an intensive programme of clinic visits and imaging of the retroperitoneum by yearly CT for the first 4 years along with 6 monthly CXR along with physical examination and tumour marker assessment every 3 months is advocated. Patients have to be committed to this extensive surveillance approach.

In addition to the above, I would warn him that while the majority of relapses occur in the first few years of follow-up about 20% of late relapses occur after 4 years [17], and hence there is a necessity for prolonged follow-up which in some cases can be lifelong, with its attendant anxiety and psychological stress that this may generate in some patients. Any relapse following a period of observation requires a more intensive treatment schedule of radiotherapy or chemotherapy.

Q. **Are there any prognostic factors that you are aware of for clinical stage I seminoma that may guide you in counselling this patient?**

A. Yes. Data from retrospective meta-analysis of surveillance studies suggest that the tumour size (>4 cm) and invasion of the rete testis represent a group of men that are at higher risk for future relapse for stage I seminoma. Together, the presence of both these factors can represent a relapse rate of 32% versus 16% for the presence of one risk factor and 12% when both these risk factors are absent [19]. For this reason the notion of a risk-adapted approach has developed where patients at higher risk of failure are encouraged to undergo adjuvant therapy and those at lower risk can safely choose surveillance as a reasonable option in the first instance. Early data of the risk-adapted approach suggest that this approach can safely be used in this setting.

Q. **What other options are available to him? What would you tell him about the other options for stage I seminoma?**

A. He can consider adjuvant radiotherapy or chemotherapy. Both radiotherapy and chemotherapy are equally effective and reduce the risk of relapse in the retroperitoneum down to 3%–4% (from the 15%–20% risk from surveillance alone).

Radiotherapy is administered in a hockey-stick fashion to the para-aortic field and ipsilateral iliac nodes to a total dose of 20 Gy over a 2-week period, and chemotherapy consists of a single dose of carboplatin (EORTC trial AUC 7, MRC trial TE 19). After a follow-up of 4 years both have been shown to be equally effective [20].

Q. **What do the oncologists in your unit generally now advise?**

A. Given the equal efficacy of single-dose chemotherapy (i.e. one cycle of carboplatin) to radiotherapy, there is a general trend in offering the former as the preferred adjuvant modality for its ease of administration, shorter time to delivery and the recognised late secondary pelvic malignancy rate with the use of radiotherapy (albeit small and unquantified).

Q. **This patient decides to have adjuvant chemotherapy. How would you then follow-up the patient?**

A. Three-monthly clinic appointments with physical examination, tumour markers and 6 monthly CXRs and yearly CT scans for the first 3 years eventually stretching out at year 5 to annual assessments. The follow-up regime is more intensive in the first 2 years as this is the time when relapses are more likely to occur.

Q. **Why do you think that follow-up needs to be extended in such cases?**

A. While most disease relapse occurs within the first few years, there remains with seminoma a 20% risk of relapse after 4 years with some cases presenting after the 10-year mark and so some would advocate a lifelong follow-up schedule.

Q. **If instead, following his staging investigations he presented with a CT as shown in Figure 2.4, what do you think this shows?**

A. Figure 2.4: This shows the presence of enlarged retroperitoneal nodes encasing the inferior vena cava highly suggestive of metastatic disease in the retroperitoneum. This indicates that the patient has stage II disease or nodal metastatic disease.

In general, metastatic disease can be classified into low-volume metastatic disease which includes stages IIA and IIB (stage II disease can be divided into A [<2 cm nodal mass] and B [2–5 cm nodal mass]) and advanced metastatic disease which encompasses stage IIC (nodal mass >5 cm) and stage III disease (supradiaphragmatic or visceral metastases).

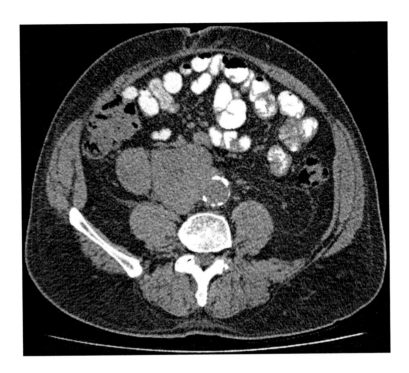

Figure 2.4

Q. **What do you want to do with this patient now?**

A. The mainstay of treatment for seminoma in this group (stage IIA/B) is three cycles of BEP chemotherapy (bleomycin, etoposide and cisplatin) or four cycles of EP (etoposide and cisplatin) for those in whom bleomycin should be avoided (age >40, smokers). There are, however, some centres that still would offer radiotherapy, 30–36 Gy, but this is not the norm in UK practice despite being popular in Europe, especially for stage IIA disease.

Treatment in metastatic germ cell tumours is based on the prognostic groups defined by the International Germ Cell Cancer Consensus Group (IGCCCG) which have validated a model for germ cell tumours that separates patients into good, intermediate and poor prognostic groups based on histology, location of primary tumour, location of metastases and post-orchidectomy tumour marker levels (Table 2.5). Treatment and specifically chemotherapy is tailored according to this classification allowing high cure rates with minimal toxicity for the good prognostic group and more aggressive chemotherapy reserved for the poor prognostic group.

Table 2.5 The International Germ Cell Cancer Collaborative Group (IGCCCG) prognostic-based staging system for metastatic seminoma

Good prognosis group	
(90% of cases)	*All of the following criteria*
5-year PFS 82%	Any primary site
5-year survival 86%	No non-pulmonary visceral metastases
Normal AFP	
Any hCG	
Any LDH	
Intermediate prognosis group	
(10% of cases)	*Any of the following criteria*
5-year PFS 67%	Any primary site
5-year survival 72%	Non-pulmonary visceral metastases
Normal AFP	
Any hCG	
Any LDH	
Seminoma	
No patients classified as poor prognosis	

Note: PFS – progression-free survival.

Q. **Following from the above he has induction chemotherapy and has a follow-up CT scan 3 months later, which shows the persistence of a retroperitoneal mass. What do you do now?**

A. I would check his tumour markers in the first instance. Seminomatous residual masses following chemotherapy or radiation therapy are not common and can be observed by serial imaging without the need to resort to immediate resection of the retroperitoneal mass irrespective of size. PET scanning has been found to be particularly useful in this group of patients in separating retroperitoneal masses that have active tumour in them. Generally it is agreed that residual masses >3 cm that do not regress after therapy should undergo this imaging modality to look for evidence of active tumour. A positive PET scan after a 4–6 week interval following the end of chemotherapy/radiotherapy is a very reliable predictor for viable tumour tissue in this group of patients. For such patients confirmation by way of biopsy may require further treatment such as retroperitoneal lymph node dissection (RPLND), salvage chemotherapy (or radiotherapy in those who did not receive this initially). In general a residual mass after primary treatment in seminoma is rare. Surgery after treatment for seminoma is generally more difficult and restricted to patients with 'globular' masses rather than a retro-peritoneal fibrosis type of picture.

Q. **If the patient presented with advanced seminoma from the outset (stage IIC and greater) what would the mainstay of treatment have been?**

A. The mainstay of treatment is three or four cycles of chemotherapy with BEP or EP if contraindications to bleomycin exist (i.e. smoker, >40 years of age, high burden of pulmonary metastases) which again is based on the IGCCCG classification grouping system (Table 2.5). The final regime that the patient receives is guided by the prognostic group he falls into. For the good prognosis group this is three cycles of BEP, for the intermediate group this is four cycles. There is no poor prognosis group for seminomatous disease.

STAGING AND TREATMENT: CLINICAL STAGE I, II NSGCT

Q. **If the tumour was an NSGCT but still stage I disease, would you do anything different compared to clinical stage I seminoma?**

A. Again, a number of options exist post-radical orchidectomy with surveillance or adjuvant chemotherapy or, for those not prepared to consider the first two options, RPLND remains an option.

Across all NSGCTs surveillance alone has a 30% relapse rate (the majority in the retroperitoneum and then the lungs) if orchidectomy is the sole treatment. The majority of such relapses occur in the first year of follow-up (~80%).

Q. **Is there anything that can guide you in determining and counselling the patient about the most appropriate option?**

A. For NSGCTs the presence of vascular invasion is the most important prognosticator for distant relapse. The presence of vascular invasion portends a 48% risk of developing metastatic disease versus 14%–22% without vascular invasion. Once again, a risk-adapted approach can be used to stratify patients into low-risk and high-risk groups based on the absence or presence of vascular invasion, respectively.

Q. **What would you advise the patient?**

A. The patient can choose adjuvant treatment but in the absence of vascular invasion we would advocate a surveillance program with regular CT scans at 0, 3 and 12 months. This means that 78%–86% of patients are cured following orchidectomy alone and do not require further treatment.

However, if there are difficulties with patient compliance with this regime, adjuvant chemotherapy with two cycles of BEP are recommended.

However, in the presence of vascular invasion, we would advise adjuvant chemotherapy with two cycles of BEP. Surveillance can be used but given the 48% risk of relapse and the anxiety this can generate adjuvant chemotherapy is advised.

Q. **Is there anything else that can be offered in clinical stage I NSGCT with vascular invasion in this group of patients?**

A. Occasionally, patients unwilling to undergo surveillance or adjuvant chemotherapy can be offered an RPLND. This exposes patients to surgery and its associated side effects in about 50% of cases who may never have relapsed. At the same time RPLND does not eliminate the possibility of late distant recurrence, often in the lungs (~10%). In such patients who undergo an RPLND ~30% have disease in the retroperitoneum that upstages their disease to pathological stage II disease and will require additional chemotherapy with two cycles of BEP to reduce the 30% risk of relapse to 2%, although in some centres surgery alone will be used. In the United States it is normal practice to offer all stage I NSGCTs an RPLND to accurately pathologically stage the disease. In the United Kingdom, first-line treatment is surveillance or two cycles of BEP chemotherapy. If the patient is unwilling to follow an intensive surveillance program or undergo chemotherapy an RPLND can be advised.

Q. **In general what would the follow-up be for these patients?**

A. The follow-up schedule differs depending on the treatment modality chosen. For those who choose surveillance this is more intensive and regimens vary but generally patients require three-monthly clinic visits with tumour marker assessment, biannual chest x-rays and biannual abdomino-pelvic CT for the first 2 years with the frequency of these tailing off with up to 10 years of follow-up. For those who choose RPLND or adjuvant chemotherapy the follow-up is less intensive with the above applicable in general but with the CT scan being undertaken annually.

Q. **If instead the patient at first presentation on his staging CT had the following appearances, Figure 2.5, with elevated tumour markers what would you do?**

A. He has clinical stage II disease and I would therefore offer the patient induction chemo-therapy based on the IGCCCG prognostic classification (Table 2.6). For the good prognosis group, they would normally receive three cycles of BEP (22 day cycle), or for those in whom bleomycin needs to be avoided, four cycles of EP. For the intermediate and poor groups, four cycles of BEP, or if bleomycin is to be avoided, then four cycles of cisplatin, etoposide and ifosfamide (PEI/VIP) with a follow-up repeat CT scan to look for regression of the retroperitoneal nodes at 4–6 weeks. Occasionally, a rare situation arises where small retroperitoneal nodes are detected, that may well be benign, without elevation of tumour markers (marker negative stage IIA disease). The difficulty is deciding whether such nodes are pathological. For marker negative stage IIA disease with small 1–2 cm nodes, a policy of surveillance especially if the nodes are shrinking on serial scans is acceptable although this depends also on the original orchidectomy histology. The EAU recommends that in clinical stage IIA disease with negative markers, patients with pure embryonal carcinoma in the orchidectomy specimen undergo immediate chemotherapy. If the histology was teratoma or mixed tumour, surveillance or an RPLND can be undertaken. In practice in the United Kingdom, most centres would give chemotherapy or an early CT and if the nodes were still present, proceed with chemotherapy. Patients with marker negative stage IIA disease who are unwilling to undergo chemotherapy have the option to have RPLND with adjuvant chemotherapy (two cycles of BEP) if nodal disease is present on RPLND histology.

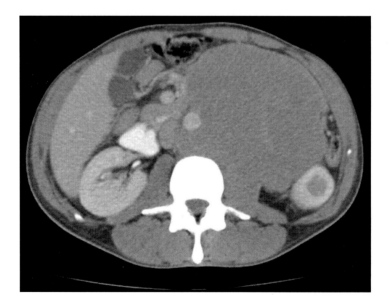

Figure 2.5

Table 2.6 The International Germ Cell Cancer Collaborative Group (IGCCCG) prognostic-based staging system for metastatic NSGCT

Good prognosis group		
(56% of cases)	*All of the following criteria*	
5-year PFS 89%	Testis/retroperitoneal primary	
5-year survival 92%	No non-pulmonary visceral metastases	
AFP < 1000 ng/mL		
hCG < 5000 IU/L (1,000 ng/mL)		
LDHz < 1.5 × ULN		
Intermediate prognosis group		
(28% of cases)	*Any of the following criteria*	
5-year PFS 41%	Mediastinal primary	
5-year survival 48%	Non-pulmonary visceral metastases	
AFP > 1000 and <10,000 ng/mL or		
hCG > 5000 and <50,000 IU/L or		
LDH > 1.5 and <10 × ULN		
Poor prognosis group		
(16% of cases)	*Any of the following criteria*	
5-year PFS 41%	Mediastinal primary	
5-year survival 48%	Non-pulmonary visceral metastases	
AFP > 10,000 ng/mL or		
hCG > 50,000 IU/L (10,000 ng/mL) or		
LDH > 10 × ULN		

Note: PFS – progression-free survival.

Q. His CT after induction chemotherapy is as shown in Figure 2.6. What would you do now?

A. There still remains a large para-aortic retroperitoneal mass that has regressed considerably following the chemotherapy. At this point I would check his tumour markers again. If these have normalised he has potentially resectable disease by way of an RPLND. However, if his markers remained elevated but at a plateau we would watch this a little further with further markers taken at variable times in the succeeding 4–12 weeks. If at this stage these remained stable we would offer him an RPLND. If they continue to rise then instead of surgery, salvage chemotherapy is needed with PEI/VIP or paclitaxel, ifosfamide and cisplatin (TIP) regimes.

There is no reliable model to predict whether such masses harbour active tumour and so RPLND is mandatory with residual masses in excess of 1 cm as the likelihood of significant residual disease rises. Unlike stage II seminoma there is no role for PET scanning in this group. In general, for those patients who undergo RPLND for a residual mass after primary induction BEP chemotherapy, the histology will show necrosis in 50% (~30% in most series), mature teratoma in 35% and viable cancer in 15%, although there are few predictors of this. Such masses have an increased risk of harbouring teratoma in the final histology if the original orchidectomy specimen had teratoma.

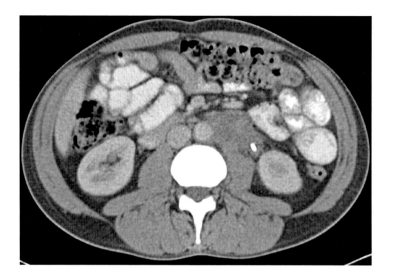

Figure 2.6

Q. A different patient had initially presented with clinical stage I NSGCT disease with vascular invasion and completed two cycles of primary BEP chemotherapy. He has a follow-up CT scan at 12 months. What do the images show – Figures 2.7 and 2.8?

A. Axial (Figure 2.7) and coronal (Figure 2.8) CT images show bulky nodes in the retroperitoneum encasing the great vessels indicating clinical relapse.

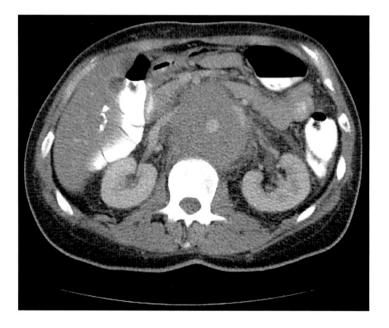

Figure 2.7

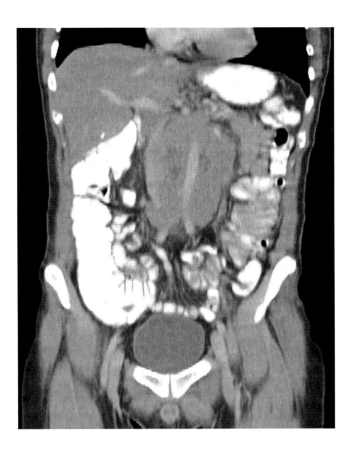

Figure 2.8

Q. What do you do now with the patient?

A. In this instance given a residual mass following induction chemotherapy, the patient needs second-line or salvage chemotherapy. This normally takes the form of four cycles of PEI/VIP (cisplatin, etoposide and ifosfamide) or four cycles of TIP (cisplatin, ifosfamide and pacli-taxel). The response to this salvage chemotherapy depends on a variety of factors such as the original histology and location of the tumour, response to first-line treatment, duration of remission and level of tumour markers at relapse. There is some early evidence that treatment of refractory germ cell tumours may benefit from a combination of Taxol and gemcitabine chemotherapy and referral to centres that have expertise in this area as well as entering such patients into clinical trials is advised.

Q. If the retroperitoneal mass persisted despite salvage chemotherapy (Figure 2.9) is there anything else that could be offered?

A. Yes, salvage RPLND 4–6 weeks after normalisation of tumour markers or achievement of their plateau could be offered. The outlook is poor for those patients who after second- or third-line chemotherapy still harbour undifferentiated tumour in the surgical specimen.

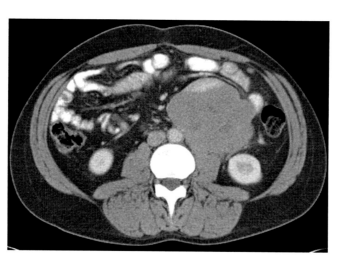

Figure 2.9 Persistent retroperitoneal mass despite salvage chemotherapy.

Q. What are the principles of post-chemotherapy RPLND surgery?

A. Through a transabdominal or thoracoabdominal approach, the retroperitoneal great vessels are completely cleared removing all lymphatic tissue out to the ureters, extending from the renal artery down to the ipsilateral external iliac vessels. Nodal tissue is dissected out in an attempt to cure the patient (if this is the only site of metastatic disease) but one must minimise morbidity and particularly attempt to preserve antegrade ejaculation, if possible. With unilateral disease it may be possible to preserve the contralateral hypogastric plexus and postganglionic sympathetic fibres (and so antegrade ejaculation). In pre-chemotherapy cases nerve-sparing RPLND can be performed leading to an antegrade ejaculation rate as high as 90%.

Q. What would you warn the patient about prior to an RPLND?

A. RPLND is a major undertaking that has an associated mortality (1%–3%) and morbidity rate (5%–25%) and with the use of modern dissection templates is designed to minimise the complications mainly associated with ejaculation and subsequent fertility in young men.
The main complications are as follows:

- Overall complication rate ~10%
- Major complications ~1%–5%
  - Chylous ascites – 1%–3%
  - Renovascular injury and nephrectomy – higher in post-chemotherapy cases – it is not 'injury' but a planned nephrectomy in around 5%–8%
  - Small bowel obstruction – 1%–3%
  - Spinal cord ischaemia – <1%
- Minor complications ~15%
  - Wound infections
  - Anejaculation
  - Paralytic ileus
  - Lymphocele
  - Transient hyperamylasemia
  - Pneumonitis/atelectasis

Q. How would you follow-up a patient after an RPLND?

A. This depends on the histology. For necrosis and mature teratoma no further adjuvant treatment is required as the relapse rate in this group of patients is low (~5%–10%) but for viable tumour further salvage chemotherapy is advised with second-line chemotherapy [21]. In completely resected tumours with viable tumour, 70% of patients remain disease free as compared to none who did not receive further chemotherapy. Furthermore, patients with complete resection, good IGCCCG prognostic grouping and less than 10% viable tumour, tend to fair well following RPLND and therefore may not need further salvage chemotherapy.

With respect to chemotherapy, caution is used in those who have already received bleomycin as this cumulative dose increases the risk of 'bleomycin lung', a pneumonitis and fibrotic condition of the lung interstitium. Occasionally if a further residual mass persists despite this, a second RPLND can be considered but this is rare.

Q. **If the patient had first presented with stage III NSGCT disease how would the treatment broadly speaking differ?**

A. Again the treatment would be similar to advanced seminoma based on the IGCCCG classification system. In essence this is three cycles of BEP chemotherapy in the first instance for the good prognosis group and four cycles for the intermediate group. For the poor prognostic group the standard remains four cycles of BEP or PEI (cisplatin, etoposide and ifosfamide) but referral to a reference centre for inclusion into trials is recommended as the optimum treatment remains to be established.

Q. **If a patient at first presentation has a CT of the brain that shows a metastatic deposit, does that confer a poor prognosis compared to a later relapse to the brain following initial successful treatment (Figure 2.10)?**

A. No. Approximately 10% of all patients with a germ cell tumour present with brain metastases and overall have a long-term survival of 30%–40%. Patients who relapse in the brain following initial treatment do so as part of a systemic relapse pattern and have a poor 5-year survival in the order of 2%–5%.

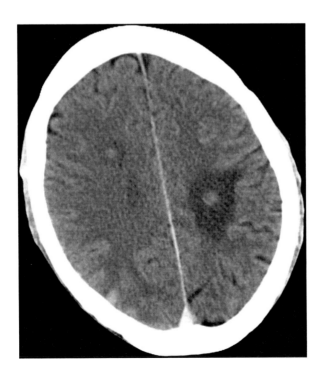

Figure 2.10

KEY FACTS AND SUMMARY

- *Relapse rates for surveillance*

Clinical stage I seminoma	Relapse after surveillance 15%–20% Relapse after adjuvant chemotherapy 3%–4% Relapse after adjuvant radiotherapy 3%–4%
Relapse with poor prognostic factors	Tumour >4 cm Rete testis involvement
Clinical stage I NSGCT	Surveillance relapse 30% (greater if vascular invasion) Adjuvant chemotherapy 2% Poor prognostic factor: vascular invasion

- *Metastatic germ cell tumour* – Treatment based on IGCCCG prognostic classification.

Stage IIA/B disease: seminoma	Chemotherapy (three cycles of BEP or four of EP) (occasionally radiotherapy)
Stage IIA/B NSGCT	Good prognosis group: three cycles of BEP Intermediate and poor group: four cycles of BEP If residual mass perform RPLND – if histology positive then salvage chemotherapy
Stage IIC and III	Based on IGCCCG grouping Good group: three cycles of BEP Intermediate group: four cycles of BEP Poor group: four cycles of BEP or PEI/VIP (recommend enrolment in trials)

- *Drainage of nodes to retroperitoneum* – Defined drainage (landing sites) to retroperitoneum is based on the site of the tumour.
  - *Right-sided testicular tumours* – First landing zone is the inter-aortocaval area, followed by the pre-caval and pre-aortic nodes and finally the right common iliac and external iliac nodes.
  - *Left-sided testicular tumours* – First landing zone is the para-aortic and pre-aortic nodes followed by the inter-aortocaval nodes and finally the left common iliac and external iliac nodes.

  Rare for left-sided tumours to have positive right-sided nodes (~1%) but more common the other way round.

ACKNOWLEDGEMENT

We are very grateful to Dr Matthew Gaskarth (Consultant Radiologist, Addenbrookes Hospital, Cambridge) and Dr Anne Warren (Consultant Pathologist, Addenbrookes Hospital, Cambridge) for providing the radiology and histopathological images to complement the chapter.

REFERENCES

1. Schottenfeld D et al. The epidemiology of testicular cancer in young adults. *Am J Epidemiol* 1980; 112: 232–246.
2. Whitaker RH. Neoplasia in cryptorchid men. *Semin Urol* 1988; 6: 107–109.

3. Berthelsen JG et al. Screening for carcinoma in situ of the contralateral testis in patients with germinal testicular cancer. *Br Med J (Clin Res Ed)* 1982; 285: 1683–1686.
4. Henderson BE et al. Risk factors for cancer of the testis in young men. *Int J Cancer* 1979; 23: 598–602.
5. Dieckmann KP et al. The prevalence of familial testicular cancer: An analysis of two patient populations and a review of the literature. *Cancer* 1997; 80: 1954–1960.
6. Westergaard T et al. Cancer risk in fathers and brothers of testicular cancer patients in Denmark. A population-based study. *Int J Cancer* 1996; 66: 627–631.
7. Marshall S. Potential problems with testicular prostheses. *Urology* 1986; 28: 388–390.
8. Dieckmann KP et al. Spermatogenesis in the contralateral testis of patients with testicular germ cell cancer: Histological evaluation of testicular biopsies and a comparison with healthy males. *BJU Int* 2007; 99: 1079–1085.
9. Harland SJ et al. Intratubular germ cell neoplasia of the contralateral testis in testicular cancer: Defining a high risk group. *J Urol* 1998; 160: 1353–1357.
10. Dieckmann KP et al. Prevalence of contralateral testicular intraepithelial neoplasia in patients with testicular germ cell neoplasms. *J Clin Oncol* 1996; 14: 3126–3132.
11. Dieckmann KP et al. Diagnosis of contralateral testicular intraepithelial neoplasia (TIN) in patients with testicular germ cell cancer: Systematic two-site biopsies are more sensitive than a single random biopsy. *Eur Urol* 2007; 51: 175–183.
12. Skakkebaek NE et al. Carcinoma-in-situ of the undescended testis. *Urol Clin North Am* 1982; 9: 377–385.
13. Classen J et al. Radiotherapy with 16 Gy may fail to eradicate testicular intraepithelial neoplasia: Preliminary communication of a dose-reduction trial of the German Testicular Cancer Study Group. *Br J Cancer* 2003; 88: 828–831.
14. Hobarth K et al. Incidence of testicular microlithiasis. *Urology* 1992; 40: 464–467.
15. DeCastro BJ et al. A 5-year followup study of asymptomatic men with testicular microlithiasis. *J Urol* 2008; 179: 1420–1423.
16. Rashid HH et al. Testicular microlithiasis: A review and its association with testicular cancer. *Urol Oncol* 2004; 22: 285–289.
17. Warde P et al. Surveillance for stage I testicular seminoma. Is it a good option? *Urol Clin North Am* 1998; 25: 425–433.
18. Groll RJ et al. A comprehensive systematic review of testicular germ cell tumor surveillance. *Crit Rev Oncol Hematol* 2007; 64: 182–197.
19. Warde P et al. Prognostic factors for relapse in stage I seminoma managed by surveillance: A pooled analysis. *J Clin Oncol* 2002; 20: 4448–4452.
20. Oliver RT et al. Radiotherapy versus single-dose carboplatin in adjuvant treatment of stage I seminoma: A randomised trial. *Lancet* 2005; 366: 293–300.
21. Donohue JP et al. Integration of surgery and systemic therapy: Results and principles of integration. *Semin Urol Oncol* 1998; 16: 65–71.

FURTHER READING

http://uroweb.org/wp-content/uploads/11-Testicular-Cancer_2017_web.pdf

CHAPTER 3
PENILE CANCER

Asif Muneer

Contents

PENILE CANCER: AETIOLOGY AND EPIDEMIOLOGY

Q. A 50-year-old man attends your outpatient clinic as he is worried about developing penile cancer as he gets older. Approximately how many cases of penile cancer are reported annually in the United Kingdom?

A. The incidence is between 1.2 and 1.4 cases per 100,000 population which amounts to approximately 500–600 new cases per year in the UK.

Q. He wants to have a circumcision performed as he believes that this will be protective and reduce the risk of penile cancer in the long term. How would you counsel him?

A. Although neonatal circumcision significantly reduces the risk of developing penile cancer later in life, adult circumcision in the presence of a normal foreskin is unlikely to change the long-term risk. However, in the presence of an abnormal foreskin or glans, e.g. features of lichen sclerosus or pre-malignant lesions on the glans, adult circumcision would be a recommendation and can reduce the long-term risk.

Q. Do you know any risk factors for penile cancer?

A. It has been shown that neonatal circumcision virtually eliminates the risk of developing penile cancer which is why there are very few cases of penile cancer in countries which practice routine neonatal circumcision for religious or cultural reasons. Therefore the presence of a foreskin is a significant risk factor. Other risk factors include increasing age, phimosis, poor penile hygiene, smoking, exposure to ultraviolet (UV) radiation and a history of HPV infection. A history of lichen sclerosus is also a risk factor.

Q. **What is the most common histological subtype?**

A. Squamous cell carcinoma (SCC) accounts for the majority of penile cancers (95%) and is classified as usual type, papillary, condylomatous, basaloid, verrucous and sarcomatoid. Basaloid and sarcomatoid subtypes tend to be aggressive subtypes and carry a poor prognosis.

Rarer penile cancers include malignant melanoma (2%), basal cell carcinoma (2%) and extra-mammary Paget's disease, which is essentially an adenocarcinoma arising in the penile skin. Sarcomas account for less than 1% of penile cancers.

Q. **What is the role of HPV status as a prognostic marker?**

A. Although high risk HPV has been found to be an aetiological factor in penile cancer, the role as a prognostic marker is still unclear. Some reports suggest that HPV-positive tumours carry a better overall prognosis [1]. However, these studies are still limited by the low number of patients included in the study.

ASSESSMENT AND MANAGEMENT OF PRE-MALIGNANT PENILE LESIONS

Q. **A 77-year-old insulin-dependent diabetic is referred to you with a non-retractile foreskin. What is the clinical term used for this condition?**

A. This is referred to as a phimosis.

Q. **What are the key points to ascertain from the history?**

A.
1. Determine the duration of the phimosis.
2. How well controlled is his diabetes?
3. Does he have problems with splitting of the foreskin or bleeding?
4. Is there any discharge from under the foreskin?
5. Are there any associated lower urinary tract symptoms?
6. Is there a smoking history?
7. Obtain sexual history including number of partners and any previous HPV-related warts.
8. What is the extent of exposure to UV radiation?

Q. **How would you conduct an examination of this patient?**

A. Initially I would conduct a general examination to assess the overall health of the patient. A more focussed examination would include an examination of the penis and scrotum in order to identify any visible skin lesions or palpable lumps under the foreskin. If the foreskin is retractable I would conduct a visual examination of the glans penis. If it is not retractable I would palpate the glans penis in order to identify any palpable lesion on the glans penis. I would then palpate both inguinal regions to determine whether there are any palpable inguinal lymph nodes.

With regards to the foreskin I would also assess for any change in colour or evidence of scarring or thickening which may indicate lichen sclerosus or pre-malignant disease on the foreskin.

Q. **The foreskin is completely non-retractile with extensive scarring and fissuring similar to that shown in Figure 3.1. What does this show and what would you advise the patient?**

A. Figure 3.1 shows a significant phimosis developing secondary to lichen sclerosus et atrophicus (referred to as lichen sclerosus and also known as balanitis xerotica obliterans, BXO) and

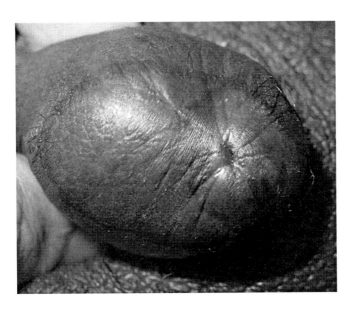

Figure 3.1

therefore I would advise the patient to undergo a circumcision. If there was a suspicion of a penile cancer related to the foreskin then surgery would need to be performed urgently.

Q. **If there was mild scarring and the foreskin was retractable, are there any other treatment options available?**

A. As long as there is no suspicion of a neoplastic lesion then a trial of ultra-potent topical corticosteroid for 4 weeks can resolve mild to moderate cases of lichen sclerosus but treatment must be under medical supervision and the patient must be reviewed after 4 weeks.

Q. **How would you consent a patient for a circumcision?**

A. The process of consent should include the risks and side effects specific for the procedure, which in this case is a circumcision, and also the general risks related to having any surgical procedure.

Specific risks and side effects for a circumcision include the following:

1. Bleeding (early or late –1%–2% require a return to theatre for wound exploration and haemostasis).
2. Infection (1%–2% require post-operative antibiotics).
3. Change in glans sensitivity due to the glans mucosa gradually being replaced by a layer of keratin after a circumcision.
4. Meatal stenosis (reported in the literature in up to 10%).
5. Need for a further biopsy if a suspicious lesion is found at the time of surgery.
6. In childhood circumcision approximately 4% of parents are unhappy with the cosmetic appearance.
7. The small risk of lymphoedema at the suture line or inner preputial remnant.

General risks which would be low in this procedure include the following (if performed under general anesthesia):

1. Deep vein thrombosis
2. Pulmonary embolism
3. Cardiorespiratory complications
4. Anaesthetic complications

Q. Following the patient consent for surgery describe how you would perform a circumcision.

A. (There are several techniques so be familiar with your own technique.)

I would ensure that the patient is consented and fully informed of the risks and expectations. I would prepare the patient in the supine position. At the beginning of the procedure I would perform a local anaesthetic penile block.

As the foreskin is completely non-retractable in this case, I would have to perform a midline dorsal slit as the initial step in order to visualise the urethral meatus and ensure that the glans penis does not have an unexpected lesion and also to ensure that there is no hypospadias present. I use a scalpel technique which involves making a circumcoronal incision of the inner prepuce and also the outer penile skin ensuring to leave adequate penile shaft skin to avoid discomfort on erection. The foreskin is dissected and removed between these two incisions. Meticulous haemostasis is ensured using bipolar diathermy or absorbable ties. I then perform either a two-layer closure of the inner dartos layer and outer skin using interrupted absorbable sutures or if there is very little dartos a single-layer closure is adequate.

Q. The foreskin is sent for histological analysis and the pathologist shows you the slide in Figure 3.2. What is the diagnosis?

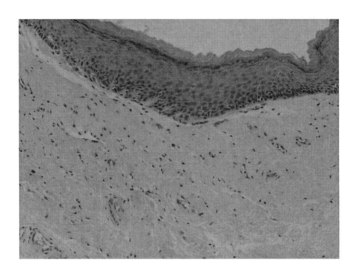

Figure 3.2

A. Figure 3.2: The histology slide shows lichen sclerosus et atrophicus otherwise known as balanitis xerotica obliterans (BXO).

Q. What are the histological features of this condition?

A. The typical pathological features of lichen sclerosus include loss of rete pegs, epidermal atrophy and chronic inflammatory changes. There is perivascular infiltration of the dermis and homogenisation of collagen in the upper dermis.

Q. Following the procedure the patient is referred again to your outpatient clinic having undergone an uncomplicated procedure. He has noticed a small red area on the dorsal aspect of the glans penis which has developed since undergoing the circumcision several months ago.

How would you manage this patient?

A. It is possible that an area of residual lichen sclerosus can persist on the glans penis despite undergoing a circumcision. Initially, I would perform a culture swab of the area and treat it with a topical steroid followed by an early outpatient review (in 2–4 weeks).

Q. The culture swab is negative. He is reviewed again and the abnormal area has increased in size as shown in this picture (Figure 3.3). What would you do now?

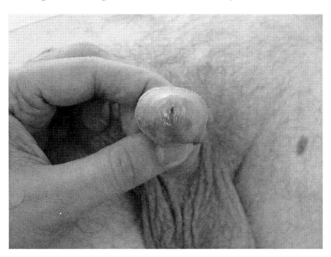

Figure 3.3 Carcinoma *in situ* of the glans penis.

A. I would arrange an urgent biopsy of this area.

Q. The biopsy is performed and the histology is shown in Figure 3.4. What is the diagnosis?

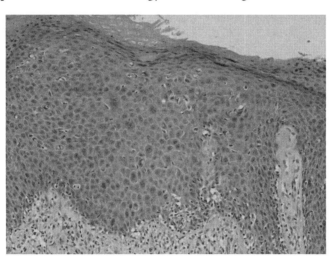

Figure 3.4

A. Figure 3.4: The histology slide shows carcinoma *in situ* (CIS) of the glans penis also known as erythroplasia de Queyrat.

> **Note:** *Erythroplasia de Queyrat is the eponym for carcinoma in situ (CIS) affecting the mucosal surface of the glans or inner surface of the prepuce (non-keratinising CIS). Bowen's disease refers to CIS affecting penile shaft or scrotal skin (keratinising CIS).*

Erythroplasia de Queyrat is 10 times more likely to progress to invasive SCC compared to Bowen's disease.

Q. What is the definition of CIS?

A. CIS refers to a lesion which has all the characteristics of malignancy except for invasion (i.e. does not cross the basement membrane). Specifically for pre-malignant penile lesions the classification now refers to PeIN (penile intraepithelial neoplasia) whereby undifferentiated PeIN refers to HPV-related disease and differentiated PeIN is independent of HPV and most likely driven by lichen sclerosus.

Q. What are the histological features characterising this lesion?

A. The mucosa is replaced by atypical hyperplastic cells. These show disorientation with multiple hyperchromatic nuclei and multilevel mitotic figures. The rete is elongated and bulbous. The submucosa shows proliferation of capillaries with an inflammatory infiltrate rich in plasma cells.

Q. Specifically with the penis which other pre-malignant lesions are you aware of?

A. Pre-malignant lesions of the penis include erythroplasia de Queyrat, Bowen's disease, Bowenoid papulosis, leukoplakia, cutaneous horns, pseudoepitheliomatous micaceous, extra-mammary Paget's disease, condyloma acuminatum.

Q. How would you treat this patient with CIS?

A. If the lesion is small I would initially prescribe topical treatment in the form of either 5-FU or imiquimod. He has already been circumcised but if he had not undergone a circumcision then I would recommend that any patient with pre-malignant disease should be circumcised.

Q. What is 5-FU and how does it work?

A. 5-FU refers to 5% 5-Fluorouracil (or %-fluoro-2,4[1H, 3H]-pyrimidinedione; chemical formula $C_2H_3FN_2O_2$) and is a pyrimidine analogue. This is an anti-metabolite chemotherapeutic agent. The mechanism of action is at the S-phase and involves non-competitive inhibition of thymidylate synthase causing cell cycle arrest and apoptosis.

Q. What are the side effects of 5-FU?

A. There is commonly discomfort on the area of application due to a local inflammatory reaction in addition to erythema, crusting and weeping of the affected area. When the inflammation is troublesome, topical corticosteroids can be used.

Q. Do you know of any other penile preserving therapies excluding surgery which have been described for the treatment of CIS?

A. A number of treatment options have been described in the literature but not gained widespread popularity due to the high local recurrence rate. These include laser therapy (CO_2, Nd-YAG or KTP), photodynamic therapy, cryotherapy and Moh's micrographic surgery.

Q. With this same patient, having been successfully treated with topical 5-FU he presents again several months later with multiple red areas affecting most of the glans penis confirmed as CIS on a further biopsy. What surgical option would you offer him?

A. An alternative topical agent is imiquimod. If there is still no response and considering that the lesion is affecting a large surface area of the glans penis, the alternative would be surgical excision by performing a total glans resurfacing procedure which excises the affected area and uses a split skin graft to cover the denuded glans. At the same time deeper biopsies of the spongiosum are taken to ensure that there is no corpus spongiosum involvement (i.e. check that it has not progressed into an invasive carcinoma).

Q. What are the advantages of penile preserving surgery?

A. Penile preserving surgery allows preservation of penile length so that the patient can void standing up as well as allow maintenance of sexual function to allow penetrative sexual

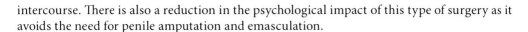

intercourse. There is also a reduction in the psychological impact of this type of surgery as it avoids the need for penile amputation and emasculation.

Q. **What is the disadvantage of undertaking penile preserving surgery?**
A. Follow-up data show that there is a higher local recurrence rate and therefore close clinical surveillance is required for patients post-operatively.

Q. **What is a Buschke-Löwenstein tumour (verrucous carcinoma, giant condyloma acuminatum)?**
A. This is a *locally* invasive penile lesion of viral aetiology. Although tumours in extragenital sites can metastasise, penile verrucous carcinoma does *not* metastasise unless there has been malignant degeneration of the primary lesion.

MANAGEMENT OF INVASIVE PENILE CARCINOMA

Q. **A 60-year-old patient who is an ex-smoker presents with a large lump on his glans penis and a palpable lump in the left groin. The lump is shown in Figure 3.5. What is the likely diagnosis?**

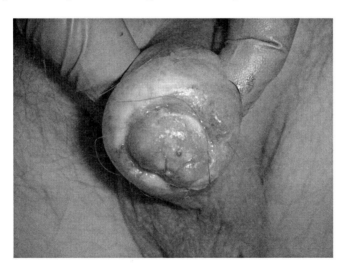

Figure 3.5

A. Figure 3.5: Penile tumour. This is an extensive carcinoma of the penis affecting the glans penis.

Q. **Which is the most common type of cancer affecting the penis?**
A. Squamous cell carcinomas (SCCs) account for over 95% of tumours.

Q. **Which region of the penis does SCC most commonly affect?**
A. SCC is commonly found on the glans penis or foreskin. The primary tumour is localised to the glans penis in approximately 48% of cases.

Q. **What are the risk factors for SCC of the penis?**
A. These include smoking, increasing age, previous HPV infection (type 16 and 18), uncircumcised males, poor penile hygiene and retained smegma. There is an association with exposure to psoralen and ultraviolet A photo chemotherapy (PUVA) and lichen sclerosus. (Premalignant lesions are mentioned in a previous question.)

Q. Which HPV subtypes are commonly implicated in penile SCC?

A. High-risk HPV subtypes 16 and 18 are most commonly associated with SCC.

Q. With this particular case what would you do next?

A. I would perform a biopsy of the lesion in order to confirm the diagnosis and organise further imaging to stage the tumour. As this is highly likely to be a penile cancer I would also ensure that the patient receives the appropriate information related to penile cancer and has access to a specialist nurse. The patient needs to be discussed at a specialist penile cancer multidisciplinary meeting with the results of the biopsy and the imaging.

Q. How would you stage the tumour?

A. The penile lesion can be imaged using penile magnetic resonance imaging (MRI) which requires an injection of intracavernosal prostaglandin (to induce an artificial erection) in order to assess whether the lesion invades the corpus cavernosum or the urethra. A computed tomography (CT) scan of the chest, abdomen and pelvis will identify enlarged or abnormal lymph nodes.

Q. Does CT imaging pick up all pathological lymph nodes?

A. No. The CT criteria for metastatic lymph nodes rely mainly on the size of the lymph nodes and abnormal features of the hilum or the shape of the lymph nodes. It will not detect small foci of metastatic disease.

Q. Describe the image presented in Figure 3.6.

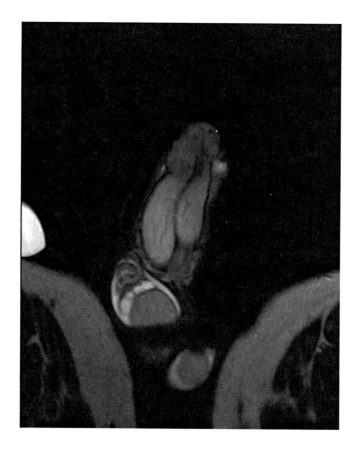

Figure 3.6

A. Figure 3.6: This is an MRI of the penis demonstrating a penile tumour on the glans penis extending into the corpus spongiosum and corpus cavernosum.

Q. **What is the likely T stage of this tumour?**
A. The tumour is extending into the corpus spongiosum and cavernosum and therefore it is at least a T3 lesion according to the 2017 AJCC TNM classification (Table 3.1). (Previously it would have been classified as T2 on the AJCC 7th Edition classification.)

Table 3.1 TNM classification of penile cancer 2017 (8th edition)

TX	Primary tumour cannot be assessed
T0	No evidence of primary tumour
Tis	Carcinoma *in situ* (penile intraepithelial neoplasia – PeIN)
Ta	Non-invasive localised squamous cell carcinoma
T1	Tumour invades subepithelial connective tissue (lamina propria)
T1a	Tumour invades subepithelial connective tissue without perineural or lymphovascular invasion and is not poorly differentiated or undifferentiated (T1G1–2)
T1b	Tumour invades subepithelial connective tissue with perineural or lymphovascular invasion or is poorly differentiated or undifferentiated (T1G3–4)
T2	Tumour invades corpus spongiosum with or without invasion of the urethra
T3	Tumour invades corpus cavernosum (including tunica albuginea) with or without invasion of the urethra
T4	Tumour invades other adjacent structures (scrotum, prostate, bone)
NX	Regional lymph nodes cannot be assessed
N0	No lymph node metastasis
N1	Metastasis in one or two unilateral inguinal lymph nodes, but without extra-nodal extension
N2	Metastasis in three or more *unilateral* inguinal lymph nodes without extra-nodal extension, *or*, any number of *bilateral* positive inguinal lymph nodes without extra-nodal extension
N3	Metastasis to any number of inguinal lymph nodes with extra-nodal extension, or, metastasis to pelvic lymph nodes
M0	No distant metastases
M1	Distant metastases

Q. **How accurate is MRI in predicting invasion into the corpus cavernosum?**
A. Penile MRI is very accurate and has been shown to predict corpus cavernosum/spongiosum invasion in all cases analysed [2].

Q. **What would be the surgical treatment option in this case?**
A. As the tumour is located distally, the tumour can be excised with clear margins by performing a partial penectomy.

Q. **Would you advise any other surgical treatment if the tumour had involved the glans without extension into the corpus cavernosum?**
A. Tumours which are limited to the glans penis can be managed by performing a glansectomy and reconstruction of the neoglans using a split skin graft. Spongiosal invasion of the glans or urethra is now classified as T2 according to the AJCC TNM 8th Edition.

Q. **How would you perform a partial penectomy?**
A. I would ensure that the patient is fully consented for the risks of surgery which include bleeding, infection, penile shortening, erectile dysfunction, spraying of urine, and graft loss if a split skin graft is being used as part of the reconstruction. The patient is placed in a supine position and the tumour is covered with a finger glove or condom. I would then mark and incise the penile shaft skin proximal to the tumour and deglove the penis.

The next step involves mobilising and ligating the neurovascular bundle followed by mobilisation of the urethra. The penis is then transected. There are several techniques described for the procedure e.g. straight transection or 'fish mouth' or urethral centralisation technique (be familiar with at least one). I would send the proximal shavings of the corpus cavernosum and urethra for frozen section analysis to ensure that they are tumour free. The corpora and Bucks fascia are oversewn with absorbable sutures. After spatulating the urethra, the neoglans can be covered either with the penile shaft skin or a split skin graft can be used to reconstruct the neoglans. I would leave a catheter *in situ* for approximately 1 week.

Q. How would you follow up a patient who has undergone penile preserving surgery with no inguinal lymph node disease?

A. Most recurrences will occur within the first 2–3 years following surgery. The EAU guidelines recommend that follow-up should be on a three-monthly basis for the first 2 years then six-monthly after that until 5 years depending on the inguinal lymph node status. At each follow up I would examine the penis and inguinal lymph nodes for any local or distant recurrence. Patients should also be encouraged to self-examine and request an urgent follow-up if any new lesion is palpable.

Q. What is the local recurrence rate following a partial or total penectomy?

A. This varies according to the initial stage of the tumour. Studies have generally reported a local recurrence rate of between 0% and 8%.

Q. How does this compare with the recurrence rates following penile preserving surgery?

A. Although early studies reported a local recurrence rate of up to 40%, more recent studies have shown a local recurrence rate of approximately 11%.

Q. How would you manage the palpable lump in the groin?

A. This is likely to be an enlarged inguinal lymph node. Bearing in mind the size and the stage of the primary penile tumour, it is likely that this is a metastatic lymph node since penile cancer will metastasise to the inguinal lymph nodes and then to the ipsilateral pelvic lymph nodes in a stepwise pattern. I would therefore confirm the diagnosis by arranging for an ultrasound of the groin combined with fine needle aspiration cytology (FNAC) of the enlarged lymph node.

Q. If the FNAC confirms SCC in the palpable inguinal node, what would be the next step in the management of this patient?

A. I would advise the patient that there is confirmed metastatic disease in the palpable lymph node and a possibility of micrometastatic disease within the other inguinal lymph nodes on the same side and recommend that he undergoes a radical inguinal lymphadenectomy.

Q. Following the radical inguinal lymphadenectomy, a single node is found to be involved with metastatic SCC in this patient, what is the N stage according to the 2017 AJCC TNM classification (8th Edition)?

A. As only one (unilateral) lymph node is involved, the nodal staging is N1.

Q. Assuming that this patient was found to have a single metastatic lymph node in both the right and left groin, what would be the N stage according to the 2017 AJCC TNM classification?

A. For inguinal nodes, regardless of the number involved, bilateral nodal involvement is classified as N2.

Q. What percentage of palpable inguinal lymph nodes is involved with metastatic disease?

A. This is controversial. In previous studies, mainly from South America, it was suggested that only 50% of palpable inguinal lymph nodes were involved with tumour and the remaining

50% were enlarged as a result of associated sexually transmitted or other infections. Therefore traditionally a short course of antibiotics was given in an attempt to differentiate between the two with the infected ones likely to reduce in size. However, recent data have suggested that over 90% of palpable inguinal nodes are involved with metastatic disease and therefore require a radical inguinal lymphadenectomy. Therefore patients should be assumed to have metastatic disease in the palpable lymph nodes and further imaging for staging using CT and ultrasound should not be delayed.

Q. What is this surgical procedure?

A. Figure 3.7 shows an open inguinal lymphadenectomy. The saphenous vein has been preserved (demonstrated with the loop).

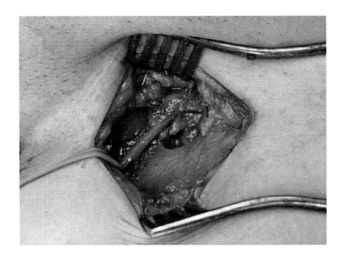

Figure 3.7

Q. What are the anatomical boundaries of the femoral triangle?

A. The femoral triangle is bordered by the inguinal ligament superiorly, medial border of the sartorius muscle laterally, lateral border of the adductor longus and adductor longus tendon medially and the floor comprises the pectineus muscle medially and iliopsoas muscle laterally together with the femoral artery and vein.

Q. What is the difference between a superficial modified and a radical inguinal lymph node dissection?

A. The modified superficial lymph node dissection uses a much smaller incision and the boundaries are reduced compared to a radical lymph node dissection. The saphenous vein is preserved and the femoral vessels do not have to be skeletonised deep to the fascia lata.

Note that if any nodes are found to be positive in a modified superficial inguinal node dissection then one proceeds to a radical inguinal node dissection. Also, if two or more inguinal lymph nodes are found to be involved on histology or there is a single metastatic node with extracapsular spread, the patient should proceed to a pelvic lymph node dissection on the ipsilateral side.

Q. What are the complications of a radical inguinal lymph node dissection?

A. The morbidity of this procedure is reported to be between 30% and 50%. The complications include early haemorrhage, wound infection, flap necrosis, lymphoedema of the lower limb, lymphocele, prolonged lymph drainage and patchy sensory loss of the thigh.

Q. **What is the advantage of performing a superficial modified inguinal node dissection compared to a radical inguinal node dissection?**

A. The superficial inguinal node dissection can only be performed for patients with impalpable lymph nodes and is a technique which reduces the morbidity of the inguinal lymphadenectomy procedure by utilising a smaller inguinal incision with less extensive dissection required to develop the skin flaps. The saphenous vein is also preserved in order to try and reduce the degree of lower limb lymphoedema. The procedure also avoids the need to use a sartorius transposition flap to cover the exposed femoral vessels.

Q. **Does superficial modified lymphadenectomy reduce the lymphoedema rate?**

A. Yes, it does. Approximately 20% of patients will suffer from lymphoedema with a very small proportion developing persistent lower limb lymphoedema.

Q. **Can you describe what has happened here? (Figure 3.8)**

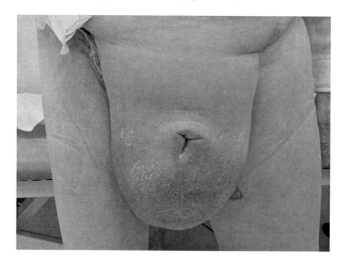

Figure 3.8

A. Figure 3.8: Extensive scrotal lymphoedema. This patient has had surgery to the penis combined with bilateral inguinal lymphadenectomy as indicated by the surgical scars in the inguinal region. This has resulted in extensive genital lymphoedema.

Q. **How would you manage the post-operative complication of genital lymphoedema?**

A. Initially conservative management includes the use of supportive underwear or specially designed compressive garments which also cover the lower limbs. Patients should ensure that they avoid trauma to the skin in areas affected by lymphoedema, e.g. scratches, pressure sores, and insect bites. Once the patient is mobile, the lymphoedema may start to reduce. However, for troublesome and persistent scrotal lymphoedema where the penis is buried, surgical excision is required which includes a scrotectomy combined with a scrotoplasty and unburying of the penis.

Q. **In patients with impalpable inguinal lymph nodes, what is the risk of lymph node metastases?**

A. The risk is approximately 15%–25%.

Q. **Would you offer a radical inguinal lymphadenectomy to every patient diagnosed with penile cancer?**

A. As the aim of radical inguinal lymphadenectomy is to remove metastatic lymph nodes from the inguinal region, subjecting everyone with impalpable inguinal nodes would result in overtreatment in approximately 75%–85% of patients. As the procedure is associated with significant morbidity including lymphoedema, wound complications, seromas and lymph fistulae, alternative techniques should be offered to minimise the complications.

Q. Do you know of any other techniques available to reduce the number of individuals undergoing inguinal lymphadenectomy in those patients with impalpable inguinal nodes?

A. In patients who have clinically impalpable inguinal lymph nodes, dynamic sentinel lymph node biopsy can be offered which will target the first draining lymph node(s) only. In centres where a dynamic sentinel lymph node biopsy programme has not been established, an alternative option would be to use a laparoscopic assisted or robot assisted inguinal lymphadenectomy. This is referred to as video endoscopic inguinal lymphadenectomy (VEIL).

Q. Which radioisotope is used for dynamic sentinel lymph node biopsy?

A. ^{99m}Tc nanocolloid.

Q. What is the false-negative rate of dynamic sentinel lymph node biopsy for penile cancer?

A. Approximately 4%–7% [3,4].

Q. Do you know of any modifications to the original technique of dynamic sentinel lymph node biopsy which has reduced the false-negative rate to 5%?

A. The false-negative rate has been reduced by incorporating pre-operative inguinal ultrasonography combined with FNAC of suspicious nodes. The rationale for this is to locate morphologically abnormal lymph nodes as well as those which are filled with extensive tumour and therefore unlikely to have normal lymphatic drainage and may not take up the ^{99m}Tc nanocolloid. Additionally the use of a blue dye (Patent Blue V) has also helped in localising the lymph nodes during inguinal explorations.

Q. Which pathological features correlate with lymph node metastases and prognosis?

A. T stage ($\geq$T2), lymphovascular and perineural invasion, histological grade of tumour, histological subtype, e.g. basaloid or sarcomatoid features. Other factors include depth of invasion of the primary tumour, positive margins following resection and the presence of corpus cavernosum invasion. Of all of these factors the most important appear to be perineural invasion, vascular invasion and high-grade tumours.

Q. An 83-year-old patient with a 2 cm primary SCC on the glans penis opts for radiotherapy to this lesion as opposed to surgical excision as he is worried about the perioperative risks and complications. What would you quote as the response rate and recurrence rate of external beam radiotherapy?

A. Radiotherapy is no longer considered a primary treatment option as the response rate is approximately 56% and the local failure rate is 40%.

Q. What are the main complications of external beam radiotherapy for penile SCC?

A. There is a risk of meatal stenosis and urethral stricture (up to 30%), telangiectasia (90%) and even radionecrosis. (Note that the patient must be circumcised prior to radiotherapy otherwise the prepuce will become fused to the glans.)

Q. Is there a role for radiotherapy for clinically impalpable nodes?

A. Currently there is no evidence to suggest that radiotherapy prevents the development of metastatic inguinal lymph nodes. However, there is a possible role in patients who have undergone inguinal lymphadenectomy for metastatic inguinal lymph nodes which show extracapsular spread.

ADVANCED PENILE CANCERS AND PRIMARY URETHRAL TUMOURS

Q. **A 55-year-old patient previously treated with a partial penectomy and superficial modified bilateral inguinal lymphadenectomy presents with a large mass in the right groin fixed to the skin. What are the surgical treatment options?**

A. A large mass in the groin presenting at follow-up after an inguinal lymphadenectomy will most likely represent metastatic disease. The prognosis is poor and the treatment is directed at palliation and improvement of the patient's quality of life. If the performance status is good then a surgical resection combined with coverage of the defect with a flap is an option. As the defect is often large, coverage can be performed using a pedicled flap, e.g. vertical rectus abdominis (VRAM) or tensor fascia latae (TFL).

Q. **He is brought in as an acute emergency as he is suffering from dehydration, feeling unsteady and confusion. Can you explain any metabolic reason for this to occur?**

A. He is likely to have developed hypercalcaemia related to the bulk of the disease as opposed to metastatic bone disease. A series from Memorial Sloan Kettering reported that approximately 20% of patients with penile cancer develop hypercalcaemia possibly due to parathyroid hormone or parathyroid-like hormone secretion.

Q. **A 67-year-old man has noticed a palpable lump in the mid-shaft of his penis which is getting progressively larger. The lump is not attached to the skin and he presents with urethral bleeding and discharge. How would you investigate this patient?**

A. Having taken a full history and undertaken a general examination, I would also examine the inguinal areas to check for any palpable inguinal lymph nodes as well as the external urethral meatus. I would then organise an urgent cystoscopy and biopsy of the lesion. My suspicion would be a neoplasm of the urethra and therefore he requires CT staging of the chest, abdomen, pelvis and inguinal regions together with an MRI scan of the penis (ideally with an artificial erection).

Q. **The cystoscopy shows an obvious tumour in the mid-urethra which is biopsied. What is the most common primary urethral tumour in males?**

A. Squamous cell carcinoma accounts for 80% of the primary urethral tumours.

Q. **Where in the urethra do these tumours most commonly arise?**

A. Sixty per cent of these tumours are located in the bulbomembranous urethra with the majority (80%) being squamous cell carcinomas.

Q. **What are the risk factors for a urethral tumour?**

A. Risk factors include chronic stricture disease, inflammatory conditions, HPV infection and sexually transmitted diseases. Proximal lesions can also be adenocarcinomas or transitional carcinomas (TCCs). If it is TCC the same risk factors for bladder TCC apply.

Q. **How would you manage this patient?**

A. As these tumours are very rare, the management involves a multimodality approach. A tumour of the mid-shaft or anterior urethra with no synchronous tumour elsewhere can be managed by performing a wide local excision of the urethra together with the adjacent tunica albuginea and the anterior urethra. Urethral reconstruction is then performed either by bringing the urethra out as a perineal urethrostomy or if the length is adequate, a hypospadiac opening can be constructed. The inguinal lymph nodes are managed as for a penile cancer although the majority of patients will undergo a radical/superficial modified inguinal lymphadenectomy rather than a sentinel lymph node biopsy.

REFERENCES

1. Muneer A et al. Molecular prognostic factors in penile cancer. *World J Urol* 2009; 27: 161–167.
2. Kayes O et al. The role of magnetic resonance imaging in the local staging of penile cancer. *Eur Urol* 2007; 51: 1313–1318.
3. Hadway P et al. Evaluation of dynamic lymphoscintigraphy and sentinel lymph-node biopsy for detecting occult metastases in patients with penile squamous cell carcinoma. *BJU Int* 2007; 100: 561–565.
4. Arya M et al. Malignant and premalignant lesions of the penis. *BMJ* 2013; 346: f1149.

FURTHER READING

Arya M, Shergill IS, Silhi N, Grange P, Bott S (eds). *Essential Urology in General Practice*, London: Quay Books; 2009.

Muneer A, Horenblas S (eds). *Textbook of Penile Cancer* 2nd edn., London: Springer; 2016.

Wein AJ, Kavoussi LR, Partin AW et al. (eds). *Campbell-Walsh Urology*, 11th edn. Philadelphia, PA: Elsevier; 2016.

CHAPTER 4
UROTHELIAL CANCER

*David Mak, Muhammad Jamal Khan, Herman S Fernando,
Ciaran Lynch and Lyndon Gommersall*

Contents

HAEMATURIA

Q. How common is haematuria?

A. Haematuria is a common finding. In the paediatric population, this is as low as 1% rising to 5% in young adults and 10% in patients over the age of 50 years. The prevalence of non-visible haematuria has been reported to be approximately 2.5% in men and between 8% and 11% in women [1].

Q. A 65-year-old woman is referred with non-visible haematuria. A midstream specimen of urine (MSU) has been sent for microscopy, culture and sensitivity. Microscopy shows a normal white cell count (WCC), 18 red blood cells (RBCs) per high-powered field and no growth has been found on culture. She has moderate irritative voiding lower urinary tract symptoms (LUTS) and is otherwise well. No other investigations have been performed. How would you assess this woman?

A. This woman would be seen in a 2-week wait haematuria clinic and assessed with a focussed urological history, examination and investigations, detailing her smoking and occupational history. Environmental carcinogen exposure confers a less than 1% risk of developing bladder cancer but is an important component of assessment. Blood pressure should be measured as well as a full abdominal and pelvic examination should be conducted. Investigations should include an MSU for culture and sensitivity, urine for cytology, routine bloods, an ultrasound scan (USS) of her renal tract and a flexible cystoscopy. Some institutions advocate performing a computed tomography urogram (CTU) as the first-line radiological investigation. Urinary molecular marker tests (e.g. NMP 22 and UroVysion) have been developed to improve diagnostic sensitivity but none of these markers are currently accepted in routine practice or clinical guidelines.

If a bladder cancer is found then further staging investigations are required in selected cases and she would be counselled for transurethral resection of bladder tumour (TURBT). If these tests are negative with high-grade malignant cells on urine cytology then a CTU should be performed if not already done (contemporary radiological practice clearly favours the CTU over intravenous urography [IVU]). If this does not reveal an upper tract tumour then an examination under anaesthetic, rigid cystoscopy with biopsies, selective ureteric urine sampling, retrograde studies and ureteroscopy should be undertaken.

Q. What is the most likely presentation of a patient with bladder cancer?

A. The most common presentation of bladder cancer is with visible painless haematuria. Almost all patients diagnosed with bladder cancer will have had either visible or non-visible haematuria. The degree of bleeding is not proportional to disease stage. Storage voiding symptoms are a worrying feature and can occur in approximately 20% of patients with either bladder cancer or carcinoma *in situ*. Urological bleeding associated with urinary infection cannot solely be attributed to inflammation as a proportion of patients will have necrotic infected elements within the bladder tumour and therefore must be investigated with equal intensity. Patients who receive imaging or a cystoscopy for another reason make up the remainder of patients.

Q. What are the causes of haematuria?

A. The causes of haematuria can be divided into urological or nephrological, benign or malignant, visible or non-visible, or based upon the anatomical location of the bleeding (i.e. renal, ureteric, bladder, prostatic or urethral). Table 4.1 demonstrates the causes of haematuria based on the anatomical location.

Table 4.1 Causes of haematuria based on anatomical location

Anatomical location	Cause
Renal	Renal cancer Renal pelvic malignancy: TCC, adenocarcinoma, SCC or other Trauma: Penetrating or blunt Nephrological: IgA nephropathy (Berger's disease), diabetes, Alport's syndrome, thin basement membrane disease Renal stones Infective: TB, pyelonephritis
Ureter	Ureteric malignancy: TCC, adenocarcinoma, SCC or other Ureteric stone Trauma: Penetrating or blunt Infective: TB
Bladder	Bladder malignancy: TCC, adenocarcinoma, SCC or other Bladder stone Trauma: Blunt or penetrating, pelvic fracture Infective: Bacterial, TB, schistosomiasis
Prostate	Prostate cancer Benign prostatic hyperplasia Infective: Bacterial prostatitis, TB prostate
Urethra	Infective: Urethritis Stricture Trauma: Blunt or penetrating and catheterisation
Other	Epididymitis Menses

Q. What is the definition of haematuria?

A. Haematuria can be divided into visible haematuria (VH) (i.e. macroscopic or gross haematuria) or non-visible haematuria (NVH) (microscopic haematuria). NVH can be further sub-classified into symptomatic non-visible haematuria (s-NVH) (i.e. with voiding LUTS) or asymptomatic non-visible haematuria (a-NVH) (i.e. without voiding LUTS).

The definition of NVH varies between guidelines (as do the recommended investigations that are suggested), and these definitions are summarised in Table 4.2. The quantification of NVH depends on two key techniques: the sediment count and the chamber count. The sediment count involves spinning urine down in a centrifuge with the supernatant removed. The pellet of cells is then re-suspended in saline and examined under the microscope. The chamber count detects the number of RBCs per millilitre of urine.

The American Urological Association (AUA) definition of haematuria utilises the sediment count and defines three or more RBCs per high-powered field as abnormal. Most nephrologists will utilise the threshold of 5 RBCs per microlitre. The *Journal of the American Medical Association* (*JAMA*) defined microscopic haematuria in 1990 as >2–3 RBCs per high-powered field [2]. Campbell's *Urology* defines haematuria as 3 or more RBCs per high-powered microscopic field. Table 4.3 shows the relationship between the dipstick positive result and the RBC count per high-powered field. A trace result is generally considered negative and 1+ and above a positive result.

Table 4.2 Summary of varying definitions of non-visible haematuria

Organisation	Definition
AUA	Three or greater RBCs per high-powered field on a spun specimen
Nephrology	>5 RBCs per microlitre
JAMA	>2–3 RBCs per high-powered field is non-visible haematuria [2]
Campbell's	Three or more RBCs per high-powered field

Table 4.3 Equivalent dipstick and microscopy results for non-visible haematuria

Dipstick result	RBCs per high-powered field
±	1–10
+	10–40
++	40–100
+++	100–200

Khadra et al. has also reported on the percentage of patients who would have had a cancer diagnosis missed for 10, 5 and 3 RBCs per high-powered field. This equates to a missed cancer diagnosis in 20%, 14.8% and 10%, respectively [3].

Q. What do you know about dipstick testing for haematuria?

A. Dipstick testing for haematuria is commonplace. It is based on the oxidation of a chromogen (orthotolidine) by the peroxidase activity of haemoglobin. This results in a colourific change that is compared to a set of known standards. Electronic strip readers remove the subjective nature of the test and eradicate reader error. False-positive results can occur with myoglobin-uria, oxidizing agents and peroxidases. A false-negative result can also occur with high levels of ascorbic acid, nitrite, pH < 5 and high specific gravity of the urine specimen. There is no substitute for urine microscopy performed by a competent laboratory.

Q. How would you set up a haematuria clinic?

A. Haematuria is an ideal symptom to be investigated with the one-stop clinic format. Each patient requires a full history and examination. This should include a detailed report of the haematuria, duration and any associated symptoms. Exposure to smoking and occupational history must be recorded. Examination should include an abdominal examination, external genital examination and a digital rectal examination in men. Blood tests including full blood count, urea and electrolytes, clotting screen and prostate-specific antigen (PSA) (after counselling) should be performed. An MSU and urine cytology are required. Radiological imaging of the urinary tract is required as well as flexible cystoscopy. CTU is increasingly being used as the first-line imaging modality although ultrasound can be used first-line. However, ultrasound cannot exclude the presence of upper tract tumours. Interpretation of this data can then lead to immediate discharge of the patient, or organisation of further investigations if indicated. For example in the patient with positive cytology, negative MSU, normal USS/CTU and normal urothelium on flexible cystoscopy, then diagnostic cystoscopy with random bladder biopsies, biopsy of prostatic urethra, retrograde studies and ureteroscopy are required to elucidate the cause of the high-grade malignant cells detected.

From a referral perspective, National Institute for Health and Care Excellence (NICE) Suspected Cancer: Recognition and Referral (2015) guidelines specify referral of patients who are aged 45 years and above, and have unexplained visible haematuria (VH) in the absence of urinary tract infection (UTI), or VH that persists or recurs after successful treatment of UTI. In addition, the guidelines stipulate that patients aged 60 years and over with unexplained symptomatic (e.g. associated with dysuria) non-visible haematuria (s-NVH) should be referred for investigation.

Q. **How do you perform urine cytology?**

A. Urine cytology is performed on a random or ideally, a mid-morning urine sample. Early morning urine samples provide degenerative specimens for cytological examination. The sample should be the whole voided urine as an MSU is the most acellular fraction. The sample needs to be rapidly transferred to the laboratory for processing. If a short delay occurs refrigeration is recommended. If longer delays are expected then prompt fixation with an equal amount of 50% alcohol can be utilised. Sensitivity of urine cytology increases with the number of specimens examined. Ideally at least three mid-morning or random specimens should be submitted for examination, but this is often impractical. Catheter specimens can be utilised but cellular changes can be seen with this method of collection. Saline washouts may also be utilised (saline barbotage) and need to be recorded on the request form. The laboratory will then centrifuge the sample, perform fixation in formalin and stain with Papanicolaou or haematoxylin and eosin dyes. The resulting slides are then analysed under the microscope for morphological changes consistent with malignancy.

Cytology is most useful in the detection of high-grade malignancy and is positive in 90% of these cases. In low-grade tumours it is positive in only 10% of patients. It is often used as a safety system for the detection of malignancy in the investigation negative group of individuals.

Q. **Can you describe any alternatives to urine cytology?**

A. Urine cytology has been the basis of urine testing for urothelial cancer for many decades. With a reported specificity of 95% and sensitivity of 30%–50% it is an adequate test for detecting high-risk disease but lacks the sensitivity for the detection of low-grade disease. Several novel urinary markers for urothelial carcinoma have been developed including NMP22 (nuclear matrix protein 22), BTA (bladder tumour associated antigen), BTA Stat, UroVysion and Telomerase. These urinary molecular markers generally have a high sensitivity but lower specificity compared to urine cytology. Currently, these markers are not accepted for diagnosis or follow-up in clinical guidelines. The specificity and sensitivity of these bladder cancer urinary markers are reviewed in Table 4.4.

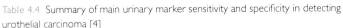

Table 4.4 Summary of main urinary marker sensitivity and specificity in detecting urothelial carcinoma [4]

	Overall sensitivity (%)	Overall specificity (%)
Cytology	49	96
UroVysion (FISH)	30–86	63–95
Microsatellite analysis	58–92	73–100
ImmunoCyt/uCyt+	52–100	63–79
NMP22 (BladderChek)	47–100	55–98
BTA stat	29–83	56–86
BTA TRAK	53–91	28–83
Cytokeratins	12–88	73–95
Telomerase (TRAP)	74	79

Source: Adapted from European Association of Urology. http://uroweb.org/wp-content/
uploads/EAU-Guidelines-on-Non-muscle-Invasive-BC_TaT1-2017.pdf

NMP22 (nuclear matrix protein 22) is promoted as the 'NMP22 BladderChek' test. It has reported increased sensitivity compared to cytology and has been used in surveillance.

The BTA stat test identifies overproduction of the complement protective peptide complement factor H related protein (CFHrp) in the urine. This is known as the BTA. BTA TRAK is a quantitative assay of BTA.

The UroVysion test utilises fluorescent *in situ* hybridisation (FISH) to test for aneuploidy of chromosomes 3, 7, 17 and loss of the 9p21. This complicated test requires intact cells, expensive equipment and a dedicated laboratory.

Telomerase is overexpressed in many cancers and can be detected in the urine with the TRAP (telomerase repeat amplification) assay. Telomerase adds telomeres to chromosomal terminal DNA sequences preventing cell senescence. ImmunoCyt is a test combining cytology and immunofluorescent assay.

Q.   What is the evidence for your haematuria investigation regime?

A.   The National Institute for Health Research reported a lack of studies analysing the efficacy of diagnostic regimes for the investigation of haematuria [5]. Not unsurprisingly, there is wide variation in adopted haematuria investigation modalities.

However, two studies are classically quoted for the investigation of haematuria. Khadra et al. studied 1930 patients who attended a haematuria clinic from 1994 to 1997 [3]. All patients underwent a history and examination, routine blood tests, urinalysis, cytology, plain abdominal radiography, renal ultrasound, intravenous pyelogram (IVP) and flexible cystoscopy. In this cohort, 61% of patients had no pathology identified, 12% were diagnosed with bladder cancer, 13% had UTI and 2% had stone disease. The key message here is that if only ultrasound or IVP had been performed a significant proportion of upper tract malignancy would have been missed (six with ultrasound alone and at least three with IVP alone) and hence the use of both imaging modalities is recommended. Overall, macroscopic and microscopic haematuria resulted in a cancer diagnosis in 24% and 9.4%, respectively. Bladder cancer was found in more patients with microscopic haematuria than the 5% or less reported within the urological literature.

Edwards et al. studied 4020 patients attending a haematuria clinic [6]. Macroscopic haematuria resulted in a fourfold increase in the diagnosis of cancer versus microscopic haematuria (19% versus 5%). In 75% no pathology was identified. Three upper tract tumours were identified after a normal USS with 46% of this cohort receiving an IVU.

IVU has now largely been replaced by CTU given the superior sensitivity and specificity of CT over IVU. Albani et al. followed 416 patients who underwent either CTU or IVU in addition to diagnostic cystoscopy [7]. A higher sensitivity for detecting upper tract pathology was reported with CT than IVU (94.1% versus 50%). However CTU had a low sensitivity for lower tract lesions. They concluded that CTU is a more sensitive alternative to IVU in haematuria investigations but CTU does not eliminate the need for cystoscopy. Presently, there is no published large series using CTU as the main radiological investigation.

Q. Is screening for bladder cancer effective?

A. In 1992, Britton et al. investigated the use of dipstick testing for haematuria in 2356 men over 60 years old [8]. And 20% (474 patients) of these patients had non-visible haematuria on recurrent testing. Overall, 319 agreed to undergo urological examination. In this cohort 17 (5.3%) asymptomatic patients were diagnosed with bladder cancer.

In a similar study, Messing et al. screened 1575 men aged 50 years and older and found 16.4% (258 patients) had haematuria [9]. Of those with haematuria 8.1% (21 patients) were diagnosed with bladder cancer. Using the Wisconsin State Tumor Registry as an unscreened cohort for comparison, they observed a smaller proportion of muscle-invasive bladder cancer in the screened men compared to non-screened men (5%–24%). At 14 years' follow-up, the cancer-specific mortality rate in screen-detected bladder cancer patients was zero compared to 20.4% in bladder cancer patients of the non-screened cohort.

Although these studies suggest that bladder cancer may be detected at an earlier stage through screening, there remains a high false-positive rate (85%–95%), i.e., haematuria positive but no cancer identified on investigations. Screening would therefore lead to large numbers of asymptomatic patients requiring investigation. The cost per bladder cancer diagnosis is prohibitively high at the present time.

The use of urinary dipstick testing with other urinary biomarkers, such as UroVysion, NMP22 (BladderChek) and ImmunoCyt, in bladder cancer screening in specific populations has been studied. Targeted screening of a population of smokers has reported a 3.3% pick of malignancy using cytology, dipstick and the urinary markers UroVysion and NMP22 (BladderChek) [10].

Q. If all her initial haematuria investigations are negative except for positive cytology – what now?

A. The patient with negative cystoscopy and imaging but positive cytology poses a diagnostic challenge. This patient should be offered a CTU if not already performed as part of the haematuria investigations. If the CTU is normal, then EAU guidelines [4] recommend that GA cystoscopy be performed with biopsies from normal-looking mucosa taken from trigone, bladder dome and right, left, anterior and posterior bladder walls to exclude carcinoma *in situ* (CIS). In men, prostatic urethra biopsies should also be taken when no tumour is seen in the bladder. Photodynamic diagnostic (PDD) cystoscopy has been shown to be more sensitive than white light cystoscopy in detecting malignant tumours, particularly CIS. If PDD equipment is available, then PDD guided bladder biopsies are recommended in positive cytology settings. Retrograde studies and ureteroscopy are also to be considered.

Q. Who should be referred to a nephrologist?

A. The Joint Consensus Statement on the Initial Assessment of Haematuria prepared on behalf of the Renal Association and British Association of Urological Surgeons (July 2008) outlined guidelines for referral to nephrology. Patients who have negative investigations from a urological perspective need nephrology referral if other factors are present:

- Evidence of declining GFR by >10 mL/min within the previous 5 years or by >5 mL/min within the last 1 year
- Stage 4 or 5 chronic kidney disease (eGFR <30 mL/min)
- Significant proteinuria (albumin-to-creatinine ratio [ACR] of ≥30 mg/mmol or protein-to-creatinine ratio [PCR] of ≥50 mg/mmol)

Primary nephrology referral should be considered in patients under 40 years old with non-visible haematuria and risk factors for severe glomerulonephritis:

- Significant proteinuria (ACR of ≥30 mg/mmol or PCR of ≥50 mg/mmol)
- Hypertension (BP ≥140/90)
- eGFR <60 mL/min

Note that the Joint Consensus Statement is currently under review.

Q. **What are common renal (nephrological) causes of non-visible haematuria?**
A. NVH from the nephrological perspective is either glomerular or non-glomerular, see Table 4.5.

Table 4.5 Nephrological disorders resulting in non-visible haematuria

Glomerular	Non-glomerular
IgA nephropathy	Cystic disease
Alport's syndrome	Inflammatory disorders of the urothelium
Thin basement membrane disease	Interstitial nephritis
Henoch-Schönlein purpura	Papillary necrosis
Vasculitis, e.g. lupus	Renal artery stenosis
Goodpasture's syndrome	
Nephrotic syndrome	
Diabetic glomerulosclerosis	

Glomerular disease is a common cause of NVH. IgA nephropathy, also known as Berger's disease, results in mesangial deposition of IgA. This is often after an upper respiratory tract infection. VH or NVH can be present. Approximately 10%–20% will develop renal failure in 10–20 years. Prognosis is worse if the patient develops hypertension or has proteinuria or fibrosis on biopsy. Treatment depends on the strict control of blood pressure and occasionally requires steroids and immunosuppression.

Alport's syndrome is an X-linked collagen mutation resulting in blindness, deafness and nephritis resulting in chronic renal failure.

Thin basement membrane disease is an asymptomatic disease resulting in a-NVH. It is non-progressive and diagnosed only on electron microscopy of a renal biopsy.

Nephrotic syndrome results from a non-inflammatory injury to the glomerulus. Patients classically have hypoalbuminaemia, hypercholesterolaemia and hyperlipidaemia due to excessive hepatic lipoprotein synthesis. Considerable proteinuria may exist. Treatment is with steroids.

Causes of non-glomerular NVH include interstitial nephritis. This results from an inflammatory infiltrate affecting nephron function. Acute interstitial nephritis occurs 4 days to 5 weeks after starting a new drug, commonly penicillin. Symptomatically the patient develops a fever and generalised rash with oliguria, increased creatinine and hypertension.

Papillary necrosis is characterised by coagulative necrosis of the renal papillae from pyelonephritis, obstructed uropathy, sickle cell, tuberculosis, trauma, cirrhosis, analgesic nephropathy, renal vein thrombosis or diabetes (the acronym POSTCARD). Urological management involves resolution of urinary obstruction, treatment of infection and resuscitation.

A renal artery stenosis can result in renin-mediated hypertension and occurs only with a stenosis greater than 70%. Clinically a bruit may be auscultated.

NON-MUSCLE-INVASIVE BLADDER CANCER

Q. What are the histological types of primary bladder carcinoma?

A. Almost 95% of patients with bladder cancer have a transitional cell carcinoma (TCC). The remaining patients have squamous cell carcinoma (4%) or rarely adenocarcinoma of the bladder.

Q. What proportion of patients present with non-muscle-invasive disease?

A. Over 80% of patients with TCC present with non-muscle-invasive Ta or T1 disease and the remaining patients present with muscle-invasive malignancy (T2 to T4).

Q. A 67-year-old man has been assessed in the haematuria clinic. Flexible cystoscopy is performed and reveals a 2 cm papillary lesion on the posterior wall of his bladder. A CTU has been performed which shows normal upper tracts. He is concerned about this diagnosis. How would you treat this man? How would the treatment differ if a solid/non-papillary lesion was found?

A. This man requires an examination under anaesthetic and transurethral resection of bladder tumour (TURBT) with a single intravesical instillation of mitomycin C. I would consent him for the risk of bleeding, infection and bladder perforation as well as further adjuvant treatment with the risk of recurrent disease. He will require catheterisation following his operation.

The European Association of Urology (EAU) guidelines [4] have outlined recommendations on performing TURBT systematically, which is performed either under general or spinal anaesthesia (Table 4.6). If the tumour is over the obturator nerve on the postero-lateral aspects of the bladder then a general anaesthetic is preferable to avoid obturator spasm and the almost inevitable risk of bladder perforation. Bimanual palpation under anaesthesia should be undertaken initially to assess for a bladder mass, which would suggest muscle-invasive disease.

The cystoscope is then inserted to examine the urethra and bladder. A 70° telescope allows

Table 4.6 Recommended steps for TURBT

Bimanual palpation under anaesthesia
Insertion of resectoscope and inspection of urethra
Inspection of whole urothelium of bladder
Resection of tumour
Prostatic urethra biopsy and cold cup biopsies if indicated

Source: Adapted from European Association of Urology. http://uroweb.org/wp-content/uploads/EAU-Guidelines-on-Non-muscle-Invasive-BC_TaT1-2017.pdf

a more complete examination of the urothelium. A continuous flow resectoscope can then be introduced to perform the operation. A monopolar (or bipolar) diathermy loop is used to resect the exophytic tumour in fractions (exophytic part, bladder tumour base with detrusor muscle and edges of resection) to obtain a histological diagnosis and fully stage the lesion. Rollerball monopolar diathermy is then utilised to provide haemostasis and fulgurate the edge of the lesion to destroy any potentially malignant urothelium. *En bloc* resection using monopolar or bipolar current, Thulium-YAG or Holmium-YAG laser is feasible in selected exophytic tumours. These provide high-quality resected specimens with the presence of detrusor muscle in 96%–100% of cases [4].

If any other abnormal areas of urothelium are seen then these sites need separate sampling with a cold cup biopsy and diathermy to detect CIS. Random biopsies of normal mucosa are rarely performed in Ta/T1 disease as the chance of detecting CIS is less than 2%. A three-way irrigating catheter can then be inserted to washout any malignant cells and blood following the procedure. Generally this can be removed the next day but with larger resections may have to wait 48 hours. Care must be taken when resecting deep lesions that a perforation of the bladder does not occur. Following the resection a further bimanual examination can then be performed to assess whether a bladder mass has resolved. A residual mass strongly suggests residual invasive disease (T3).

In the operation note, it is important to document tumour characteristics (size, location, number and appearance), all steps of the procedure undertaken and the extent and completeness of resection.

The EAU recommends additional biopsies from normal-looking mucosa when high-risk exophytic (i.e. solid/non-papillary) tumour is visualised. Prostatic urethra biopsies are indicated when a tumour arises from the bladder neck, abnormal areas are seen at the prostatic urethra or if bladder CIS is suspected.

Note: *Conversely NICE guidelines recommend that no additional biopsies of normal-looking urothelium be taken unless there is a specific indication, such as unexplained positive cytology.*

There is a significant risk of residual disease after TURBT with some studies reporting rates of up to 27% and 53% in those patients with Ta and T1 tumours, respectively. In those patients with T1 disease, upstaging to T2 disease occurs in approximately 21%–25% of patients following a second resection. Second resection is thus recommended 4–6 weeks later in all T1 and high-grade tumours (high-grade G2 and G3). Re-resection is also indicated after incomplete initial TURBT or if there is a lack of muscle in the initial resection (except in G1pTa tumours and primary CIS).

Post-operatively clinically superficial lesions should receive adjuvant intravesical mitomycin C. A meta-analysis by Sylvester et al. has shown a decrease in the relative risk of recurrence by 39% [11].

Q. What do you know about fluorescence cystoscopy?

A. Fluorescence cystoscopy, photodynamic diagnosis (PDD) or blue light cystoscopy relies on the molecular handling of 5-aminolaevulinic acid (5-ALA) by tumour cells. 5-ALA is instilled into the bladder at least 1 hour prior to cystoscopy and taken up by the urothelium. 5-ALA is converted to protoporphyrin, which is preferentially taken up by malignant cells. When blue light (375–440 nm) is used to illuminate the bladder, red fluorescence from abnormal mucosa is seen compared to the surrounding normal bladder mucosa.

In a systematic review by Kausch et al., PDD had a 20% higher detection rate in non-muscle-invasive tumours and 39% increase diagnosis of CIS when compared to white light cystoscopy [12]. However, a higher detection rate in patients with positive cytology was not observed in a prospective randomised trial [13]. Although PDD has been shown to be more sensitive than white light cystoscopy, PDD has lower specificity.

Fluorescence cystoscopy, as compared to white light cystoscopy, has also been shown to reduce recurrence rates (<10% absolute reduction within 12 months) [14]. No benefit of PDD on progression rates or disease-specific survival has been demonstrated to date.

A prospective multicentre randomised trial comparing PDD guided bladder tumour resection with standard white light resection in patients with newly diagnosed non-muscle-invasive bladder cancer is currently under way with the objective of establishing the effect of PDD on time to recurrence and cost effectiveness (PHOTO trial).

Q. What factors predispose this man to non-muscle-invasive bladder cancer?

A. The main risk factors for bladder cancer are cigarette smoking (increases risk by threefold particularly in slow hepatic acetylators), industrial carcinogens in rubber and paint industries (aniline dyes, α-naphthylamine), phenacetin, and cyclophosphamide (used in chemotherapy of many haematological cancers). Carcinogenesis in bladder cancer has been extensively reported. The main karyotypic changes involve aberrations of chromosome 9 (>50% tumours), chromosome 17 (p53 loci) and chromosome 13 (retinoblastoma gene loci). A loss of retinoblastoma gene expression, H-ras activation and overexpression of telomerase are early genetic changes in non-muscle-invasive bladder cancer with p53 mutations, FGF and VEGF overexpression leading to invasive or metastatic disease.

Two key theories govern the development of bladder cancer. The clonal theory argues that multifocal and recurrent tumours evolve from one single transformed cell from which all cells share identical genetic mutations. The field change or oligoclonal theory suggests a global change in the urothelium. Genetically pre-malignant cells then transform into clinically detectable tumours, which are genetically unrelated.

Q. Can you name any lesions that predispose a patient to bladder cancer?

A. Several clinically detected lesions can predispose to malignancy. These are summarised in Table 4.7.

Table 4.7 Lesions arising from the urothelium and their malignant potential

Keratinising squamous metaplasia	This is seen in exstrophy, chronic bladder inflammation and schistosomiasis. It is pre-malignant.
Non-keratinising squamous metaplasia	Not pre-malignant.
Urothelial dysplasia	A flat non-invasive lesion typified by nuclear clustering. Can be seen with or without malignancy.
Cystitis cystica	Non pre-malignant enfolding of normal bladder lining cells.
Cystitis glandularis	Associated with adenocarcinoma.
Papillary urothelial neoplasm of low malignant potential	Difficult to define. Histology reveals exaggeration of normal glandular rests in bladder urothelium.
Leucoplakia	Clinically seen as thick and raised white plaques of squamous metaplasia on bladder surface. It is associated with chronic urinary infections. There is a weak association with malignancy. Histology shows keratinising squamous metaplasia.
Malakoplakia	Similar if not the same as leucoplakia. Malakoplakia histologically is characterised by Michaelis-Gutmann bodies with distinctive basophilic inclusions and foamy histiocytes. Clinically seen as yellow soft plaques on the urothelium.

Q. This 67-year-old man mentioned earlier attended for a TURBT. Examination under anaesthesia (EUA) revealed no mass. A 2 cm papillary looking tumour was resected from the posterior wall of his bladder. Deep muscle samples were sent separately. He received a single dose of MMC intravesical chemotherapy post-operatively. The histology shows grade 1 disease invading sub-epithelial tissue. The deep muscle biopsies are clear of tumour. He attends clinic to have the histology explained to him. At what TNM stage is this man?

A. This man has G1 pT1 disease. The TNM bladder cancer staging system is reproduced in Table 4.8.

Q. Do you know of any risk stratification for bladder cancer?

A. Several authorities have proposed a risk stratification of non-muscle-invasive bladder cancer (NMIBC).

The NICE bladder cancer: Diagnosis and management guidelines 2015 risk classification outline three risk groups as detailed in Table 4.9. This risk stratification incorporates time to recurrence unlike the risk stratification proposed by the EAU.

The European Organisation for Research and Treatment of Cancer – Genito-urinary Cancer Group (EORTC-GUCG) have also published risk categories (Table 4.10) based on a scoring system utilising the following pathological features: number of tumours (i.e. multifocality), tumour diameter, prior recurrence rate, stage, concomitant CIS and grade. This scoring system is derived from seven trials in non-muscle-invasive bladder cancer organised by the EORTC [15]. It calculates a percentage risk of recurrence and progression at 1 and 5 years as well as defining scores for low-, intermediate- and high-risk disease (Tables 4.11 and 4.12).

Table 4.8 TNM classification of urinary bladder cancer 2017 (8th edition)

Tx	Primary tumour cannot be assessed
Ta	Non-invasive papillary carcinoma
Tis	Carcinoma *in situ*
T1	Tumour invades subepithelial connective tissue
T2	T2a: Tumour invades superficial muscularis propria (inner half)
	T2b: Tumour invades deep muscularis propria (outer half)
T3	T3a: Tumour invades perivesical tissue microscopically
	T3b: Tumour invades perivesical tissue macroscopically (extravesical mass)
T4	T4a: Tumour invades prostate stroma, seminal vesicles, uterus or vagina
	T4b: Tumour invades pelvic wall or abdominal wall
Nx	Regional lymph nodes cannot be assessed
N0	No regional lymph node metastasis
N1	Metastasis in a single lymph node in true pelvis (hypogastric, obturator, external iliac or presacral)
N2	Metastasis in multiple lymph nodes in true pelvis (hypogastric, obturator, external iliac or presacral)
N3	Metastasis in common iliac lymph node(s)
Mx	Distant metastasis cannot be assessed
M0	No distant metastasis
M1	M1a: Non-regional lymph nodes
	M1b: Other distant metastases

Table 4.9 NICE bladder cancer risk classification in NMIBC 2015

Low risk	• Solitary G1/2 (low-grade) pTa tumour <3 cm • Any papillary urothelial neoplasm of low malignant potential (PUNLMP)
Intermediate risk	Urothelial cancer that is not low or high risk including: • Solitary G1/2 (low-grade) pTa tumour > 3 cm • Multifocal G1/2 (low-grade) pTa tumours • High-grade G2pTa tumour • Any low-risk NMIBC recurring within 12 months
High risk	• G3 tumour • G2/G3 pT1 tumour • CIS • Aggressive variant tumour (e.g. micropapillary or nested variant)

Table 4.10 EAU bladder cancer risk group stratification 2017 [4]

Low risk	• Primary, solitary Ta, G1 (PUNLMP/low grade), <3 cm, no CIS
Intermediate risk	• All tumours not defined in low- or high-risk groups
High risk	Any of the following: • T1 tumour • G3 (high-grade) tumour • carcinoma *in situ* (CIS) • Multiple, recurrent and large (>3 cm) TaG1G2/low grade tumours (all features must be present) *Subgroup of highest risk tumours:* T1G3/high grade associated with concurrent bladder CIS, multiple and/or large T1G3/high grade and/or recurrent T1G3/high grade, T1G3/high grade with CIS in the prostatic urethra, some forms of variant histology of urothelial carcinoma, lymphovascular invasion.

Source: Adapted from European Association of Urology. http://uroweb.org/wp-content/uploads/ EAU-Guidelines-on-Non-muscle-Invasive-BC_TaT1-2017.pdf

Table 4.11 EORTC-GUCG scoring system

Factor	Recurrence	Progression
Number of tumours		
Single	0	0
2–7	3	3
≥8	6	3
Tumour diameter		
<3 cm	0	0
≥3 cm	3	3
Prior recurrence rate		
Primary	0	0
≤1 recurrence/year	2	2
>1 recurrence/year	4	2
Stage		
Ta	0	0
T1	1	4
Concurrent CIS		
No	0	0
Yes	1	6
Grade		
G1	0	0
G2	1	0
G3	2	5
Total score	0–17	0–23

Source: European Association of Urology. http://uroweb.
org/wp-content/uploads/EAU-Guidelines-on-
Non-muscle-Invasive-BC_TaT1-2017.pdf

Table 4.12 EORTC-GUCG probability of recurrence and disease progression

Recurrence score	Probability of recurrence at 1 year		Probability of recurrence at 5 years	
	%	(95% CI)	%	(95% CI)
0	15	(10–19)	31	(24–37)
1–4	24	(21–26)	46	(42–49)
5–9	38	(35–41)	62	(58–65)
10–17	61	(55–67)	78	(73–84)
Progression score	Probability of progression at 1 year		Probability of progression at 5 years	
	%	(95% CI)	%	(95% CI)
0	0.2	(0–0.7)	0.8	(0–1.7)
1–4	1	(0.4–1.6)	6	(5–8)
5–9	5	(4–7)	17	(14–20)
10–17	17	(10–24)	45	(35–55)

Source: European Association of Urology. http://uroweb.org/wp-content/uploads/EAU-Guidelines-on-Non-
muscle-Invasive-BC_TaT1-2017.pdf

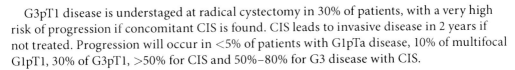

G3pT1 disease is understaged at radical cystectomy in 30% of patients, with a very high risk of progression if concomitant CIS is found. CIS leads to invasive disease in 2 years if not treated. Progression will occur in <5% of patients with G1pTa disease, 10% of multifocal G1pT1, 30% of G3pT1, >50% for CIS and 50%–80% for G3 disease with CIS.

Q. **Are you aware of the histological grading of non-muscle-invasive bladder cancer?**

A. The 1973 World Health Organisation (WHO) classification of urothelial carcinomas, stratifies tumours histologically into groups of urothelial papilloma, grade 1 (well differentiated), grade 2 (moderately differentiated) and grade 3 (poorly differentiated).

In 2004, the WHO and International Society of Urological Pathology (ISUP) produced a new histological classification consisting of groups of urothelial papilloma (benign), papillary urothelial neoplasm of low malignant potential (PUNLMP), low-grade and high-grade lesions.

The 2004 WHO classification has been updated in 2016, which includes additional categories of urothelial proliferation of uncertain malignant potential and urothelial dysplasia. Current management guidelines are still based on the 2004 WHO classification.

Although the prognostic values of both 1973 and 2004 WHO classifications have been demonstrated, neither has been shown to be superior and are thus both used in current practice.

Q. **What is the evidence for using mitomycin C intravesical chemotherapy in non-muscle-invasive bladder cancer and how do you consent a patient for and administer Mitomycin C?**

A. Mitomycin C (MMC) is an anti-tumour antibiotic, which causes DNA cross-linking in bladder tumour cells. It has been extensively investigated in the treatment of Ta/T1 bladder cancer. Following on from work in the United Kingdom for the MRC by Parmar and Tolley in the late 1980s [16], a meta-analysis in 2004 by Sylvester et al., reported on seven trials studying the use of single-dose intravesical chemotherapy post TURBT. This showed a 39% decrease in the relative risk of recurrence with adjuvant treatment [11]. Its use is therefore 'standard of care' post TURBT. In the latest meta-analysis by Sylvester et al., benefit from a single instillation of chemotherapy after TURBT was evident only in patients with a prior recurrence rate ≤1 recurrence per year and those with an European Organisation for Research and Treatment of Cancer (EORTC) recurrence score <5 [17].

Sylvester et al. have published four meta-analyses for adjuvant treatment of bladder cancer, which are summarised in Table 4.13.

Table 4.13 Summary of the four meta-analyses published by Sylvester et al. for the use of adjuvant intravesical treatment following TURBT in NMIBC and bladder CIS

1. Meta-analysis comparing TURBT plus single-dose adjuvant chemotherapy versus TURBT [11]	7 randomised controlled trials involving 1476 patients with NMIBC. Resulting in an absolute risk reduction of recurrence of 12% (NNT 8.5) and relative risk reduction of recurrence of 39%. Therefore single-dose MMC reduces the risk of recurrence.
2. Meta-analysis comparing single instillation of chemotherapy after TURBT with TURBT alone [17]	11 randomised controlled trials involving 2278 patients with NMIBC. Resulting in an absolute risk reduction of recurrence of 13.7% and relative risk reduction of recurrence of 35%. NNT to prevent one recurrence within 5 years was 7. Only patients with a recurrence rate of ≤1 recurrence per year or EORTC recurrence score <5 benefited. No effect on progression was observed.
3. Meta-analysis of TURBT plus BCG versus TURBT alone or another adjuvant treatment [18]	24 randomised controlled trials involving 4863 patients with NMIBC. Resulting in an absolute risk reduction of progression of 4% and relative risk reduction of progression of 27%. Therefore BCG reduces the risk of progression.
4. Meta-analysis comparing intravesical chemotherapy and BCG in CIS of the bladder [19]	9 randomised controlled trials involving 700 patients with NMIBC. Resulting in an absolute risk reduction in recurrence of 20.5% and relative risk reduction in recurrence of 59%. Therefore BCG is more effective than intravesical chemotherapy in CIS.

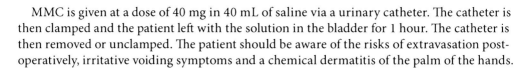

MMC is given at a dose of 40 mg in 40 mL of saline via a urinary catheter. The catheter is then clamped and the patient left with the solution in the bladder for 1 hour. The catheter is then removed or unclamped. The patient should be aware of the risks of extravasation post-operatively, irritative voiding symptoms and a chemical dermatitis of the palm of the hands.

Q. Tell me about BCG?

A. BCG or bacillus Calmette-Guérin was first used by Morales in 1976 [20]. It is live attenuated mycobacterium bovis. Connaught, OncoTice and RIVM are the three strains used. No difference in efficacy has been reported between these strains. The mechanism of action of BCG is still poorly understood. What is known is that it attaches to the urothelium via the fibronectin receptor and is internalised within the cell. Glycoproteins remain on the surface membrane of the cell and these antigens mediate the immune response by macrophage chemotaxis and cytokine production. Histologically BCG granulomas consist of epithelioid cells, Langerhans' giant cells and lymphocytes.

In the setting of adjuvant intravesical treatment of bladder cancer, BCG has been shown to reduce the risk of recurrence and progression.

A meta-analysis by Sylvester et al. analysed data from 4863 patients enrolled in 24 RCTs observed an absolute risk reduction in progression of 4% (13.8% versus 9.8%) and a relative risk reduction in progression of 27% in patients with non-muscle invasive (stage Ta, T1 or carcinoma *in situ*) bladder cancer. It must be noted that the median follow-up was short (2.5 years) and most tumours recurring were of low or intermediate risk (only 7.6% were G3 recurrence) [18].

Malmström et al. conducted a meta-analysis of 2820 patients from nine RCTs comparing MMC and BCG, observed a 32% reduction in risk of recurrence in patients treated with maintenance BCG (compared to MMC). However, a 28% increase in recurrence risk occurred in patients treated with BCG without maintenance BCG [21]. Another RCT by Sylvester et al. comparing BCG to epirubicin demonstrated between overall and disease-specific survival in patients with intermediate- and high-risk Ta T1 disease treated with BCG [22].

Q. How do you consent a patient for and administer BCG intravesical immunotherapy?

A. Patients who receive intravesical BCG must be at least 2 weeks post TURBT or bladder biopsy. The instillation is performed via a catheter, which is immediately removed, and the BCG is held within the bladder for up to 2 hours. Precautions such as sitting down to void in order to avoid splashing, hand washing after voiding as well as rinsing the toilet with undiluted bleach, are recommended. Patients should be encouraged to increase their fluid intake and void regularly.

Common side effects include dysuria, frequency and malaise with a mild fever for up to 24 hours. More serious symptoms of a high fever for 48 hours, arthralgia, headaches, rash and increased malaise suggest BCG sepsis. This requires hospitalisation, resuscitation, blood cultures and commencement of anti-tuberculous treatment. Steroids should be considered. Expert help should be sought and medication continued for a period of at least 6 months. Many of the agents used are hepatotoxic, which requires regular monitoring.

Absolute contraindications of BCG instillation include recent TURBT within 2 weeks, visible haematuria, traumatic catheterisation and symptomatic urinary tract infection.

The treatment regime involves once weekly instillations for 6 weeks followed by a 6-week break and three further instillations once a week for 3 weeks. If maintenance treatment is instigated, once weekly instillations for 3 weeks every 6 months for up to 3 years is given. This is the basis of Lamm's regime [23].

Thus the complete BCG treatment consists of

- Initial post TUR – 6 week course
- At 3 months – 3 week course
- At 6 months – 3 week course
- Then every 6 months thereafter a 3 week course up to 3 years

The complete course entails 27 doses of BCG, however poor compliance to complete the entire 3 year course was reported (only 16% achieved 27 doses). Quinolones have some anti-tuberculous activity and should be avoided to maintain efficacy.

Instillation of a reduced dose of BCG has been proposed to reduce toxicity. However, a full dose of BCG is more effective in multifocal tumours. The CUETO study compared one-third dose (27 mg) to full dose BCG (81 mg) and demonstrated no difference in efficacy. The EORTC randomised study by Oddens et al., comparing one-third dose to full dose BCG, found no difference in toxicity but in high-risk patients, 3 year is associated with a reduction in recurrence only when given at full dose [24].

Q. Do you know any alternatives to intravesical BCG?

A. In patients who fail a course of BCG, intravesical immunotherapy combination with 50 mega-units of interferon alpha with one-third dose of BCG has shown an increased response rate of 50%. Electromotive MMC has also been used in combination with BCG and shown to improve recurrence-free interval and reduce progression rates. The inflammatory reaction induced by BCG is thought to increase the absorption of MMC into the transformed urothelium. The effect of hyperthermia and MMC is currently being studied in the HIVEC II trial, which is comparing hyperthermia and MMC with MMC alone in patients with intermediate-risk NMIBC.

Q. When do you offer patients re-resection and what is the evidence for this practice?

A. Residual disease after TURBT has been reported in T1 tumours (33%–55%) and G3Ta tumours (41.4%). Understaging of tumours by initial resection has been observed in 4%–25% of T1 tumours and up to 45% if no muscle was included in the initial resection.

In a meta-analysis by Brausi et al., of 2410 patients from seven EORTC trials, in patients with T1 disease, 15%–35% had residual tumour and disease upstaging occurred in 30% [25]. Herr et al. evaluated 710 patients with re-resection and reported only 39% had no evidence of disease on re-TUR. Upstaging of tumour was observed in high-grade Ta (9%) and G3T1 tumours (23%). 76% of patients with residual T1 tumour on re-resection were found to progress in stage or grade compared with 14% of patients who had other than T1 tumours on re-resection [26]. Re-resection therefore improves staging accuracy, which is critical as the treatment of T1 disease differs significantly from T2 disease.

Re-resection has also been demonstrated to increase recurrence-free survival. Grimm et al. conducted an observational study of patients undergoing re-resection and primary TUR alone and found lower recurrence rates at 3 years in the re-resection group (33% versus 61%) [27].

Based on the described evidence, recommendations for re-resection are outlined in EAU guidelines [4]. Re-resection should be performed in the following situations:

- After incomplete initial TURBT
- If there is no muscle in the specimen of the initial resection (with exception of G1Ta tumours and primary CIS)
- In all T1 tumours
- In all high-grade/G3 tumours (except primary CIS)

The NICE guidelines recommend re-resection within 6 weeks of initial resection for those patients with high-risk NMIBC.

Q. How do you manage G3pT1 disease?

A. High-grade T1 bladder cancer presents significant difficulties in management. For G3pT1 disease, 30% of patients will never have a recurrence, 30% will undergo deferred cystectomy and 30% will die of metastatic disease. Based on the EORTC-GUCG risk tables, G3 disease has a 25%–75% risk of disease progression. Aggressive management is thus warranted in G3pT1 disease.

Given the high risk of residual disease and 23% risk of upstaging of G3T1 tumours [26], re-resection is recommended in the EAU and NICE guidelines within 6 weeks of the first resection to accurately stage the tumour.

After discussion at the uro-oncology MDT, treatment options including adjuvant intravesical immunotherapy (BCG) or primary radical cystectomy (especially in the highest risk group) should be offered. Radiotherapy has shown no increase in progression-free interval, progression-free survival or overall survival. Patient and disease factors should be taken into account when deciding on treatment with intravesical immunotherapy or primary radical cystectomy (e.g. patient fitness, life expectancy, pathological variants and large tumours).

If intravesical strategies fail, consideration of radical cystectomy in carefully chosen individuals results in a 5-year survival rate of 90%, however, 5%–10% of patients will still have positive lymph nodes.

Follow-up should be tailored to the risk of recurrence. Table 4.14 summarises the investigation, treatment and follow-up of NMIBC from the NICE guidelines.

Table 4.14 NICE guidelines for the investigation, treatment and follow-up of NMIBC by risk group

Risk group	Investigation	Treatment	Follow-up
Low			
• Solitary G1/2 (low grade) pTa tumour <3 cm • Any PUNLMP	Cystoscopy Cytology or urinary biomarker test Histopathology	Single dose of intravesical MMC at time of TURBT	Cystoscopic follow-up at 3 and 12 months after diagnosis Discharge if no recurrence within 12 months
Intermediate			
Urothelial cancer that is not low or high risk including • Solitary G1/2 (low grade) pTa tumour > 3 cm • Multifocal G1/2 (low grade) pTa tumours • High-grade G2pTa tumour Any low-risk NMIBC recurring within 12 months	Cystoscopy Histopathology Cytology	Single dose of intravesical MMC at time of TURBT. Offer a course of at least six doses of intravesical MMC	Cystoscopic follow-up at 3, 9 and 18 months, and once a year thereafter Discharge after 5 years of disease free follow-up
High			
• G3 tumour • G2/G3 pT1 tumour • CIS • Aggressive variant	Cystoscopy Histopathology CTU (CT staging if radical treatment considered) Cytology Re-resection	Single dose of intravesical MMC at time of TURBT. Offer another resection within 6 weeks of initial TURBT. Offer choice of intravesical BCG or radical cystectomy	For patients treated with intravesical immunotherapy cystoscopic follow-up: • Every 3 months for the first 2 years then • Every 6 months for the next 2 years then • Once a year thereafter

The EAU guidelines recommendations for follow-up in NMIBC patients do differ from the NICE guidelines in some respects:

- Low-risk Ta tumours should undergo cystoscopy at 3 months, 12 months and then yearly for 5 years.
- Surveillance of high-risk tumours should entail cystoscopy and cytology. Yearly upper tract imaging is recommended.
- Random biopsies or PDD-directed biopsies should be considered after intravesical treatment in patient with CIS.

Q. How do you manage carcinoma *in situ* (CIS) of the bladder?

A. CIS is a histological diagnosis and is a flat, non-invasive (i.e. not crossing the basement membrane), high-grade malignancy of the bladder (Figure 4.1).

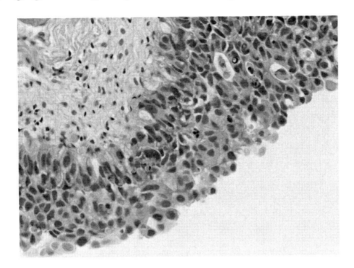

Figure 4.1 Haematoxylin and Eosin staining of carcinoma *in situ* of bladder displaying flat, non-invasive full thickness disordered proliferation of atypical cells with loss of cell polarity and cell cohesion (changes do not cross the basement membrane). (Thanks to Dr Rupali Arora, Consultant Histopathologist, University College Hospitals, London, UK, for providing this image.)

CIS leads to invasive disease in 2 years if not treated. Additionally, if untreated progression occurs in >50% of patients with CIS alone and in 50%–80% of patients of for G3 disease with CIS.

Primary CIS of the bladder is defined as CIS without any concomitant or previous TCC. Secondary CIS is defined as CIS with a TCC of the urothelium. Concurrent CIS is defined as CIS in the presence of any other urothelial bladder tumour.

Primary disease represents about 5% of CIS diagnosed. It occurs most commonly in men over the age of 50 years old. Secondary disease often occurs in association with high-grade invasive lesions. Urine cytology is very sensitive and specific for the detection of CIS (94% and 96%, respectively). Fluorescence cystoscopy has been used to detect carcinoma *in situ* but does have a 35% false-positive rate on biopsy. CIS cells show a high percentage of p53 mutations. The mainstay of treatment of CIS is with intravesical immunotherapy with BCG. A meta-analysis by Sylvester et al. shows that BCG is superior to MMC in the treatment of CIS [19]. With maintenance BCG up to 3 years, 75% of patients have an initial complete response with 50% remaining disease free at 5 years and 30% at 10 years. Response to intravesical BCG is a prognostic factor for progression and death with 10%–20% of complete responders progressing to muscle-invasive disease compared with 66% of non-responders.

For BCG refractory disease other novel approaches have been used, including BCG with electromotive MMC, combination BCG with interferon alpha and photodynamic therapy.

Upper tract CIS is a very dangerous condition and BCG treatment is associated with a higher degree of BCG-related complications due to increased systemic absorption.

Q. What do you know about squamous cell carcinoma of the bladder?

A. Squamous cell carcinoma of the bladder accounts for 3%–7% of all bladder tumours. It is often associated with long-term inflammation and irritation of the bladder from catheterisation, stone disease or schistosomiasis (in sub-Saharan Africa). It generally presents with haematuria in advanced stages and carries a poor prognosis. Cystoscopy reveals an invasive ulcerative lesion often on the trigone or lateral walls of the bladder. Treatment is with cystectomy for loco-regional control. At presentation only 8%–10% of patients will have metastatic disease. Five-year survival is 50% in those whose aetiology is schistosomiasis.

Q. **What do you know about adenocarcinoma of the bladder?**

A. Adenocarcinoma of the bladder is rare and accounts for less than 1% of all bladder tumours. It is either primary (de novo carcinoma often on the trigone or posterior wall of the bladder) or secondary (metastatic or associated with an urachal remnant). There is an association with cystitis glandularis rather than with CIS. Adenocarcinoma also has an increased incidence in bladder exstrophy patients and bowel augmentation/bladder substitution into the urinary tract (after 10–20 years).

In urachal adenocarcinoma, the urachal remnant is patent in one-third of patients. These patients often present with both haematuria and a mucous discharge. Histology shows mucous-secreting cells in a glandular, colloid or signet ring pattern. Clinically an important consideration is to identify a colonic tumour extending into the bladder. The treatment is with radical cystectomy with excision of the urachus and umbilicus but with aggressive management the 5-year survival rate is only 40%. There is no proven role for chemotherapy in this rare tumour, which often presents with muscle-invasive disease at diagnosis.

MUSCLE-INVASIVE BLADDER CANCER

Q. **A 70-year-old man has been seen in the haematuria clinic. His renal tract has been imaged with a CTU, which shows normal upper tracts, a filling defect in his bladder and no lymphadenopathy (Figure 4.2).**

Flexible cystoscopy shows a large invasive looking bladder tumour on the posterior wall of the bladder. He has attended for his TURBT. Outline how you would stage bladder cancer if you thought at TURBT it was muscle invasive?

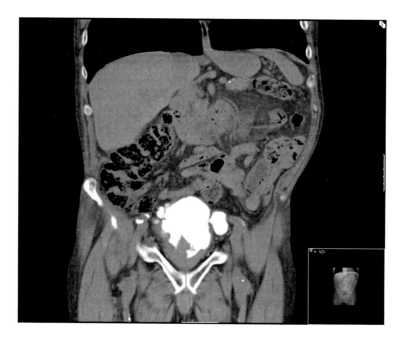

Figure 4.2 CTU (coronal view) demonstrating large filling defect in base of bladder (bladder diverticulae also present).

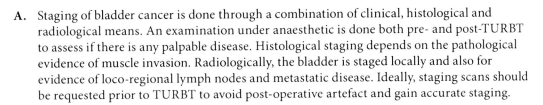

A. Staging of bladder cancer is done through a combination of clinical, histological and radiological means. An examination under anaesthetic is done both pre- and post-TURBT to assess if there is any palpable disease. Histological staging depends on the pathological evidence of muscle invasion. Radiologically, the bladder is staged locally and also for evidence of loco-regional lymph nodes and metastatic disease. Ideally, staging scans should be requested prior to TURBT to avoid post-operative artefact and gain accurate staging.

Q. **Outline how you would do a TURBT on a solid, 6 cm tumour that looked muscle invasive?**

A. As outlined by the EAU recommendations, having obtained appropriate consent, I would begin with a bimanual examination of the bladder under anaesthesia. Following detailed visual inspection of the whole urethra and bladder, I would resect the tumour separately in parts including the exophytic portion and edges of resection, and send it as the superficial specimen. I would then resect the underlying muscle to assess muscle invasion and send this separately. For tumours <1 cm *en bloc* resection can be performed. Prostatic urethra biopsies are indicated if there is bladder neck tumour, if bladder CIS is present or suspected, or if abnormalities of the prostatic urethra are seen. Some authorities advocate prostatic biopsies if radical treatment and orthotopic neobladder construction are considered. After tumour resection, I would complete haematosis and perform a post-resection bimanual EUA. A three-way irrigating catheter should be inserted.

Q. **What is N1 disease? What is N2 disease? What is N3 disease?**

A. The 2017 TNM classification of bladder cancer is reproduced in Table 4.8. N1 disease is metastasis in a single lymph node within the true pelvis (hypogastric, obturator, external iliac or presacral), N2 disease is a metastasis in multiple lymph nodes in the true pelvis, and N3 disease is metastasis in one or more common iliac lymph nodes.

Q. **What criteria are used to differentiate normal from involved lymph nodes on imaging (CT or MRI)?**

A. Lymph nodes are measured in maximum short axis diameter (MSAD). Pelvic nodes >8 mm and abdominal node >10 mm in the short axis are taken as significant. However, size criteria alone are inaccurate, ranging from 50%–80% overall accuracy in detecting metastatic disease.

Q. **How is muscle-invasive bladder cancer staged? For local staging do you use CT/MRI or both? Is there any advantage to one or the other?**

A. NICE and EAU guidelines recommend performing a CT scan of the chest, abdomen and pelvis with urographic phase to stage muscle-invasive bladder cancer. MRI abdomen and pelvis can be used as an equivalent alternative to CT abdomen and pelvis for local staging and metastatic disease within the abdomen. A bone scan to look for distant metastatic disease can be considered but is not routinely required unless there are specific symptoms or signs. Bone scans can be positive in 5%–15% of patients with muscle-invasive TCC.

   With respect to local staging, CT and MRI are generally equivalent. MRI has better soft tissue contrast resolution but CT has higher spatial resolution. MRI is superior to CT in determining depth of bladder wall involvement as CT is not able to differentiate between the layers of the bladder wall and thus cannot distinguish between tumours invading the lamina propria from those invading superficial and deep muscle. MRI and CT are both of similar accuracy in detecting perivesical extension, i.e. differentiating T2 from T3 disease.

   CT and MRI have similar accuracy in detection of lymph node metastasis. There is little evidence to support routine use of positron emission tomography (PET)-CT but in MIBC patients where there are equivocal findings on CT or MRI or have high risk of metastatic disease, PET-CT can be considered to aid radical treatment decisions (NICE recommendation).

Q. At TURBT the 70-year-old man previously mentioned has a palpable mass, and histology confirms high-grade (G3) muscle-invasive disease. A bone scan was negative and CT scan of his pelvis, abdomen and chest is normal except for the bladder mass, which suggests T2 disease. You are about to see this man in your clinic. What is his TNM staging?

A. He is stage pT2 at least N0 M0.

Q. Is this man suitable for radical treatment and how would you decide between radical treatment options?

A. Following MDT discussion with radiological and oncological colleagues, an agreed management plan based on the available information should be formulated. The patient should be seen along with a specialist nurse and preferably a family member.

An assessment of his fitness, including cardiac and respiratory status and exercise tolerance, should be made and a recent eGFR obtained. His treatment options are radical cystectomy (with ileal conduit or neobladder formation) or radical radiotherapy.

A Cochrane review demonstrated a better overall survival benefit with surgery in comparison to radical radiotherapy at 5 years (36% versus 20%) [28]. Although the 5-year survival rates appear better with radical cystectomy, this may be because radical radiotherapy is likely to be given to patients with significant comorbidity. More importantly, no direct randomised comparisons are available between these two treatment options and therefore the patient should have the opportunity to discuss each treatment option in detail including the risk profile of each procedure.

Manual dexterity is essential if a neobladder is being considered in order to be able to perform intermittent self-catheterisation. Table 4.15 summarises the benefits, risks and outcomes of radical treatment options for muscle-invasive bladder cancer.

Table 4.15 Benefits, risks and outcomes of radical treatment options for muscle-invasive bladder cancer

	Radiotherapy	Cystectomy
Benefits	Avoids major surgery Preserves functioning bladder	Full staging available with bladder and lymph node histology
Risks	Irritative voiding symptoms Dysuria Small bladder capacity Lethargy Nausea Proctitis Second malignancy	Major surgery Bleeding Chest infection Wound infection Deep vein thrombosis Pulmonary embolism Collection Anastomotic leak Stomal stenosis Anastomotic stricture Hyperchloraemic metabolic acidosis
Outcome	Better 5-year survival rates reported with radical cystectomy but this may be because radical radiotherapy is likely to be given to patients with significant comorbidity. No RCTs comparing two modalities to date. There is a proven survival benefit for neoadjuvant chemotherapy in both groups.	

Q. In which situations is radical cystectomy the treatment of choice as compared to radical radiotherapy?

A. In the following situations radical cystectomy is advocated as compared to radical radiotherapy:

- Presence of CIS (radiotherapy does not treat CIS)
- Upper tract obstruction
- Presence of inflammatory bowel disease

- Presence of severe irritative urinary symptoms
- Previous extensive abdominal surgery
- Previous pelvic radiotherapy
- Young patient

Q. How do you consent for radical cystectomy?

A. Cystectomy is associated with mortality in 3% of patients and morbidity in 30%. It has a significant risk of bleeding requiring blood transfusion. Infection in the surgical wound, chest and pelvis can occur. Complications, such as ileo-ileal anastomotic leak, uretero-ileal anastomotic leak, deep vein thrombosis, pulmonary embolus, stroke, myocardial infarction and death, must be discussed with the patient as well as disease recurrence. Patients requiring an ileal conduit need to be aware of the late complications, including risks of stomal stenosis, anastomotic stricture, herniation and metabolic sequelae, such as a hyperchloraemic metabolic acidosis.

For a patient receiving an ileal neobladder the operation carries risks of impotence, incontinence or retention. Female surgical candidates should be aware of the risk of shortening and narrowing of the vagina. A rare risk of rectal injury should also be conferred to the patient.

Q. Is there any advantage to lymphadenectomy and to what extent should it be carried out?

A. Lymphadenectomy is an important step in radical cystectomy, providing accurate staging and therapeutic effect. Lymph node (LN) status is a strong predictor of cancer-specific survival (CSS). Tarin et al. reported that the presence and number of positive LNs were significantly associated with increased risk of cancer-specific death (5-year CSS 81% with N0 versus 40% with N+ve) [29]. Mapping studies demonstrate that regional LNs consist of all pelvic LNs below the aortic bifurcation and that nodal spread from MIBC is predictable (i.e. that there are rarely positive nodes outside the pelvis if the pelvic nodes are uninvolved).

There is currently no consensus to the extent of LN dissection (LND). The limits of differing extents of lymphadenectomy are detailed below:

- *Standard LND* – Nodal tissue up to common iliac bifurcation, with ureter as medial border, including internal iliac, presacral, obturator fossa and external iliac nodes.
- *Extended LND* – Standard LND and nodal tissue in region of aortic bifurcation, and presacral and common iliac vessels medial to ureters. The limits of LND include genitofemoral nerves laterally, and circumflex iliac vein, lacunar ligament and lymph node of Cloquet caudally.
- *Super-extended LND* – Limit of LND extends cranially to level of inferior mesenteric artery.

A systematic review on the impact of extent of LND reported improved oncological outcome for LND compared with no LND being performed. Improved outcomes were observed with super-extended LND when compared with limited or standard LND [30]. Currently there are two RCTs studying the effect of extent of lymphadenectomy – SWOG 1011 and AUO trials. Early data from the AUO trial report a trend but no significant difference with extended LND in CSS.

The number of LNs excised during LND has been reported to be associated with progression-free and overall survival. Cohort studies have suggested that removal of >10 LNs is associated with increased overall survival [31]. There is presently no data from RCTs to draw any conclusions on the optimal number of LNs that should be removed.

Q. Is there any advantage to laparoscopic or robotic-assisted laparoscopic radical cystectomy?

A. There is still controversy as to the optimal technique to radical cystectomy. Published evidence suggests that oncological outcomes were comparable with the robotic-assisted laparoscopic cystectomy (RALC) or open radical cystectomy (ORC) approaches. RALC and laparoscopic radical cystectomy (LRC) have the advantage of reduced blood loss and shorter length of hospital stay than ORC but longer operative times were observed. Complication rates also appeared less with LRC and RALC in comparison to ORC. Although the benefits of RALC and LRC appear to be similar, there are ergonomic advantages to RALC but at the detriment of high expense. It has been noted that the critical factor for outcome is not the technique but rather the surgeon experience and institutional volume.

Q. What proportion of men will have prostate cancer detected in a cystoprostatectomy sample?

A. Incidentally found prostate cancer is detected in 25%–46% of male patients undergoing a cystoprostatectomy. Of these 20% are Gleason 7 or more. The implications of incidental prostate cancer in such circumstances are not clear but careful follow-up of these patients with PSA testing is required.

Q. Is there any evidence for the use of adjuvant or neoadjuvant chemotherapy in muscle-invasive (non-metastatic) bladder cancer?

A. The evidence for adjuvant chemotherapy in muscle-invasive (non-metastatic) bladder cancer is limited and is not advocated for routine use. However, adjuvant chemotherapy is recommended to patients with muscle-invasive disease and/or lymph node positive disease.

The role of neoadjuvant chemotherapy has been established. The advanced bladder cancer (ABC) meta-analysis of data from 11 trials demonstrated a significant benefit of 5% absolute improvement in 5-year survival and 14% reduction in the risk of death [32]. This is a modest increase in survival, and the numbers are relatively small in the relevant trials. Therapeutic benefit has only been observed with cisplatin-based combination chemotherapy.

The disadvantages of neoadjuvant chemotherapy are the associated morbidity and the potential delay in cystectomy in chemotherapy non-responders, which may affect outcome.

Q. Do you know of any trials relating to the treatment of muscle-invasive bladder cancer?

A. The SPARE trial was initiated by Cancer Research UK and involves randomising patients with non-metastatic bladder cancer (T2 or T3) to radical external beam radiotherapy or radical cystectomy after neo-adjuvant chemotherapy. If there has been a good response to chemotherapy in the radiotherapy arm, they will have radiotherapy, and if not, they will have cystectomy. This trial should hopefully help to answer several questions about the relative efficacy of radiotherapy and cystectomy as well as the benefits of neoadjuvant chemotherapy.

The BOLERO trial also supported by Cancer Research UK is multicentre study that aims to determine the feasibility of randomisation to open versus laparoscopic or robotic-assisted laparoscopic cystectomy. The secondary outcomes include comparing the safety, efficacy and outcomes of the different techniques.

Q. Tell me what options are available for urinary diversion following radical cystectomy?

A. The most commonly used method of diversion in the United Kingdom is the ileal conduit. This is formed by anastomosing the ureters to an isolated piece of distal ileum 20 cm from the ileo-caecal valve. The distal end is brought out as a stoma on the right side of the abdomen. This is then managed with a stoma bag.

Uretero-colonic diversion, such as uretero-rectosigmoidostomy, is less commonly used in the United Kingdom particularly as there was a long-term risk of developing colon malignancy. The Mainz II pouch involves opening the sigmoid longitudinally and closing it transversely with a tunnelled ureterosigmoid anastomosis. The Mansoura rectal pouch entails intussusception of the sigmoid to prevent reflux of urine into the colon and augmentation of the sigmoid with ileum to reduce intraluminal pressure. It is proposed that this method reduces the contact between urine and colonic mucosa and lowers the risk of malignancy.

Continent cutaneous urinary diversion requires formation of a low-pressure reservoir and a continence mechanism. Many types require self-catheterisation. Usually a detubularised ileal segment is used but gastric, and ileo-caecal pouches have been described. Examples include the Kock pouch (ileal reservoir with catheterisable conduit), Mainz I and Indiana pouches (caecal reservoir with ileal catheterisable conduit).

Ureterocutaneostomy involves either directly anastomosing both ureters to the skin separately or attaching one ureter, to which the other ureter is attached (end-to-side trans-ureteroureterostomy) to the skin. Although it is the simplest technique of diversion, higher stenosis rates have been observed with ureterocutaneostomy compared with intestinal diversions and is thus rarely used.

Orthotopic bladder substitution or neobladder formation is the favoured bladder substitution method. Many techniques have been described, such as the Studer bladder. Most patients are dry with some requiring self-catheterisation. Voiding occurs by Valsalva and pelvic floor relaxation.

Q. **What are the potential problems with ileal conduit formation?**

A. The complications have already been outlined in the consent for cystectomy section but they can be classified in a number of ways: early or late, mechanical and metabolic. Early complications include those associated with any bowel operation, such as ileus, bowel obstruction, UTI, anastomotic leak, stenosis or ischaemia of the conduit. Up to 48% of patients develop early complications. Late complications include stomal stenosis or para-stomal herniation (24%) and uretero-ileal stenosis. Some of these complications are due to chronic ischaemia. Metabolic problems are less common with an ileal conduit than with a neobladder (as the ileal conduit does not act as storage reservoir for urine) but can include absorption of acid and chloride leading to a hyperchloraemic metabolic acidosis. This responds well to sodium bicarbonate (1 g od). Macrocytic anaemia can be a consequence of vitamin B12 deficiency or from a loss of iron absorption from the terminal ileum.

Q. **What are the advantages and disadvantages of neobladder construction?**

A. Neobladder formation is increasingly being offered to patients, particularly the young, at the time of cystectomy. It has the advantage of dispensing with the need for a stoma and approximately 90% of patients are continent by day and approximately 70%–80% by night. The disadvantages are that it requires a larger segment of small bowel as compared to an ileal conduit, which can lead to increased risk of vitamin B12 deficiency and metabolic complications (15 cm versus 60 cm in the Studer neobladder). Morbidity of approximately 22% is reported. The oncological outcomes have been shown to be similar. There is still debate as to whether neobladder affords a better quality of life then other types of urinary diversion.

Q. **Under what circumstances would a primary urethrectomy be considered?**

A. Traditionally, urethrectomy in females formed a routine part of radical cystectomy. In men, cystectomy with urethrectomy used to be offered. With the growing use of neobladders, this approach was questioned. It appears that the risk of urethral recurrence is lower with the use of a neobladder compared to an ileal conduit with reported decreases from 8% to 4% in the incidence of urethral recurrence if a neobladder is anastomosed to the native urethra, suggesting that urine is protective in this setting to the development of recurrent disease. It is recommended to preserve the urethra if margins are negative. If urethrectomy is not performed at the time of cystectomy then long-term follow-up of the urethra is required if no neobladder is formed.

A urethrectomy should be considered if there are positive margins at the urethral resection margin (frozen section can be performed), if the primary tumour is located at the bladder neck or in the urethra (in women), if tumour extensively infiltrates the prostate or if there is extensive CIS/multifocal disease.

Q. **What treatment options are available for patients who present with metastatic bladder cancer?**

A. Approximately 10% of patients will present with metastatic bladder cancer. The mainstay of treatment, after thorough assessment, is with a debulking TURBT to gain histology and decrease the risk of further haematuria and voiding symptoms. After discussion at the MDT, the patient should then be offered palliative chemotherapy if of good performance status and adequate renal function. The current gold standard is cisplatin-based combination chemotherapy (e.g. gemcitabine and cisplatin or MVAC). The overall response rate is 38%–73% with long-term disease-free survival in 15%. A median survival of up to 14 months has been reported.

TRANSITIONAL CELL CANCER OF RENAL PELVIS AND URETER

Q. **What percentage of urothelial malignancies does cancer of the renal pelvis and ureter constitute?**

A. Urothelial cancer of the renal pelvis and ureter is an uncommon finding accounting for 5% of urothelial malignancies and <10% of renal malignancies.

Q. **A 65-year-old woman presents to your haematuria clinic with macroscopic haematuria. Her cytology shows high-grade malignant cells and flexible cystoscopy is normal. A CT urogram has been performed which shows a filling defect in the right renal pelvis and right ureter. She has no other co-morbidities and a normal glomerular filtration rate (GFR). How would you assess this patient?**

A. I am concerned that this woman has a TCC of her renal pelvis and ureter. A full urological history including cigarette-smoking exposure is required. The case should be discussed at the local multidisciplinary team meeting (MDT) seeking the opinion of a radiologist.

The need for pre-operative histological diagnosis of upper tract urothelial TCC prior to nephroureterectomy is still under debate. A review of the BAUS nephroureterectomy database revealed 81% of nephroureterectomies were performed without pre-operative histological diagnosis, from which malignancy was found in 96.2% [33]. Although the incidence of benign histology is low in patients whether a pre-operative biopsy was performed or not, diagnosis ureteroscopy should be considered. EAU guidelines [4] recommend performing diagnostic ureteroscopy and biopsy where there is diagnostic uncertainty, if kidney-sparing treatment is considered or in a solitary kidney.

Q. **What are the risk factors and genetics for the development of ureteric cancer?**

A. The aetiology is similar to bladder cancer including exposure to cigarette smoking, industrial carcinogens, phenacetin and cyclophosphamide. Smoking has a long latent period of up to 20 years whereas cyclophosphamide has a much shorter latent period of around 12 years. Phenacetin is a historically used non-steroidal anti-inflammatory agent. Its use with cocaine has been reported.

Aristolochic acid, which is commonly used in Chinese herbal medicine, is also associated with upper tract urothelial cancer. Mutation in the p53 gene occurs with derivatives of aristolochic acid.

The genetic aberrations for ureteric cancer are similar to bladder cancer, i.e. chromosome 9, chromosome 17 (p53 loci), and chromosome 13 (retinoblastoma gene loci). However, in upper ureteric TCC a higher level of microsatellite instability compared to bladder tumours is reported.

Q. What treatment options does the patient have?

A. Treatment options for this woman include open or laparoscopic radical nephroureterectomy (RNU) with excision of a cuff of bladder tissue at the ureteric orifice. This is essential as a high rate of ipsilateral ureteric recurrence occurs with nephrectomy alone due to the whole of the urothelium being susceptible to recurrent lesions.

The traditional approach for the open technique is the loin incision. A second Pfannenstiel or lower midline incision can be used to facilitate excision of the bladder cuff. The entire renal unit and collecting system can be removed through a midline abdominal incision.

A laparoscopic RNU can be performed with either a transperitoneal or retroperitoneal approach. Hand-assisted and robotic-assisted laparoscopic techniques are recognised.

Both approaches must tackle the distal ureter, ureteric orifice and bladder cuff. This can be performed through a variety of incisions. The ureter can be dissected free either with an intravesical or extravesical technique. With the extravesical approach care must be taken to complete the ureteric resection to the UO. The intravesical approach is the most precise in terms of ureteric resection but requires an extra cystotomy.

In addition to formal open ureteric excision, the 'rip and pluck' technique is also described. This involves the resection or cystoscopic dissection of the distal ureter to perivesical fat. The ureter is then 'plucked' during the distal ureteric dissection. Concern remains over tumour cells extravasating into the retroperitoneum. The approach avoids the morbidity of a second incision.

Laparoscopic and open RNU have been shown to be comparable in outcome and safety in a prospective randomised trial [34]. In T3 and/or high-grade upper tract urothelial carcinoma (UTUC), open RNU was shown to have better oncological outcomes over the laparoscopic approach. Due to insufficient data on the robotic-assisted laparoscopic approaches, no recommendations have been made on its use.

As the risk of lymph node positivity is low in Ta/T1 disease, lymphadenectomy is recommended by EAU in invasive tumours. There is no evidence to support routine lymph node dissection in all UTUCs.

The rate of bladder recurrence after RNU has been reported to be 22%–47%. The ODMIT-C trial analysed the effect of a single post-operative administration of Mitomycin C after RNU, and reported a relative risk reduction in bladder tumour recurrence within the first year after RNU of 40% [35]. Based on such data, offering a post-operative bladder instillation to lower risk of bladder tumour recurrence is included in the EAU guidelines [4].

Q. Do you know of any kidney-sparing treatment options for upper tract transitional cell carcinoma?

A. Kidney-sparing surgery should be offered in all low-risk cancers as it avoids the morbidity associated with RNU. Where there is risk of renal insufficiency or solitary kidney, kidney-sparing surgery can be considered in high-risk tumours.

The ureteroscopic approach involves tissue sampling with cold cup biopsy forceps or a stone basket. Fulguration of the tumour base can then be achieved with either the Holmium:YAG laser (0.5 mm tissue penetration) or neodymium:yttrium aluminum garnet YAG laser (5 mm tissue penetration). Retrograde stenting is required as part of the procedure. The perforation rate is less than 10% in large series and can be treated with the placement of a retrograde ureteric stent. The stricture rate is also in the region of 10%.

The percutaneous approach is more invasive and disrupts urothelial integrity. It does however allow excellent access to the renal pelvis with a 30 Fr sheath and the use of biopsy forceps, loop resection and base sampling to fully stage the lesion resected. The tract can also serve as a conduit for delivering adjuvant therapy following initial resection. Complications from this approach include bleeding, infection and injury to adjacent organs or pleura and potentially seeding along the tract.

For both approaches, patients must be counselled for the need for long-term surveillance after treatment with imaging and direct visual inspection with repeated ureteroscopy.

Using these approaches recurrence rates of 33% for pelvic tumours and 31% for ureteric tumours are reported. The most common site of recurrence is in the bladder.

EAU guidelines outline the indications for kidney-sparing treatment:

- Low-risk tumours and two functional kidneys
- Solitary kidney and/or impaired renal function
- High risk distal ureteric tumours in imperative cases (solitary kidney and/or impaired renal function)

Note that low-risk tumours classified as

- Unifocal tumour
- Tumour <1 cm
- Low-grade tumour
- Non-invasive disease on CTU

Adjuvant instillation of bacillus Calmette-Guérin (BCG) or Mitomycin C antegrade via percutaneous nephrostomy after kidney-sparing treatment has been shown to be a feasible treatment option [36].

Q. What options are available for an isolated distal ureteric tumour (Figure 4.3)?

A. The gold standard for this lesion would be either an open or laparoscopic RNU with excision of a cuff of bladder tissue. However, segmental resection has a role in high-risk tumours where renal preservation is paramount (e.g. solitary kidney of renal insufficiency) or in an elderly patient with significant co-morbidity. This can be performed as a direct excision and spatulated tension-free uretero-ureteral anastomosis or in the lower one-third of the ureter with a Boari flap and psoas hitch. Comparable oncological failure rates to RNU are reported.

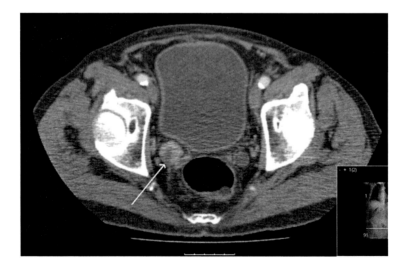

Figure 4.3 CTU (axial view) demonstrating right ureteric tumour.

Q. The 65-year-old patient mentioned previously is treated with an uncomplicated laparoscopic NU with open excision of a cuff of bladder urothelium. The pathologist reports that the lesion is a grade 3 transitional cell carcinoma invading into the renal parenchyma, and the nodes removed are negative for tumour spread. The surgical margins are clear of tumour. What is the TNM stage for this patient?

A. The tumour, node and metastasis (TNM) stage for this patient is pT3N0Mx. The TNM staging of renal pelvic and ureteric cancer is reproduced in Table 4.16.

Table 4.16 TNM classification for upper tract urothelial carcinoma 2017 (8th edition)

Tx	Tumour not assessed
T0	No tumour
Ta	Non-invasive papillary carcinoma
Tis	Carcinoma *in situ*
T1	Invades subepithelial connective tissue
T2	Tumour invades muscularis propria
T3	Renal pelvis – tumour invades beyond muscularis into peripelvic fat or renal parenchyma Ureter – tumour invades beyond muscularis into periureteric fat
T4	Tumour invades into adjacent organs or through kidney into perinephric fat
Nx	Lymph nodes not assessed
N0	No nodes
N1	Metastasis in a single lymph node 2 cm or less in the greatest dimension
N2	Metastasis in a single lymph node more than 2 cm, or multiple lymph nodes
Mx	Distant metastasis not assessed
M0	No distant metastasis
M1	Distant metastasis

Q. What is the prognosis of TCC of the renal pelvis?

A. Hall et al. have reported the 5-year survival rates for upper tract TCC [37]. The results can be seen in Table 4.17.

Table 4.17 Actuarial disease-specific 5-year survival rates by grade

Stage	Actuarial disease specific 5-year survival rates (%)
Ta/CIS	100
T1	91.7
T2	72.6
T3	40.5
T4	<5

Q. How does upper tract TCC differ from bladder cancer at presentation and what percentages of patients develop bladder cancer following upper tract TCC?

A. The majority of UTUCs are invasive at presentation (60%) unlike bladder tumours (15%–25%). Bladder tumour recurrences after treatment of UTUC occur in 22%–47% of patients [38]. If high-grade upper tract malignancy is resected then the patient has a higher chance of high-grade bladder cancer at recurrence.

Concurrent bladder tumour is seen in 17% of UTUC patients [39]. Although synchronous bladder tumours are uncommon, 46% were found to be invasive [40].

Q. What percentage of patients develop synchronous and metachronous upper tract TCCs?

A. Synchronous tumours of the upper tract have been reported in 2%–3% of patients. Metachronous upper tract TCC has been reported in approximately 2%–6% of patients. This highlights the importance of cystoscopic, ureteroscopic and radiological surveillance of these patients following definitive treatment.

Q. Is there a role for adjuvant chemotherapy in invasive upper tract urothelial tumours?

A. No randomised trials on the effect of adjuvant chemotherapy for UTUC have been published to date. A recent meta-analysis observed a beneficial effect of adjuvant chemotherapy with cisplatin-based adjuvant chemotherapy on both overall survival and disease-free survival (51% risk reduction) [41]. The POUT trial is a multicentre, randomised controlled trial that aims to determine the effect of adjuvant chemotherapy after radical nephroureterectomy, which is currently ongoing.

Q. How would you follow up a patient after an upper tract TCC had been treated (with nephroureterectomy)?

A. Close follow-up of upper tract TCC is essential to monitor for metachronous bladder and contralateral ureteric recurrence. Flexible cystoscopy, urine cytology and radiological imaging are the main surveillance investigations.

EAU guidelines [4] suggest surveillance protocols for at least 5 years based on tumour invasiveness and type of treatment undertaken.

Flexible cystoscopy and urine cytology are suggested 3 months after RNU, and then annually. CT urogram should be performed annually for non-invasive tumours and every 6 months for 2 years and then annually for invasive tumours.

For those patients treated with kidney-sparing surgery, a more intense surveillance regime is required. Urine cytology and CT urogram at 3 and 6 months, and then annually should be performed along with ureteroscopy at 3 and 6 months, and then every 6 months for 2 years, and then annually.

Q. Several years later this woman returns with weight loss, anorexia and loin pain. A repeat CT scan is performed and shows a local recurrence in the renal bed (Figure 4.4). How would you assess this patient?

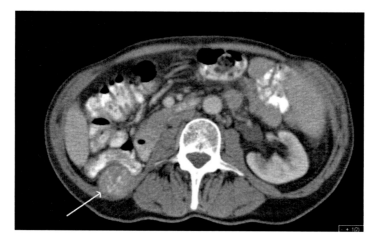

Figure 4.4 CT (axial view) showing recurrence of tumour in right renal bed.

A. This woman needs re-staging with a CT scan of her chest, abdomen and pelvis. In addition a bone scan is required. She is symptomatic and clearly needs further treatment. Palliative chemotherapy with cisplatin and gemcitabine should be discussed at the MDT meeting. Palliative care involvement will aid symptom control and support for this patient through this phase of her illness.

Most of the data concerning the use of chemotherapy in upper ureteric and renal pelvic TCC have been translated from bladder cancer TCC trials such as the ABC meta-analysis group. Chemotherapy is occasionally used in high-risk patients after consideration of the patient at the MDT as well as patients with symptomatic recurrent and metastatic disease.

No randomised controlled trials have reported on using chemotherapy in this setting. Trial design is limited by the low numbers of patients developing this disease.

ACKNOWLEDGEMENT

With thanks to Mr DMA Wallace for his help and advice with the preparation of this chapter.

REFERENCES

1. Tomson C et al. Asymptomatic microscopic or dipstick haematuria in adults: Which investigations for which patients: A review of the evidence. *BJU Int* 2002; 90: 185–198.
2. Sutton JM. Evaluation of hematuria in adults. *JAMA* 1990; 263: 2475–2480.
3. Khadra MH et al. A prospective analysis of 1,930 patients with hematuria to evaluate current diagnostic practice. *J Urol* 2000; 163: 524–527.
4. European Association of Urology (EAU). http://uroweb.org/wp-content/uploads/EAU-Guidelines-on-Non-muscle-Invasive-BC_TaT1-2017.pdf
5. Rodgers M et al. Diagnostic tests and algorithms used in the investigation of haematuria: Systematic reviews and economic evaluation. *Health Technol Assess* 2006; 10: iii–v, xi–259.
6. Edwards TJ et al. A prospective analysis of the diagnostic yield resulting from the attendance of 4020 patients at a protocol-driven haematuria clinic. *BJU Int* 2006; 97: 301–305.
7. Albani JM et al. The role of computerized tomographic urography in the initial evaluation of haematuria. *J Urol* 2007; 177: 644–648.
8. Britton JP et al. A community study of bladder cancer screening by the detection of occult urinary bleeding. *J Urol* 1992; 148: 788–790.
9. Messing EM et al. Long-term outcome of haematuria home screening for bladder cancer in men. *Cancer* 2006; 107: 2173–2179.
10. Steiner H et al. Early results of bladder-cancer screening in a high-risk population of heavy smokers. *BJU Int* 2008; 102: 291–296.
11. Sylvester RJ et al. A single immediate postoperative instillation of chemotherapy decreases the risk of recurrence in patients with stage Ta T1 bladder cancer: A meta-analysis of published results of randomized clinical trials. *J Urol* 2004; 171: 2186–2190.
12. Kausch I et al. Photodynamic diagnosis in non-muscle invasive bladder cancer: A systematic review and cumulative analysis of prospective studies. *Eur Urol* 2010; 57: 595–606.
13. Neuzillet Y et al. Assessment of diagnostic gain with hexaminolevulinate (HAL) in the setting of newly diagnosed non-muscle invasive bladder cancer with positive results on urine cytology. *Urol Oncol* 2014; 32: 1135–1140.

14. Burger M et al. Photodynamic diagnosis of non-muscle invasive bladder cancer with hexaminolevulinate cystoscopy: A meta-analysis of detection and recurrence based on raw data. *Eur Urol* 2013; 64: 846–854.

15. Sylvester RJ et al. Predicting recurrence and progression in individual patients with stage Ta T1 bladder cancer using EORTC risk tables: A combined analysis of 2596 patients from seven EORTC trials. *Eur Urol* 2006; 49: 466–475.

16. Parmar MK et al. Prognostic factors for recurrence and followup policies in the treatment of superficial bladder cancer: Report from the British Medical Research Council Subgroup on Superficial Bladder Cancer (Urological Cancer Working Party). *J Urol* 1989; 142: 284–288.

17. Sylvester RJ et al. Systematic review and individual patient data meta-analysis of randomized trials comparing a single immediate instillation of chemotherapy after transurethral resection with transurethral resection alone in patients with stage pTa-pT1 urothelial carcinoma of the bladder: Which patients benefit from the instillation? *Eur Urol* 2016; 69: 231–244.

18. Sylvester RJ et al. Intravesical bacillus Calmette-Guérin reduces the risk of progression in patients with superficial bladder cancer: A meta-analysis of the published results of randomized clinical trials. *J Urol* 2002; 168: 1964–1970.

19. Sylvester RJ et al. Bacillus Calmette-Guérin versus chemotherapy for the intravesical treatment of patients with carcinoma *in situ* of the bladder: A meta-analysis of the published results of randomized clinical trials. *J Urol* 2005; 174: 86–91.

20. Morales A et al. Intracavitary bacillus Calmette-Guérin in the treatment of superficial bladder tumors. *J Urol* 1976; 116: 180–183.

21. Malmström PU et al. An individual patient data meta-analysis of the long-term outcome of randomised studies comparing intravesical Mitomycin C versus bacillus Calmette-Guérin for non-muscle invasive bladder cancer. *Eur Urol* 2009; 56: 247–256.

22. Sylvester RJ et al. Long-term efficacy results of EORTC genito-urinary group randomized phase 3 study 30911 comparing intravesical instillations of epirubicin, bacillus Calmette-Guérin, and bacillus Calmette-Guérin plus isoniazid in patients with intermediate- and high-risk stage Ta T1 urothelial carcinoma of the bladder. *Eur Urol* 2010; 57: 766–773.

23. Lamm DL et al. Maintenance bacillus Calmette-Guérin immunotherapy for recurrent TA, T1 and carcinoma *in situ* transitional cell carcinoma of the bladder: A randomized Southwest Oncology Group Study. *J Urol* 2000; 163: 1124–1129.

24. Oddens J et al. Final results of an EORTC-GU cancers group randomized study of maintenance bacillus Calmette-Guérin in intermediate- and high-risk Ta, T1 papillary carcinoma of the urinary bladder: One-third dose versus full dose and 1 year versus 3 years of maintenance. *Eur Urol* 2013; 63: 462–472.

25. Brausi M et al. Variability in the recurrence rate at first follow-up cystoscopy after TUR in stage Ta T1 transitional cell carcinoma of the bladder: A combined analysis of seven EORTC studies. *Eur Uol* 2002; 41: 523–531.

26. Herr HW et al. A re-staging transurethral resection predicts early progression of superficial bladder cancer. *BJU Int* 2006; 97: 1194–1998.

27. Grimm MO et al. Effect of routine repeat transurethral resection for superficial bladder cancer: A long-term observational study. *J Urol* 2003; 170: 433–437.

28. Shelley MD et al. Surgery versus radiotherapy for muscle invasive bladder cancer. *Cochrane Database Syst Rev* 2002; 1: Cd002079.

29. Tarin TV et al. Lymph node-positive bladder cancer treated with radical cystectomy and lymphadenectomy: Effect of the level of node positivity. *Eur Urol* 2012; 61: 1025–1030.

30. Bruins HM et al. The impact of extent of lymphadenectomy on oncologic outcomes in patients undergoing radical cystectomy for bladder cancer: A systematic review. *Eur Urol* 2014; 66: 1065–1077.

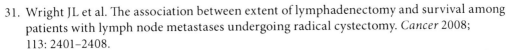

31. Wright JL et al. The association between extent of lymphadenectomy and survival among patients with lymph node metastases undergoing radical cystectomy. *Cancer* 2008; 113: 2401–2408.

32. Advanced Bladder Cancer (ABC) Meta-analysis Collaboration. Neo-adjuvant chemotherapy in invasive bladder cancer: Update of a systematic review and meta-analysis of individual patient data. *Eur Urol* 2005; 48: 202–205.

33. Malki M et al. The role of pre-operative histology in nephroureterectomy: The UK experience. *BJU Int* 2015; 115(S7): 45.

34. Simone G et al. Laparoscopic versus open nephroureterectomy: Perioperative and oncologic outcomes from a randomised prospective study. *Eur Urol* 2009; 56: 520–526.

35. O'Brien T et al. Prevention of bladder tumours after nephroureterectomy for primary upper urinary tract urothelial carcinoma: A prospective, multicentre, randomised clinical trial of a single postoperative intravesical dose of mitomycin C (the ODMIT-C Trial). *Eur Urol* 2011; 60: 703–710.

36. Giannarini G et al. Antegrade perfusion with bacillus Calmette-Guérin in patients with non-muscle invasive urothelial carcinoma of the upper urinary tract: Who may benefit? *Eur Urol* 2011; 60: 955–960.

37. Hall MC et al. Prognostic factors, recurrence, and survival in transitional cell carcinoma of the upper urinary tract: A 30-year experience in 252 patients. *Urology* 1998; 52: 594–601.

38. Seisen T et al. A systematic review and meta-analyses of clinicopathologic factors linked to intravesical recurrence after radical nephroureterectomy to treat upper tract urothelial carcinoma. *Eur Urol* 2015; 67: 1122–1133.

39. Cosentino M et al. Upper urinary tract urothelial cell carcinoma: Location as a predictive factor for concomitant bladder carcinoma. *World J Urol* 2013; 31: 141–145.

40. Palou J et al. Multivariate analysis of clinical parameters of synchronous primary superficial bladder cancer and upper urinary tract tumor. *J Urol* 2005; 74: 859–861.

41. Leow JJ et al. A systematic review and meta-analysis of adjuvant chemotherapy and neoadjuvant chemotherapy for upper tract urothelial carcinoma. *Eur Urol* 2014; 66: 529–554.

FURTHER READING

European Association of Urology (EAU). http://uroweb.org/wp-content/uploads/EAU-Guidelines-on-Non-muscle-Invasive-BC_TaT1-2017.pdf

Lamm DL et al. Maintenance bacillus Calmette-Guérin immunotherapy for recurrent TA, T1 and carcinoma *in situ* transitional cell carcinoma of the bladder: A randomized Southwest Oncology Group Study. *J Urol* 2000; 163: 1124–1129.

Sylvester RJ et al. A single immediate postoperative instillation of chemotherapy decreases the risk of recurrence in patients with stage Ta T1 bladder cancer: A meta-analysis of published results of randomized clinical trials. *J Urol* 2004; 171: 2186–2190.

Sylvester RJ et al. Systematic review and individual patient data meta-analysis of randomized trials comparing a single immediate instillation of chemotherapy after transurethral resection with transurethral resection alone in patients with stage pTa-pT1 urothelial carcinoma of the bladder: Which patients benefit from the instillation? *Eur Urol* 2016; 69: 231–244.

CHAPTER 5
RENAL CANCER

Emma Bromwich, Ahmed Qteishat, Herman S Fernando and Dominic Hodgson

Contents

RENAL MASS PRESENTATION

Q. What does the computed tomography (CT) in Figure 5.1 show?

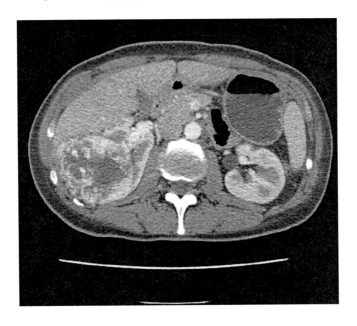

Figure 5.1

A. This is an axial post-contrast abdominal CT scan. There is a heterogeneous mass arising from the right kidney which is most likely to be a renal carcinoma. Ideally, I would like to review all the images which should include a triple-phase renal CT and a chest CT. I would look for the presence and the morphology of the contralateral kidney; assess the primary tumour, extra-renal spread, and venous, adrenal, liver and lymph node involvement.

With CT imaging, enhancement in renal masses is determined by comparing Hounsfield units (HUs) before and after contrast administration. A change of 15 or more HUs demonstrates enhancement – renal cancers demonstrate increased enhancement in comparison to normal renal parenchyma.

Q. How does renal cell cancer (RCC) present?
A. Over 50% of cases are found incidentally. The classic triad of flank pain, gross haematuria, and palpable abdominal mass is rare (6%–10%) and correlates with aggressive histology and advanced disease.

Paraneoplastic syndromes are found in approximately 30% of patients with symptomatic RCCs. Some symptomatic patients present with symptoms caused by metastatic disease, such as bone pain or a persistent cough.

Q. What are the risk factors for RCC?
A. Renal cell cancer represents 2%–3% of all cancers, with the highest incidence in Western countries. Smoking, obesity and hypertension have been strongly linked to the development of RCCs. Having a first-degree relative also increases the risk. Patients on dialysis (with their native kidneys *in situ*) are at a 3–6x increased risk. Heredity RCC accounts for 5%–8% of all cases. These include VHL syndrome, hereditary papillary renal carcinoma (HPRC), hereditary leiomyomatosis and papillary RCC (HLRCC), Birt–Hogg–Dubé syndrome and familial non-syndromic ccRCC.

Q. How would you assess a fit 55-year-old man presenting with a large renal mass on USS?
A. I would take a full medical history from him.

I would examine him for a palpable mass and for lymph nodes, a non-reducing varicocele (for left-sided renal tumours) and bilateral lower limb oedema, suggestive of venous involvement.

I would send blood samples to look for anaemia/polycythaemia, a raised ESR, abnormal liver function tests (Stauffer syndrome), and calcium and creatinine levels.

Q. What further imaging would you request?
A. A triple-phase renal CT and chest CT should be performed for initial staging unless the patient has a contrast allergy or is pregnant in which case a renal mass MRI protocol should be performed. If there is a history of renal impairment, then a non-contrast renal MRI (with diffusion) (with or without a contrast ultrasound if available) should be considered.

The EAU Guidelines recommend that split renal function should be estimated using DMSA scan in the following situations:

- When renal function is compromised (significantly decreased GFR)
- When knowledge of relative renal function is clinically important – e.g. in patients with multiple or bilateral tumours

In these situations referral to a nephrology unit prior to the surgery would be advisable due to the potential need for post-operative renal support (either in the immediate post-operative period or in the long term).

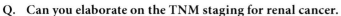

Q. Can you elaborate on the TNM staging for renal cancer.

A. The 2017 TNM staging for renal cancer is as shown in Table 5.1.

Table 5.1 The TNM classification system for renal cancer 2017

Tx	Primary tumour cannot be assessed
T0	No evidence of primary tumour
T1	Tumour <7 cm in greatest dimension, limited to the kidney
	T1a: Tumour ≤4 cm in greatest dimension, limited to the kidney
	T1b: Tumour >4 cm but ≤7 cm in greatest dimension
T2	Tumour >7 cm in greatest dimension, limited to the kidney
	T2a: Tumour >7 cm but ≤10 cm in greatest dimension
	T2b: Tumours >10 cm limited to the kidney
T3	Tumour extends into major veins or perinephric tissues but not into the ipsilateral adrenal gland and not beyond Gerota's fascia
	T3a: Tumour extends into the renal vein or its segmental branches, or tumour invades the pelvicalyceal system or tumour invades perirenal and/or renal sinus (peripelvic) fat but not beyond Gerota's fascia
	T3b: Tumour extends into the vena cava (VC) below the diaphragm.
	T3c: Tumour extends into vena cava above the diaphragm or invades the wall of the vena cava
T4	Tumour invades beyond Gerota's fascia (including contiguous extension into the ipsilateral adrenal gland)
Nx	Regional LNs cannot be assessed
N0	No regional LN metastasis
N1	Metastasis in regional LN
M0	No distant metastasis
M1	Distant metastasis

Q. What prognostic factors are there for RCC patients?

A. *Anatomical factors* – Are those of the TNM staging system.

Histological factors – High Fuhrman grade is associated with worsening prognosis. Clear cell tumours have a worse outcome than chromophobe which themselves have a poorer prognosis than papillary type. Sarcomatoid features, microvascular invasion, tumour necrosis and invasion of the collecting system all confer a poorer prognosis. Risk stratification of clear cell RCCs using the Leibovich (Mayo) scoring system takes into account a number of these histological features.

Clinical factors – Cachexia, a poor performance status, anaemia, and a low platelet count all are associated with greater risk. Numerous molecular markers such as carbonic anhydrase IX (CaIX), vascular endothelial growth factor (VEGF), hypoxia-inducible factor (HIF), Ki67 (proliferation), p53, PTEN (phosphatase and tensin homolog) (cell cycle), E-cadherin, C-reactive protein (CRP), osteopontin and CD44 (cell adhesion) [5,6] have been investigated. However, none of these markers has reliably improved the predictive accuracy of current prognostic systems and their use is not recommended in routine practice.

Q. What paraneoplastic syndromes are associated with RCC?

A. Paraneoplastic syndromes are found in 30% of patients with RCC. The kidney produces 1,25-dihydroxycholecalciferol, renin, erythropoietin and various prostaglandins, all of which can precipitate symptoms.

Hypercalcaemia secondary to the production of parathyroid-like peptides has been reported in 13% of cases. Osteolytic breakdown in metastatic disease may also play a role.

Hypertension secondary to renin production by the primary tumour is more common than polycythaemia due to erythropoietin production. Anaemia is seen in over 30% of patients.

Stauffer's syndrome is non-metastatic hepatic dysfunction in RCC patients, and is seen in approximately 5% of cases. Thrombocytopenia, neutropenia, fever, weight loss and discrete regions of hepatic necrosis are seen. Elevated serum levels of IL-6 and other cytokines may be implicated. Hepatic function will normalise in the majority of cases post-nephrectomy.

Systemic symptoms of cachexia, weight loss and pyrexia are recognised in 15%–30% of RCC patients.

Q. **This man has no significant history comorbidity. His renal function is normal and he has opted for surgery after a thorough discussion with yourself. He requires a laparoscopic radical nephrectomy. How would you consent him for this?**

A. I would review the imaging prior to consent to confirm the suspected pathology and operative side. I would introduce myself and check the patient's name and date of birth. I would then describe the procedure and explain that the intended benefit was to remove the kidney which is thought to contain cancer, but explain that there is a chance that the lesion may be benign.

I would describe and explain the potential complications of the procedure, including bleeding, wound infection, the potential need to convert to an open procedure, damage to adjacent organs, chest infection and the small chance of complications from the pneumo-peritoneum (namely impaired venous return and gas embolism, leading to thrombosis or respiratory compromise).

I would state that follow-up is required and further therapy may be indicated. The patient would be told that he might have a catheter after the procedure and possibly a drain, and that the operation would take place under general anaesthetic. I would sign the consent form and ask the patient if he had any further questions. I would then ask him to read and sign the document.

Policies on marking patients differ between departments, but it is my practice to draw a cross with indelible ink on the side for surgery.

Q. **When would you perform an ipsilateral adrenalectomy concurrently with a radical nephrectomy (RN)?**

A. Current evidence suggests that ipsilateral adrenalectomy need only be performed in those patients in whom pre-operative imaging suggests adrenal involvement or in those in whom *intra-operatively* the tumour appears to involve the adrenal in contiguity.

Q. **Would you perform a concurrent lymph node dissection?**

A. I would not routinely perform a lymph node dissection with a radical nephrectomy as there is no improved cancer-specific or overall survival benefit. However, in patients with clinically enlarged lymph nodes, I may consider a lymph node dissection for staging purposes and/or local control.

Q. **The patient undergoes the surgery and has an uneventful post-op period. His histology is shown in Figure 5.2. What features are you interested in when the histopathologist presents the case at the MDT?**

A. I would aim to ascertain the following:

- The histological type of cancer
- The Fuhrman nuclear grade
- The presence of necrosis
- The involvement of nodes
- The pathological T stage

Tumour composed of clear cells and arranged in nests

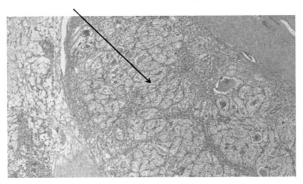

×20 magnification

Fuhrman nuclear grade 2 tumour cells have prominent nucleoli
(dot within nuclei) visible at ×400 magnification

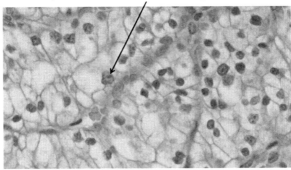

×400 magnification

Figure 5.2 H&E of clear cell renal cell carcinoma showing tumour composed of clear cells and arranged in nests. The higher magnification shows the tumour cells having prominent nucleoli. (Images courtesy of Dr Karthik Kalyanasundaram, Consultant Histopathologist, University Hospital of North Midlands NHS Trust, Stoke on Trent, UK.)

Q. **His histology is reported as clear cell carcinoma, Fuhrman grade 2, pT2a N0 with no evidence of tumour necrosis. Based on these factors, how would you risk stratify this patient and why do you need to do this?**

A. Risk stratification of these patients is necessary in order to aid in prediction of the patient's prognosis and to plan follow-up imaging. There are many risk stratification programmes and the one we use in our cancer network is the Leibovich (Mayo) scoring system (Table 5.2), which is used for clear cell renal cell carcinoma [1].

Table 5.2 The Leibovich (Mayo) score

Pathological T stage	0–4
Nodal status	0–2
Tumour size: <10 cm	0
Tumour size: >10 cm	1
Nuclear grade	0–3
Histological tumour necrosis	0–1

Source: Adapted from Leibovich BC et al. *Cancer* 2003; 97(7): 1663–1671.
Total scores vary from 0 to 11: Low risk = 0–2; Intermediate risk = 3–5;
High risk = 6 or more.

The metastasis-free survival at 10 years is approximately 90%, 60% and 25%, respectively for low-, intermediate- and high-risk disease (Figure 5.3).

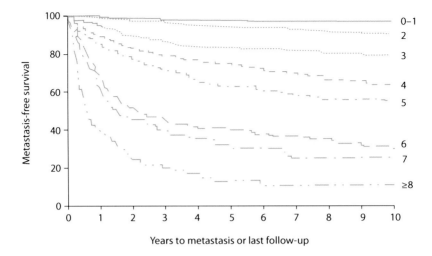

Figure 5.3 Metastasis-free survival from the time of surgery stratified by the Leibovich scoring system in patients with clear cell carcinoma. (Adapted from Leibovich BC et al. *Cancer* 2003; 97(7): 1663–1671.)

This man would therefore be in the intermediate-risk category. The EAU guidelines have proposed the following surveillance schedule based on the risk profile and I would follow this man up as per the intermediate-risk profile (Table 5.3). However, one must appreciate that local protocol for follow-up may vary and I would discuss this at my uro-oncology meeting.

Table 5.3 Proposed surveillance schedule following treatment for RCC, taking into account patient risk profile and treatment efficacy

Risk profile	Treatment	Surveillance						
		6 months	1 year	2 year	3 year	4 year	5 year	>5 years
Low	RN/PN only	US	CT	US	CT	US	CT	Discharge
Intermediate	RN/PN/cryo/RFA	CT	CT	US	CT	CT	CT	CT/2 years
High	RN/PN/cryo/RFA	CT	CT	CT	CT	CT	CT	CT/2 years

Source: Adapted from EAU guidelines 2017. https://uroweb.org/guideline/renal-cell-carcinoma/; Escudier B et al. *NEJM* 2007; 356: 125–134.

Cryo = cryotherapy; CT = CT scan of chest, abdomen and pelvis; PN = partial nephrectomy; RFA = radiofrequency ablation; RN = radical nephrectomy; US = ultrasound abdomen.

The purpose of follow-up after radical nephrectomy is to assess complications, renal function and monitor for local recurrence and metastases. The risk of local recurrence is rare (<5%), but early detection of these (and metastatic disease) increases the chance of these being surgically resectable. Additionally, if novel systemic treatments are to be used a lower tumour burden potentially increases their efficacy.

Individual follow-up protocols such as the Leibovich scoring system reflect the risk of recurrence. A low-risk patient would not necessarily need annual CT follow-up unless symptomatic, and ultrasound and chest x-ray should suffice. Intermediate- and high-risk patients will require chest, abdomen and pelvis CT imaging regularly. The benefits of an intense and prolonged follow-up needs to be balanced with the radiation exposure of the scans.

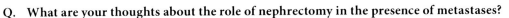

Q. What are your thoughts about the role of nephrectomy in the presence of metastases?

A. Based on data from prospective randomised trials, cytoreductive nephrectomy appears to significantly improve overall survival in patients with metastatic renal cancer treated with interferon immunotherapy, independent of patient performance status, the site of metastases and the presence of measurable disease. A European Organisation for Research and Treatment of Cancer (EORTC) study showed that median survival with interferon-a (IFN-a) and nephrectomy (18 months) was significantly better than that with IFN-α alone (11 months) [2]. The Southwest Oncology Group (SWOG) also reported that nephrectomy followed by interferon therapy resulted in significantly longer median survival among patients with metastatic renal-cell cancer than interferon therapy alone (11 months versus 8 months) [3]. Subsequently, a combined analysis of the SWOG and EORTC trials was published [4]. Data were available for 331 patients randomised to nephrectomy followed by interferon as opposed to interferon alone. The median survival rates were 13.6 and 7.8 months, respectively. This difference represented a 31% decrease in the risk of death ($p = .002$).

Thus in most patients with metastatic disease, cytoreductive nephrectomy is with a palliative intent and further systemic treatment is necessary. However, in very few patients with renal tumour and single or oligo-metastatic resectable disease, cytoreductive nephrectomy is considered curative if in addition all metastatic tumour deposits are also excised. In these cases, such surgery may improve survival and delay the need for systemic treatment.

MANAGEMENT OF SMALL RENAL MASSES

Q. A 70-year-old man is found to have a 2.5 cm exophytic right renal mass which is enhancing on CT imaging. He has normal renal function and wants to know his options. What would you advise him?

A. I would complete his staging and discuss his case in the uro-oncology MDT. I would see this patient in my clinic along with the cancer specialist nurse and review the images with him. His options are

1. Active surveillance of his small renal mass (SRM)
2. Surgery: partial nephrectomy or radical nephrectomy
3. Minimally invasive therapy: radiofrequency ablation or cryotherapy

Q. If the patient opts for active surveillance, how would you follow-up these patients in your practice?

A. Active surveillance of SRM can be defined as the initial monitoring of tumour characteristics by serial abdominal imaging with delayed intervention reserved for tumours showing clinical progression during follow-up. It has been shown that in the elderly and co-morbid patients with incidental SRM the cancer-specific mortality is low.

In Jewett's series of active surveillance, SRMs had low growth rate and the progression to metastatic disease was reported in a small number [5]. Lane reported no overall survival advantage in between the two treatments (AS and surgery) in patients more than 75 years after adjusting for other variables [6].

Therefore, short- and intermediate-term oncological outcomes indicate that in selected patients active surveillance is appropriate, and can be followed by treatment for progression if required.

Q. What is your opinion on the role of biopsy for SRMs?

A. The role of ultrasound or CT-guided percutaneous biopsies for T1a tumours has gained popularity over the past decade. This is mainly due to the increased detection of SRMs (<4 cm). A biopsy should be considered if there is

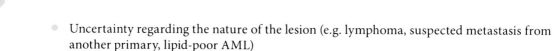

- Uncertainty regarding the nature of the lesion (e.g. lymphoma, suspected metastasis from another primary, lipid-poor AML)
- Prior to systemic therapy (i.e. for metastatic RCC)
- Prior to ablative therapy (radiofrequency ablation [RFA] or cryotherapy)
- Prior to tumour surveillance

Richard et al. have recently published their 13 years' experience on biopsies for SRMs and recommend that renal tumour biopsy (RTB) should be considered the initial step in the management of patients with radiographically indeterminate SRMs in whom a therapeutic approach is being considered. The first biopsy was diagnostic in 90% of cases and a repeat biopsy in 83% of non-diagnostic biopsies. When both were combined, RTBs yielded an overall diagnostic rate of 94%. Tumor size and exophytic location were significantly associated with biopsy outcome. RTB histology and nuclear grade were highly concordant with final pathology (more than 90%). Except for one, all adverse events (8.5%) were self-limiting [7].

In conclusion the current evidence points to the increasing use of renal tumour biopsies in indeterminate SRMs and I use this in my practice.

Q. **If the patient is now considering surgery which modality would you offer him and why?**
A. The EAU guidelines recommend that a partial nephrectomy should be offered to all patients with T1 tumours who do not have significant co-morbidity – hence I would offer this patient a partial nephrectomy (PN). This may be performed by either the open, laparoscopic or robotic-assisted technique.

Based on current available oncological and quality of life outcome studies, localised renal cancers are better managed by nephron-sparing surgery rather than radical nephrectomy (RN), irrespective of the surgical approach. The estimated 5-year cancer-specific survival (CSS) rates are comparable using these surgical techniques. In addition, PN was demonstrated to better preserve general kidney function, thereby lowering the risk of development of metabolic or cardiovascular disorders. However, the patient should be counselled that a PN is associated with a higher percentage of positive surgical margins (PSMs) (8%) compared to RN. This may increase the risk of disease recurrence with the subsequent need for further intervention (local or systemic).

Q. **What are the indications for nephron-sparing surgery?**
A. Absolute indications are bilateral synchronous RCC, and an anatomical or functionally solitary kidney.

Relative indications are unilateral RCC with a reduced or poorly functioning contralateral kidney, unilateral RCC in patients with comorbidity associated with potential renal impairment (diabetes, renovascular disease), and patients with an increased risk of a second renal malignancy (hereditary RCC such as von Hippel–Lindau [VHL] disease).

Elective indications include localised unilateral RCC with a normal contralateral kidney.

Q. **How would you consent a patient for laparoscopic partial nephrectomy?**
A. I would explain that the aim of the procedure is to remove cancer while at the same time preserving kidney function.

I would use the British Association of Urological Surgeons (BAUS) procedure specific consent form which explains the procedure, the risks, the benefits and the alternatives. The procedure-specific complications include the need to convert to open, conversion to a radical nephrectomy, need for a second procedure or vascular intervention in the post-op period to control bleeding and chance of a urine leak needing further intervention (ureteric stent insertion).

I would explain that the risk of local recurrence is about 8% and complications (including bleeding and urinary leakage) are greater than with radical nephrectomy (this is particularly so with larger tumours).

Q. How does the follow-up following partial nephrectomy differ from the radical nephrectomies?

A. It is interesting to note that EAU guidelines recommend similar follow-up of patients who had partial nephrectomy for tumours less than 4 cm to those who underwent radical nephrectomy. I would discuss the case in my uro-oncology MDT and follow-up these patients based on their risk and status of their surgical margins as per my local cancer network guidelines.

Q. Are you aware of any alternative therapeutic approaches to surgery?

A. I am aware that both cryoablation and RFA have been used to treat T1a tumours (<4 cm). Both cryoablation and RFA can be performed using either a percutaneous or laparoscopic-assisted approach. When comparing cryoablation versus RFA, there is no significant difference for overall survival (OS), CSS or recurrence-free survival (RFS). Other ablative techniques such as microwave ablation, laser ablation and high-intensity ultrasound ablation have been used but are considered experimental.

Q. How do ablative techniques compare to partial nephrectomy?

A. Comparative studies looking at cryoablation and RFA versus partial nephrectomy have shown mixed results. Some studies have shown a higher local tumour recurrence rate in the RFA group when compared to PN but no difference regarding the occurrence of distant metastasis. Others have reported the metastasis-free survival was superior after PN and cryoablation compared to RFA for cT1a patients. The EAU guidelines recommendation is to offer surveillance, RFA or cryoablation to elderly and/or co-morbid patients with SRMs. Surgery should therefore be offered to younger/fit patients.

VHL CASE PRESENTATION

Q. A 28-year-old man with a history of cerebellar surgery has an abdominal CT. What is the diagnosis (Figure 5.4a and b)?

(a)

(b)

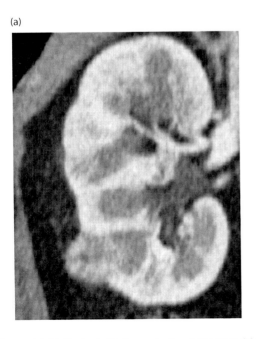 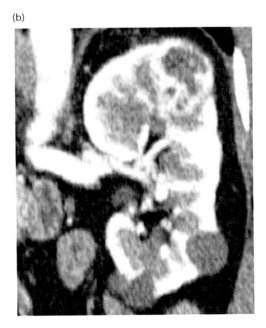

Figure 5.4 (a) Contrast CT demonstrating right kidney. (b) Contrast CT demonstrating left kidney.

A. There are multiple bilateral renal cysts with a malignant looking lesion in the upper pole of the left kidney and possibly the lateral aspect of the lower pole of the right kidney. Given this and the history of cerebellar surgery I suspect that he has von Hippel–Lindau disease.

Q. What is von Hippel–Lindau (VHL) disease?

A. This is an autosomal dominant disorder with an incidence of 1:36,000 live births which affects males and females equally. The average age of the patient at diagnosis is 26 years and is characterised by the development of various benign and malignant tumours and cysts. The VHL tumour suppressor gene is located on the short arm of chromosome 3 and the inactivation of this leads to the development of the disease. The major tumours and cysts are haemangioblastoma in the central nervous system, retinal haemangioblastoma, phaeochromocytoma, renal cell carcinoma, renal cysts, pancreatic neuro-endocrine tumours, and pancreatic and epididymal cystadenomas. Owing largely to the high incidence of ccRCC associated with VHL disease, the average life expectancy in affected individuals is 49 years with RCC being the leading cause of death. However, diligent surveillance enabling early treatment interventions can increase life expectancy.

Q. Explain how this leads to the development of renal (and other) carcinoma?

A. Inactivation of the VHL suppressor protein results in a subsequent loss of function of the VHL protein and the VBC complex. This complex normally targets transcription factors such as hypoxia-inducible factor (HIF-1α), resulting in their destruction. As such, in cells lacking VHL function, or in hypoxic conditions, HIF-1α accumulates, resulting in overexpression of many genes, in particular those related to angiogenesis, such as VEGF and platelet-derived growth factor (PDGF), as well as cell division, via transforming growth factor-α and PDGF. Importantly, the VHL gene has also been demonstrated to be inactivated in sporadic renal cell carcinomas.

Q. What new drug therapies are you aware of in VHL and renal cancer?

A. The VHL/HIF-1α growth factor pathway has become a major area for drug development targets.

Sunitinib is a tyrosine kinase inhibitor (TKI) that inhibits all three isoforms of the VEGF receptor. In a recent phase III trial, 750 patients, previously untreated, with metastatic renal cancer were randomised to Sunitinib or IFN-α. Sunitinib had significantly longer progression-free survival (11 months versus 5 months) and higher response rates (31% versus 6%) than those receiving IFN-α [8]. Pazopanib is an oral angiogenesis inhibitor and is comparable to Sunitinib in outcomes, but with better quality of life. Sorafenib is another TKI, which has been shown to prolong progression-free survival in patients with advanced renal cancer, in whom previous therapy has failed. This was demonstrated in a randomised phase III study, comparing Sorafenib to placebo [9]. Further high-quality studies have potentially shown the benefit of Temsirolimus and everolimus, mammalian target of rapamycin (mTOR) inhibitors [10,11], and Bevacizumab, a humanised monoclonal antibody to VEGF-A [12], as medical therapies in advanced renal cell cancer. Although, not a uniform policy, one approach to medical therapy is initially to stratify patients according to favourable, intermediate, and poor risk, depending upon whether they possess zero, one or two or more of the following risk factors: Karnofsky performance status $\leq$80%, anaemia, elevated serum calcium, absence of prior nephrectomy, and elevated lactate dehydrogenase [13]. Good and intermediate-risk patients should be initially treated with Sunitinib or Bevacizumab plus IFNα. Selected high-performance status patients with clear cell tumours can be considered for high-dose IL-2. Second-line therapy after progression could include Sorafenib, everolimus, or a different VEGF pathway inhibitor. Poor risk patients, especially those with non-clear-cell histology, should initially be considered for treatment with Temsirolimus. Importantly, with several ongoing clinical trials in progress, treatment options are likely to change.

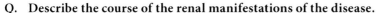

Q. Describe the course of the renal manifestations of the disease.

A. Typically RCC evolves in multiple sites in the kidney after 20 years of age. Kidneys usually develop a spectrum of small benign cysts through to large renal cell cancers. Smaller lesions are difficult to evaluate but a cut-off at 2–3 cm is thought to represent increasing risk of malignant transformation.

Q. Describe the management of RCC in VHL patients.

A. Initially urological management is in the form of surveillance with annual USS. Once cysts or lesions reach 2 cm, intensive CT/MRI follow-up, either 6 or 12 monthly depending on size and or number and growth rate of lesions will be required.

All management should aim to maintain nephrons and reduce the risk of metastasis. Cryo-ablation or radio-frequency ablation should be considered for treating smaller lesions (<3 cm). Once lesions are >3 cm partial nephrectomy may be more appropriate. For larger lesions nephrectomy is indicated.

Ultimately as the disease progresses the patient may need renal replacement therapy. The evidence for the role of transplantation and subsequent immuno-suppression in this population of patients is limited.

Q. Are you aware of any other hereditary disorders associated with RCC?

A. There are a number of other cancer susceptibility syndromes that are associated with an increased risk of renal cancer. These include the following:

- Hereditary papillary RCC (HPRCC) which is associated with papillary type 1 RCC and has an autosomal dominant transmission. Mutation of the C-MET proto-oncogene is encountered on chromosome 7. It usually has an early onset and presents with bilateral multifocal tumours.
- Hereditary leiomyomatosis and renal cell cancer (HLRCC) is a papillary type 2 RCC and is the most aggressive inherited RCC cancer syndrome. It is also known as Reed's syndrome and has an autosomal dominant transmission and is associated with a mutation of the fumarate hydratase (FH) gene on chromosome 1. Cutaneous leiomyomas and uterine fibroids are non-neoplastic findings. The mean age of diagnosis is 40 years and metastatic renal cancer can present in the teens.
- Birt–Hogg–Dubé (BHD) disease is also autosomal dominant and the BHD gene is identified on chromosome 17. It is characterised by the development of fibrofolliculomas (dysplastic hair follicles), lung cysts and spontaneous pneumothorax and renal cancer (papillary RCC, ccRCC, chromophobe, mixed and oncocytomas – even in the same kidney). The most common type of tumour is an unusual hybrid oncocytic tumour (mixed oncocytoma and chromophobe).
- Tuberous sclerosis complex is an autosomal dominant genetic disorder characterised by the formation of hamartomas in multiple organs including the brain, kidney, skin and lung. This leads to neurological disorders including epilepsy, mental retardation and autism as well as dermatological manifestations such as facial angiofibromas. Although the renal manifestations are mainly benign (AMLs and oncocytomas), renal cell cancer can occur in <5% of patients (chromophobe RCC).

BENIGN KIDNEY MASSES

Q. A 55-year-old presents with symptoms suggestive of biliary colic. A USS in addition to gallstones reveals a large right renal cyst. What would be the initial urological management of this patient?

A. After confirming normal renal function, I would arrange a pre- and post-contrast CT scan.

Q. What features are you looking for in relation to the renal cyst on the CT (Figure 5.5a and b)?

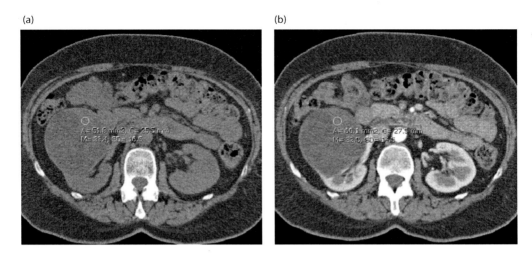

(a)   (b)

Figure 5.5 (a) Non-contrast axial CT abdomen. (b) Contrast axial CT abdomen.

A. The relevant radiological features include calcification, septations, irregular margins, solid elements and evidence of contrast enhancement. The classification is based on CT appearances and is used to determine the follow-up as well as to predict the risk for malignancy (Bosniak classification of renal cysts Table 5.4). The cyst shown does not enhance with contrast and is therefore a type II.

Table 5.4 Bosniak classification of renal cysts

Bosniak cyst type	Features	Follow-up
I	Simple benign cyst with a hairline-thin wall without septa, calcification, or solid components. Same density as water and does not enhance with contrast medium.	Benign
II	Benign cyst that may contain a few hairline-thin septa. Fine calcification may be present in the wall or septa. Uniformly high-attenuation lesions <3 cm in size, with sharp margins without enhancement.	Benign
IIF	These may contain more hairline-thin septa. Minimal enhancement of a hairline-thin septum or wall. Minimal thickening of the septa or wall. The cyst may contain calcification, which may be nodular and thick, with no contrast enhancement. No enhancing soft-tissue elements. This category also includes totally intrarenal, non-enhancing, high attenuation renal lesions >3 cm. Generally well-marginated.	Follow-up. Some are malignant.
III	These are indeterminate cystic masses with thickened irregular walls or septa with enhancement.	Surgery or active surveillance as around 50% are malignant
IV	Clearly malignant containing enhancing soft-tissue components.	Surgery. Most are malignant.

Q. What is the significance of contrast enhancement?

A. Enhancement suggests the presence of vascular tissue or communication with the collecting system. It is measured by the difference in Hounsfield units pre- and post-contrast and can point towards a malignant diagnosis (an approximate increase in enhancement of 15 or more Hounsfield units is considered significant).

Q. How does the Bosniak classification impact on clinical management?

A. Type I cysts are benign and require no follow-up. Type II cysts (as a group) require follow-up to look for change in size or development of new features as there is 10%–20% risk of malignant transformation. Surgical intervention should be considered for type III cysts as 40%–50% will be malignant. Greater than 90% of type IV cysts will be malignant and nephrectomy should be considered.

Q. What are type IIF renal cysts?

A. Type IIF cysts have an increased number of hairline-thin septae with possible minimal thickening of the septae or wall. There is no contrast enhancement or enhancing soft tissue elements. These definitely need close follow-up as they have a greater malignant potential than conventional type II cysts.

Q. What differential diagnosis would you consider for cystic renal lesions?

A. Simple renal cysts, renal cell carcinoma, autosomal dominant polycystic kidney disease, multicystic dysplastic kidney, multilocular cyst and VHL syndrome.

Q. What is the difference between autosomal dominant polycystic kidney disease, autosomal recessive polycystic kidney disease and acquired renal cystic disease?

A. Autosomal dominant polycystic kidney disease (ADPKD) is an inherited condition, with an incidence of 1:200–1:1000, leading to development of multiple, expanding renal parenchymal cysts, 95% of which are bilateral, with symptoms presenting in the fourth decade leading to end-stage renal failure. ADPKD is responsible for 5%–10% of all cases of end-stage renal failure. Diagnosis is normally on USS as an incidental finding or with investigations for haematuria, flank pain or an abdominal mass. Treatment is expectant with blood pressure control a priority.

Autosomal recessive polycystic kidney disease is distinct from ADPKD presenting in childhood, and has an incidence of 1:10,000–1:40,000. Diagnosis is often made *in utero* with the development of bilateral enlargement of renal parenchyma which is replaced by radially orientated cysts. Oligohydramnios may occur and, if severe, termination is often considered in the second trimester.

Neonates have a typical Potter's facies and a palpable mass. There is associated biliary dysgenesis leading to hepatic fibrosis. Management is supportive including good blood pressure control, dialysis and consideration of transplantation. Prognosis however, is poor particularly if pulmonary hypoplasia present. If not, with renal replacement therapy approximately half will survive childhood.

Acquired renal cystic disease (ARCD) was first described in the 1970s in patients with renal failure. It is now recognised as a feature of end-stage renal disease (ESRD) rather than a response to treatment. Uraemic toxins are implicated and cyst regression after transplantation and recurrence after transplant failure are seen.

Patients may suffer pain and haematuria which can require embolisation. A spectrum of renal adenoma to carcinoma is seen with a 3 cm cut-off usually considered for a malignant diagnosis. Most RCCs that develop in ESRD are associated with ARCD. Compared with the general population, RCC occurs on average 5 years earlier, has a 7:1 male predominance and is three to six times more common.

Q. How might a multicystic dysplastic kidney present?

A. Unilateral multicystic dysplastic kidney has an incidence of 1:2500–1:4000 and presents as an incidental finding or as an irregular flank mass. Bilateral disease is lethal with an incidence of 1:25,000. Where inherited, it is an autosomal dominant disorder, although sporadic cases are more common.

Pathologically, an irregular collection of tense non-communicating cysts lined with cuboidal or flattened tubular epithelium and dysplastic renal parenchyma is seen. There is proximal ureteric atresia secondary to ureteric bud and metanephric mesenchymal defects.

Most unilateral cases are undetected at birth, and involution commonly occurs in early childhood which may account for the recognised association with renal agenesis. And 5%–10% have a contralateral pelvi-ureteric junction obstruction (PUJO) and more still contralateral reflux.

Management is expectant. Rarely nephrectomy will be performed for uncontrolled hypertension. There is a fourfold increased risk of malignancy (Wilm's tumour). However prophylactic nephrectomy is not recommended.

Q. What do you understand by the term *multilocular cyst* or cystic nephroma?

A. This is a spectrum of multilocular cysts seen in children and adults varying from a benign multilocular cyst, to a cystic Wilm's tumour or cystic renal cell carcinoma.

Multilocular cysts tend to be bulky with thick capsules containing highly echogenic septae with loculi sometimes containing debris suggesting solid elements. Aspiration yields clear to yellow fluid.

Distribution is bimodal, with 2:1 male:female predominance under 4 years, and 8:1 female predominance above 30 years. Children present with an asymptomatic flank mass, adults with abdominal pain or haematuria.

Surgery is the treatment of choice in both children and adults. Nephron-sparing surgery should be considered.

Q. A 43-year-old female presented acutely to the accident and emergency with loin pain. She was clinically stable. An initial USS demonstrated a 4 cm, well-circumscribed, hyperechoic lesion in the cortex with posterior acoustic shadowing in the right kidney. How would you manage this patient?

A. I would arrange a pre- and post-contrast CT scan.

Q. CT reveals a fatty lesion of less than 10 Hounsfield units in the upper pole of the right kidney. What is the diagnosis and is this lesion associated with any inherited conditions?

A. The diagnosis is an angiomyolipoma (AML). 80% of AML are sporadic with 4:1 female predominance. These typically present in middle age, 80% are right sided with a recognised growth rate of 5% per year. The remainder are associated with tuberous sclerosis (TS) which has a 2:1 female predominance. These tumours tend to be smaller, bilateral and multicentric with a mean age of presentation at 30 years and a growth rate of 20% per year. TS is an autosomal dominant disorder characterised by mental retardation, epilepsy and adenoma sebaceum. There is incomplete penetrance and half of patients with TS develop AMLs.

Q. The pain settles and the patient has a normal contralateral kidney and no significant co-morbidity. What would your management plan be?

A. Four centimeters is usually recognised as a cut-off at which point an AML is more likely to become symptomatic (though this is currently being debated with some centres using 3 cm as a cut-off). For most AMLs, active surveillance is considered as the first option. If the AML is more than 4 cm and/or the patient is symptomatic at diagnosis then delaying intervention increases the risk of spontaneous bleeding. Women of child-bearing age, lipid-poor AMLs with significant vascularity or solid components are also at increased risk of spontaneous haemorrhage. Selective embolisation is usually considered as the first line of intervention especially in the acute setting. This woman's treatment options are selective arterial embolisation (given the non-incidental presentation) or close radiological surveillance.

Significant increase in size or further haemorrhage would indicate the need for intervention during follow-up. The volume of AML can be reduced by the mTOR inhibitor everolimus, which is usually reserved for AMLs >3 cm not requiring surgical intervention (EAU 2017 guidelines). Depending on the size and the centre's experience RFA or cryotherapy are also options. Alternatively, nephron-sparing surgery dependent on the location of the tumour or otherwise a nephrectomy should be considered in high-risk patients with large AMLs.

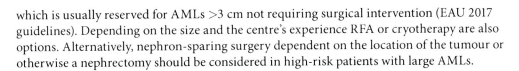
Q. What is Wunderlich syndrome?

A. Wunderlich syndrome (WS) is a rare condition characterised by a non-traumatic spontaneous acute renal haemorrhage into the subcapsular and perirenal space. It is characterised by Lenk's triad: acute abdominal pain, mainly in the flank, palpable mass and hypovoleamic shock. Renal angiomyolipoma (AML) is the most prevalent cause, however malignant renal neoplasm, vascular disorders (vasculitis, arteriosclerosis, rupture of a renal artery aneurysm), kidney infection, anticoagulant therapy and undiagnosed blood dyscrasia must be ruled out. Treatment depends on the clinical state of the patient, the degree of rupture of the kidney and the size of the retroperitoneal bleeding. If the patient is responsive to resuscitation and the haemorrhage is self-contained, a conservative approach may be adapted with/without arteriography and embolisation, otherwise the patient may require an emergency nephrectomy – if clinically indicated.

Q. What is an oncocytoma?

A. It is the most common benign solid renal tumour, representing approximately 5% of all primary renal neoplasms with a 2:1 male-to-female predominance. It affects mainly elderly patients often in the seventh decade of life.

Q. How do they present?

A. They are commonly asymptomatic and are discovered incidentally by imaging, but up to one-third of patients have signs and/or symptoms and can present with flank/abdominal pain, haematuria and/or a flank mass.

Q. Describe the clinical, radiological and pathological differences between an oncocytoma and a renal cell cancer.

A. Clinically it is not possible to differentiate between an oncocytoma and a renal cell cancer. The age of presentation and male predominance are the same for the two conditions.

Radiologically it can be impossible to differentiate the two but a central stellate scar commonly seen on CT and MRI scan and a spoke-wheel pattern of feeding arteries on angiography/magnetic resonance angiography (MRA) can suggest an oncocytoma, but this may also be seen in cases of RCC as central necrosis may mimic this scar.

Macroscopically oncocytomas are well-circumscribed, homogenous, tan-coloured lesions. Microscopically uniform eosinophilic cells are seen packed with mitochondria originating from the intercalated cells of the collecting ducts while RCC originates from the proximal tubules. Calcifications, necrosis and haemorrhage are rare with oncocytomas. Malignant features such as invasion or infiltration into the perinephric fat, collecting system or vessels are absent as is regional lymphadenopathy and metastases.

Cytogenetically loss of the first and Y chromosomes, rearrangements of 11q13, loss of hetero-zygosity on chromosome 14q are seen. Rarely are chromosome 3 abnormalities seen. These genetic alterations are characteristic and distinct from RCC subtypes.

Absolute confirmation of the diagnosis of oncocytoma is histological, therefore nephron-sparing surgery or radical nephrectomy are indicated in most cases. Once histological diagnosis is confirmed, oncocytomas do not require follow-up due to their benign nature.

Q. Describe the role for renal biopsy in the management of oncocytoma?

A. A renal biopsy is unreliable in accurately diagnosing an oncocytoma and this is best achieved by surgical excision. (It is difficult to distinguish between oncocytoma and an eosinophilic variant of chromophobe RCC on biopsy, and there is also a recognised coexistence of RCC and oncocytoma within the same lesion and at other locations within the kidney.)

Q. Describe two inherited or familial conditions associated with oncocytomas?

A. Birt–Hogg–Dubé syndrome is an autosomal dominant, inherited condition due to a mutation on chromosome 17. Features include fibrofolliculomas (neoplastic proliferation of the fibrous sheath of the hair follicle), pulmonary cysts, colonic lesions, oncocytomas and rarely malignant renal lesions.

Familial renal oncocytomatosis is a rare condition and has been described with multi-centric, bilateral tumours, with an early age of onset seen, although the genetic basis for the condition is unknown. Histological features include renal oncocytoma, hybrid oncocytic tumour and occasionally chromophobe RCC.

REFERENCES

1. Leibovich BC et al. Prediction of progression after radical nephrectomy for patients with clear cell renal cell carcinoma: A stratification tool for prospective clinical trials. *Cancer* 2003; 97(7): 1663–1671.
2. Mickisch GH et al. for the European Organisation for Research and Treatment of Cancer (EORTC) Genitourinary Group. Radical nephrectomy plus interferon-alfa-based immunotherapy compared with interferon-alfa alone in metastatic renal-cell carcinoma: A randomised trial. *Lancet* 2001; 358: 966–970.
3. Flanigan RC et al. Nephrectomy followed by interferon alfa-2b compared with interferon alfa-2b alone for metastatic renal-cell cancer. *NEJM* 2001; 345: 1655–1659.
4. Flanigan RC et al. Cytoreductive nephrectomy in patients with metastatic renal cancer: A combined analysis. *J Urol* 2004; 171: 1071–1076.
5. Jewett MA, Mattar K, Basiuk J et al. Active surveillance of small renal masses: Progression patterns of early stage kidney cancer. *Eur Urol* 2011; 60(1): 39–44.
6. Lane BR et al. Active treatment of localized renal tumors may not impact overall survival in patients aged 75 years or older. *Cancer* 2010; 116(13): 3119–3126.
7. Richard PO et al. Renal tumor biopsy for small renal masses: A single-center 13-year experience. *Eur Urol* 2015; 68(6): 1007–1013.
8. Motzer RJ et al. Sunitinib versus interferon alfa in metastatic renal-cell carcinoma. *NEJM* 2007; 356: 115–124.
9. Escudier B et al. Sorafenib in advanced clear-cell renal-cell carcinoma. *NEJM* 2007; 356: 125–134.
10. Hudes G et al. Temsirolimus, interferon alfa, or both for advanced renal-cell carcinoma. *NEJM* 2007; 356: 2271–2281.
11. Motzer RJ et al. Efficacy of everolimus in advanced renal-cell carcinoma: A double-blind, randomised, placebo-controlled phase III trial. *Lancet* 2008; 372: 449–456.
12. Escudier B et al. Bevacizumab plus interferon alfa-2a for treatment of metastatic renal-cell carcinoma: A randomised, double-blind phase III trial. *Lancet* 2007; 370: 2103–2111.
13. Motzer RJ et al. Survival and prognostic stratification of 670 patients with advanced renal-cell carcinoma. *J Clin Oncol* 1999; 17: 2530–2540.

FURTHER READING

EAU guidelines 2017. https://uroweb.org/guideline/renal-cell-carcinoma/.
Wein AJ et al. (eds). *Campbell-Walsh Urology*, 11th edn. Philadelphia, PA: Elsevier; 2016.

CHAPTER 6
PAEDIATRIC UROLOGY

Aruna Abhyankar and Arash K Taghizadeh

Contents

FORESKIN – PHIMOSIS AND CIRCUMCISION

Q. **A 5-year-old patient is referred by the GP who is concerned that the boy's foreskin does not yet retract and that the boy may require circumcision. What is phimosis?**

A. Phimosis is the inability to retract the prepuce. It is derived from the Greek word for 'muzzle.' It may be pathological or physiological. The term does not indicate whether the condition is pathological or physiological and so when it is used it is helpful to qualify which applies.

Q. **Why is it not possible to retract the prepuce in a physiological non-retractile foreskin?**

A. The preputial opening is too narrow and there are adhesions between the prepuce and the glans, i.e. the epithelial lining of the inner preputial layer is fused with the epithelium covering the glans penis. Epithelial desquamation, spontaneous erections and penile growth eventually lead to the separation of these two layers of skin.

Q. What is the cause of a pathological phimosis?

A. Balanitis xerotica obliterans or BXO (also known as lichen sclerosis et atrophicus). It is a chronic skin condition with some evidence suggesting an autoimmune aetiology. BXO is rare in children, affecting less than 1% of boys (more commonly seen in middle-aged men). The process can affect the glans, foreskin, external urethral meatus and occasionally the urethra. This may result in phimosis, difficulty voiding and even very rarely retention. Examination often reveals a thickened, scarred, fissured prepuce with pale white patches and with no pouting/flowering upon retraction.

It has been suggested *controversially* that BXO may have a later association with the development of penile cancer in adults, at least 17 years after initial presentation.

Q. How is a physiological non-retractile prepuce distinguished from a pathological phimosis?

A. In a physiological phimosis, when an attempt is made to retract the foreskin by gently pulling it back, the inner mucosa of the foreskin pouts through the preputial opening, looking a little like a carnation flower (Figure 6.1). When a similar attempt is made in BXO, the pouting does not occur; instead a scarred white ring appears around the preputial opening.

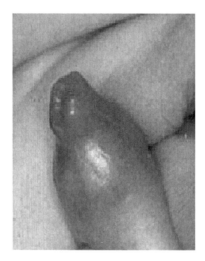

Figure 6.1 Physiological phimosis demonstrating 'flowering' of prepuce on retraction.

Q. How should pathological phimosis be managed?

A. Circumcision.

Q. How commonly are boys circumcised in the United Kingdom? How has this changed in the last 60 years?

A. About 5.6% of boys are currently circumcised in the United Kingdom [1]. In 1949 Gairdner [2] estimated a national incidence of 20%. The more startling fact from this paper was that between 1942 and 1947 about 16 boys a year were dying as a result of complications of circumcision.

Q. What is the natural history of physiological non-retractile foreskin?

A. Øster made 9,545 serial observations on the state of the prepuce in 1968 Danish schoolboys from 1957 until 1965 [3]. Phimosis was present in 8% of 6- to 7-year-olds, 6% of 10- to 11-year-olds and 1% of 16- to 17-year-olds. Preputial adhesions were even more common affecting 63% of 6- to 7-year-olds, 48% of 10- to 11-year-olds and 3% of 16- to 17-year-olds. The message from his paper is that a non-retractile foreskin is a common observation in boys, and will usually correct itself.

Physiological phimosis can safely be managed conservatively with parental reassurance and advice on bathing and maintaining proper foreskin hygiene.

Q. The boy's parents report that the foreskin 'balloons' when he voids. Should they be concerned?

A. Ballooning of the foreskin is very common and in itself, not a cause for concern. However, it is worth being alert to the unusual possibility of buried penis megaprepuce. In this condition the parent will report that urine collects in the foreskin and that squeezing the foreskin then 'milks' urine out. When the penis is examined in a boy with buried penis megaprepuce, the outer preputial skin seems to meet directly with the abdominal wall skin dorsally, and the scrotum ventrally; the penile shaft skin is deficient. Within the prepuce there are copious folds of inner preputial skin. A standard circumcision is to be avoided in these boys. Surgical correction involves removing the inner preputial skin and excising the fibrotic tissue associated with it, and then re-applying the outer preputial skin to the shaft as a substitute for the penile shaft skin.

Q. The boy's mother is worried; a family friend the same age as him has had balanoposthitis. What is this?

A. This is an acute condition characterised by redness and swelling of the foreskin, and associated with purulent discharge from the preputial opening. It is often associated with painful voiding. It may be related to separation of preputial adhesions. Frequently *Escherichia coli* or *Proteus vulgaris* may be grown, although culture often proves sterile in up to 30%. It is reasonable to treat these boys with analgesics and antibiotics. The condition is common. Because it is self-limiting it is not usually an indication for circumcision. However, if the episodes of balanoposthitis are recurrent, frequent and very bothersome, a circumcision may be warranted.

Q. Are there other clinical indications for circumcision?

A. The most common medical indications for circumcision are for BXO and recurrent balanoposthitis. Circumcision may also be performed to reduce the boy's risk of urinary tract infection (UTI). However, the evidence for this is based on observational studies, which suggest that in otherwise healthy males, 111 boys would have to be circumcised to prevent one UTI. The numbers needed to treat improve to 11 in those with recurrent UTI and 4 in high-grade vesico-ureteric reflux (VUR). Although circumcision may be justified in these last two groups, it would have to be part of a broader treatment plan to manage these conditions.

Q. What are the important steps in performing a circumcision?

A. In a suitably prepared and anesthetised child, lying supine on the operating table,

- Retract the foreskin. This may require stretching of the preputial opening or a dorsal slit. This allows inspection of the urethral meatus, so that its appearance can be documented as normal (e.g. no evidence of hypospadias).
- Preputial adhesions are completely separated.
- The prepuce is excised.
- Haemostasis is achieved with a bipolar diathermy or absorbable ties.
- The skin is closed with sutures.

Q. What risk specific to the operation should the parent be warned about?

A. The incidence of post-operative complications following circumcision varies between 0.034% and 7.4%.

- Infection requiring antibiotics (2%)
- Post-operative bleeding requiring return to theatre (1%–2%)
- Dissatisfaction with cosmetic result (4%)
- Meatal stenosis (reported at rates between 0% and 11%)

Other less common complications include inclusion cysts, abnormal rotation or chordee of the penis and very rarely formation of urethra-cutaneous fistula and partial penile amputation.

If circumcision is performed for BXO, the parents should be warned about the future small possibility of BXO affecting the glans, external meatus and/or urethra.

Q.   Are there alternatives to circumcision?

A.   In patients in whom the foreskin is slow to release, a short course of topical steroid such as 0.1% triamcinolone or betamethasone valerate 0.1% (Betnovate) twice daily for 6–8 weeks has been shown to accelerate the release of a physiological phimosis in up to 70%–80% of boys. The use of topical steroids has been shown to have no significant side effects or systemic toxicity.

Preputioplasty is where a longitudinal preputial incision is closed transversely in order to widen the preputial opening. It is ineffective in BXO and requires a motivated patient who will practice regular retraction of the foreskin post-operatively.

Q.   What are the contraindications to circumcision?

A.   A child with hypospadias should avoid circumcision as the prepuce if often used in future surgical reconstruction. Buried penis is another contraindication. The procedure should be avoided in those with an acute local infection. Other contraindications would include children with co-existing pathology in whom it would be unsafe to perform such an operation (e.g. coagulopathy). However, where medical conditions co-exist it would be prudent to carefully consider parents' request for a cultural circumcision; the child may be at higher risk if the parents press ahead with a circumcision in a more uncontrolled situation with a circumcision in the community.

Hypospadias

Q.   You are asked to see a 6-month-old boy with hypospadias. What are the features of hypospadias?

A.   Features include a ventrally situated urethral meatus, a hooded foreskin and ventral curvature, or chordee.

Q.   How might you categorise its severity?

A.   Typically hypospadias is described in terms of the situation of the urethral meatus: a distal hypospadias would have a meatus situated on the glans or at the corona; a moderate hypospadias would have a meatus on the distal or mid-penile shaft; a proximal hypospadias would have a meatus sited on the proximal penile shaft, scrotum or perineum. This, however, provides a very limited characterisation of the abnormality and does not necessarily define which patients need which operation. The underlying problem in hypospadias is a failure of normal development of the ventral aspect of the penis. As well as a meatus that is too proximal, the urethral groove, extending from the meatus to the end of the glans may be flattened, and the urethra, glans and corpora may be hypoplastic to varying degrees.

Q.   Is it worthwhile to examine the testes at this age?

A.   Absent or impalpable testes raise the possibility of disorders of sexual differentiation, especially where both testes are impalpable. If there are impalpable testes (in conjunction with hypospadias) it may be worth checking the child's chromosomes (karyotype).

Q.   What are the principles of surgical repair?

A.   Correction of curvature, re-siting the urethral meatus and dealing with the hooded foreskin. There are a very large number of operations described for correction of hypospadias, and the ultimate choice of operation will depend on the surgeon's preference and expertise.

A hypospadias does not mandate a surgical correction. Thus surgical counselling ought to include no surgery/surgery at a later date/early surgical correction.

In a very distal hypospadias without any chordee, a modified circumcision with careful attention to the distal urethra or a foreskin reconstruction are alternative surgical options to the hypospadias repair which aims to achieve correction of the meatal position.

Correction of curvature is functionally probably the most important part of the operation; often it is because the ventral skin is short and is corrected with de-gloving and re-distribution of penile skin. In more severe cases it may be necessary to mobilise the urethra, excise ventral fibrotic tissue (confusingly also called chordee), or even perform a Nesbitt's procedure.

Re-siting the meatus will involve creating a new urethra running from the original site to the tip of the glans. If there is adequate tissue, the existing urethral plate is used in a tubularized incised plate (TIP) or Snodgrass hypospadias repair. In the Snodgrass repair a longitudinal incision is made in the urethral plate. If the ventral tissues are insufficient to tubularise, then a two-stage repair is done where a free graft of preputial skin is applied to the ventral surface of the penis, and tubularised at the second operation when the graft has become fully established. The new tubularised urethra is protected with a vascular flap placed over it, usually of the dartos layer.

The hooded foreskin may have been used as a source of dartos layer, or taken to be used as a free graft, or redistributed to help correct skin-level curvature. In these cases the remainder will be excised to give the penis a circumcised appearance. Some surgeons may offer to re-construct the foreskin to give the penis an un-circumcised appearance.

Most surgeons would manage their hypospadias repairs with catheter drainage and a dressing.

Q. At what age would you attempt repair?

A. Practice varies widely. My practice is to operate at about 1 year of age, which gives a balance between the size of the patient, anaesthetic risk and how easy it will be to manage his catheter and dressing, which become more difficult between the ages of 2 and 3 years.

Q. What are the potential long-term complications of hypospadias repair?

A. These relate to the neo-urethra, and for a single-stage hypospadias repair, approximately 10% will need re-operation for fistula, stenosis or dehiscence of the urethral repair.

DISORDERS OF SEXUAL DIFFERENTIATION

Q. You are asked to go to the neonatal ward where the staff are not able to elucidate whether a term newborn baby is a boy or a girl. What should be the broad principles in managing such a baby?

A. This is a stressful situation for everyone concerned. Despite enormous pressure from the family there should be no rush to assigning sex, which may need to be done in a specialist unit with an appropriate multidisciplinary team. This may involve tests which will require time. The Registry Office makes provision for this; this is one of the few situations where full registration of the child may be delayed. It is wise to advise the parents not to give their child a first name until the sex of rearing has been formally decided upon.

One of the most commonly presenting causes of disorders of sexual differentiation is congenital adrenal hyperplasia (CAH – resulting in virilization of external genitalia in girls). Deficiency of the enzyme 21-hydroxylase accounts for 90% of cases of CAH. In this condition two-thirds of children will be in a salt-losing state due to aldosterone deficiency – *this is a neonatal emergency*. Therefore one must immediately assess the state of hydration of the child and ensure the serum electrolytes are being checked (if in salt losing state, aggressive treatment with intravenous fluids, potassium-lowering agents, mineralocorticoid and glucocorticoid supplements will be necessary).

Examination of the baby requires an assessment of the genitals as well as looking for other abnormalities. This will include an assessment of whether gonads were palpable or present in the scrotum, the size and shape of the phallus, the appearance of the labia/scrotum and the number of openings present in the perineum.

Complex investigation includes 17-hydroxy progesterone levels, chromosomal analysis and pelvic imaging (initially pelvic ultrasound scan [USS]).

Ultimately, a child in whom there is ambiguity about the genitals will need management in a specialist centre with a full multidisciplinary team including paediatric urology, endocrinology and psychology teams.

Undescended testis

Q. **What is the embryological basis of testicular differentiation and descent?**

A. Until the sixth week the gonads remain undifferentiated. Between weeks 6 and 7, under the influence of the *SRY* gene, the testes differentiate.

Testicular descent follows and occurs in two phases:

1. The first is under the influence of Müllerian inhibiting substance occurring by 12 weeks, taking the testis down from the urogenital ridge to the internal inguinal opening.
2. The second phase occurs between weeks 25 and 30 and is under the influence of testosterone, taking the testis from the inguinal canal down to the scrotum.

Q. **Describe the stages of spermatogenesis.**

A. This begins with the neonatal gonocytes. Between the ages of 3 and 12 months they will give rise to adult dark spermatogonia. These then develop into adult pale spermatogonia. Meiosis I transform these into primary spermatocytes, then meiosis II into secondary spermatocytes. These progress to spermatids which then give rise to spermatozoa.

Q. **You see a newborn baby boy whose parents are concerned that he is missing a testis. Are there any aspects of the history that are helpful?**

A.

- Are there any risk factors for undescended testis? For example, prematurity, low birth weight, neuro-muscular disorders, family history (14% of boys with undescended testis have a family history) or hypospadias.
- Are there any concurrent medical conditions that may affect your potential decision to offer surgery?

Q. **What findings are helpful in examination?**

A. In addition to a full examination, looking at the baby's overall health and the existence of other abnormalities, the following should be specifically noted:

- Is the missing testis palpable? If so what is its location? Can it be brought down without pain or tension to the fundus of the scrotum? Answering these questions will distinguish between a retractile testis, an ectopic testis and an undescended testis.
- If the testis is impalpable: Is the contralateral testis normal or hypertrophic? Is the scrotum on the side of the missing testis hypoplastic? This gives a clue that an impalpable testis might not be present. An impalpable testis carries important surgical implications (discussed later).

Q. **How would you manage this particular boy?**

A. A large proportion of testes that are not in the scrotum at birth will continue to descend. However this will stop after a couple of months. By 3 months of age, testes that are going to descend spontaneously will have done so; those that remain high will not come down any further.

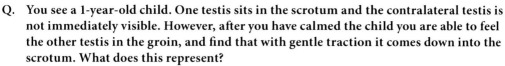

Q. You see a 1-year-old child. One testis sits in the scrotum and the contralateral testis is not immediately visible. However, after you have calmed the child you are able to feel the other testis in the groin, and find that with gentle traction it comes down into the scrotum. What does this represent?

A. This is a retractile testicle.

Q. What is the difference between a retractile and a gliding testis?

A. A retractile testis can be brought into the fundus of the scrotum, and when released, remains there. A gliding testis will only come down under tension, and/or the traction required to pull it down causes pain. A retractile testis does not require surgery; a gliding testis does.

Q. The parents are still worried about the retractile testis. What plan of management would you offer for their son?

A. The testis is retractile because of an active cremasteric reflex. This would be expected to settle with time. There is a possibility that a *small* proportion of retractile testes may become 'ascending testes' at a later age, i.e. develop a position that is higher than the scrotum (requiring surgery). It would make sense to keep the boy under review until the testis is no longer retractile, or declares itself as an ascended testis.

Q. The next 8-month-old boy you see in the clinic by coincidence has an inguinal testis on one side and a normal testis on the other side. The parents ask if this is a common problem.

A. In premature boys the incidence of undescended testes is up to 30% at birth.

In boys with a normal birth weight, the incidence of undescended testes at birth is about 3%–4%. The incidence is considerably higher in low birth weight babies. By the age of 3 months this figure has gone down to 1.5% with little change in this figure at 1 year. It is interesting, however, that the cumulative orchidopexy rate for boys is 3%.

(Note that in approximately 20% of boys the condition is bilateral.)

Q. Having assessed and examined this baby, how do you plan to manage him?

A. He has an undescended testis. Although some testes that are undescended at birth will continue to descend, it is unlikely that there is going to be very much more descent after the age of 3 months. You would be safe in deciding that this boy needed an orchidopexy.

Q. At what age would you perform this?

A. There is a possibility that orchidopexy may promote the transition of neonatal gonocytes to dark adult spermatogonia which should normally occur at 3–12 months of age. The British Association of Paediatric Urologists (BAPU) suggests that orchidopexy should ideally be performed at 3–6 months of age. However, early orchidopexy, with more delicate vas and testicular vessels is technically challenging; anaesthesia in younger infants is a more significant undertaking. BAPU state that orchidopexy at the age of 6–12 months is acceptable. There is no randomised control trial to verify true effect on fertility of the varied ages of orchidopexy.

Q. The parents do not like the idea of an operation. Why should undescended testes be corrected?

A. There are several reasons, as follows:

- To preserve fertility – Note that later paternity rates are 80%–90% if the patient has had unilateral inguinal orchidopexy (figure similar to that of the normal population) before the age of 2 years and 50% if the procedure was performed bilaterally. However, there is still some degree of subfertility in unilateral cases with 11% failing to achieve paternity within 1 year compared to only 5% of controls.
- Because of the increased risk of malignancy, which may be as high as 10 times the normal risk – Bringing the testis into the scrotum will most importantly allow the boy to perform

testicular self-examination when he becomes at risk after puberty. There is now some evidence to suggest that orchidopexy may reduce the risk of germ cell malignancy.

- Cosmesis.
- Undescended testes are at higher risk of torsion.
- Orchidopexy would abolish the small risk of hernia arising from a patent processus vaginalis that is often present.

Q. What are the main steps in inguinal orchidopexy?

A. In a suitably prepared and anesthetised child, lying supine on the operating table,

- Examine under anaesthesia to confirm the position of the testis.
- Make a skin crease incision.
- Open the external oblique to get access to the inguinal canal.
- Identify the testis.
- Divide the gubernaculum, taking care not to injure a vas that may be looping below the testes.
- Separate the lateral bands that may be fixing the testis close to the inguinal canal.
- The most important step is to carefully mobilise the vas and testicular vessels from the processus vaginalis.
- Once this is free, the processus may be transfixed and divided at the level of the internal inguinal ring.
- Mobilise vas and vessels to gain length.
- Create a dartos pouch in the scrotum and pass the testis into it without twisting the cord.
- Close the wounds.

Q. What are the risks of inguinal orchidopexy for undescended testes?

A. The risks are as follows:

- Bleeding, infection and wound complications
- Unable to bring down the testis to a satisfactory position
- Testis later ascends: this is iatrogenic ascent, where scar around the cord holds it at a fixed length, so that the testis is pulled up as the boy grows
- An approximately 5% risk of injury to the testicular vessels or vas (injury to the former results in testicular atrophy)

Q. You see a 15-month-old boy in clinic. He has a normal scrotal testis on one side. Despite your very best efforts in this co-operative infant, you are unable to palpate the other testis. What percentage of undescended testes are impalpable?

A. Approximately 20% of undescended testes are impalpable (therefore 80% are palpable). Of these 20% impalpable testes approximately 40% are intra-abdominal; in 30% the vas and vessels end blindly deep to the internal inguinal ring; in 20% the vas and vessels end blindly in the inguinal canal and 10% have a testis within the inguinal canal which was not palpated on examination (ideally this examination should be under anaesthesia in cases of impalpable testes – see later discussion).

Q. Will imaging help in locating the one impalpable testis in the child in the previous question?

A. It would seem helpful to use imaging to identify the positions of the testes before making any decisions. However, ultrasound has a significant false-negative rate, and magnetic resonance imaging (MRI) is likely to require a general anaesthetic. Radiology will not help decide whether this child needs an operation, and will not reliably help plan the operation. Thus, there is no value in organising any imaging and the patient should be taken to theatre for examination under anaesthesia +/− proceeding to inguinal orchidopexy/laparoscopy.

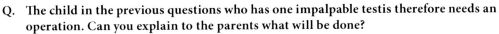

Q. The child in the previous questions who has one impalpable testis therefore needs an operation. Can you explain to the parents what will be done?

A. An impalpable testis requires that treatment decisions will have to be taken in the operating theatre. An examination under anaesthesia is performed. When the child is asleep and relaxed assessment can be easier and it may be possible to locate a previously impalpable testis in the groin.

If the testis is palpable in the groin, then inguinal orchidopexy is performed.

If the testis is impalpable under anaesthesia, then an immediate laparoscopy is performed to look for an intra-abdominal testis.

If an intra-abdominal testis is found, then a laparoscopic orchidopexy is performed. If the testis is close to the internal ring of the inguinal canal then it may be possible to do this as a single-stage procedure. However a higher testis will require the first stage of a two-stage Fowler-Stephens procedure. The testicular artery is divided, leaving the testis to survive on the artery of the vas (a branch of the inferior vesical artery). The second stage, performed 6 months later, is to mobilise the testis into the scrotum. This two-stage operation carries an approximately 20% risk of testicular loss.

If the vessels, and especially the vas, are blind ending or end in a poor nubbin of tissue a diagnosis of vanishing testes is made. The nubbin of tissue should be removed. A possible explanation for this phenomenon is prior testicular torsion. For this reason it is worth considering performing an orchidopexy on the contralateral testis to prevent that one undergoing torsion.

If the testis has been impalpable, but vas and vessels are seen entering the internal inguinal ring, the subsequent decision is controversial. Some would argue that if a testis is found then they usually do not contain germ cells, so they are not at risk of malignancy, and therefore nothing further needs to be done. One would have to be confident of examination findings, to be certain that an ectopic testis or an inguinal testis in a more chubby boy had not been missed.

HYDROCELE AND PATENT PROCESSUS VAGINALIS (PPV)

Q. A 9-month-old boy presents with unilateral scrotal swelling that is non-tender, fluctuant and trans-illuminable. What is the most likely diagnosis?

A. Hydrocele.

Q. What are the differential diagnoses and features of these conditions?

A.

- *Indirect inguinal hernia* – This is an inguino-scrotal swelling, which is usually reducible (with a gurgle sound). One cannot get above a hernia. A hernia, despite what some textbooks say, may trans-illuminate.
- *Hydrocele of the cord/encysted hydrocele* – This is fixed in the line of the cord. The testis is separate to it. Its origin relates to the processus vaginalis. It may be confused with a non-reducible hernia, but it is non-tender, and one can get above it.
- *Testicular tumour* – These are rare in infancy and so easily missed. They may be associated with a hydrocele. They cause a solid intra-testicular lump. It is therefore important to be able to palpate the underlying testis when a boy presents with an apparent hydrocele.

Q. What is the usual cause of a hydrocele in an infant?

A. A patent processus vaginalis.

Q. **How would you manage a hydrocele?**

A. Most will resolve by the age of 1 year and so require no surgery. If they persist as a problem beyond 2 years of age then they could be treated surgically. This would involve ligation and division of the processus vaginalis, similar to a herniotomy.

Acute scrotum

Q. **You are called to accident and emergency to assess a 2-year-old boy with acute scrotal swelling. When you examine him, you find redness and oedema of a hemi-scrotum, extending into his perineum and inguinal area. The testes are not tender. What is this likely to be?**

A. Idiopathic scrotal oedema.

Q. **How will you manage it?**

A. It is self-limiting. There is no association with any urinary pathology.
It can be treated with expectant observation and oral anti-inflammatory agents. Ampicillin is frequently prescribed as treatment despite there being no proven infective aetiology.

Q. **Accident and emergency are busy. They ask you to see a 12-year-old boy with a swollen painful left scrotum. On examination, there is a bluish tender lump at the upper pole of his testis. What might this be?**

A. This represents torsion of the hydatid of the testis. The hydatid sits at the upper pole of the testis, and when twisted and infarcted, can be seen as a bluish lump under the scrotal skin.

Q. **How should it be managed?**

A. If there is any doubt about the diagnosis, then the child should undergo a surgical exploration to exclude testicular torsion. Expectant or medical management of this condition is sometimes suggested (with analgesics and anti-inflammatory medication); however, it would be important that there is absolutely no doubt about the possibility of testicular torsion.

Q. **What are the indications for USS of an acutely painful scrotum?**

A. Ultrasound is of no value in acute scrotal pain of less than 48 hours duration. It will not reliably diagnose or exclude torsion. Doppler flows may be present despite the testicle undergoing venous infarction. Where the pain is of longer duration there may be value in obtaining a Doppler USS; it may help in distinguishing a necrotic testis from an infected one.

Mumps orchitis

Q. **A GP calls you for advice. One of his patients, a 6-year-old boy, has mumps. The child's mother has done a search on the Internet and is concerned that it may affect his testes. What advice could you offer?**

A. Mumps may be associated with orchitis. It is rare for mumps to affect the testes in *pre-pubertal* boys. In adolescents and adults, epididymo-orchitis may affect 15%–30% of patients who have mumps, in general following 4–8 days after their parotitis. Following mumps orchitis, a reduced testicular size is seen in up to half of post-pubertal patients, with abnormalities of semen analysis seen in about a quarter (may be a result of pressure necrosis). Sterility is rare. Effect on endocrine function has been difficult to establish.

URINARY INCONTINENCE

Q. Describe the broad categories for the causes of urinary incontinence in children.

A.

- Functional
- Structural
- Neurogenic

Q. What features would raise the possibility of neurogenic urinary incontinence?

A. Maternal diabetes during pregnancy, which is a risk factor for sacral agenesis

- A history of neurological disease, e.g. spina bifida
- Continuous urinary incontinence
- Straining to void
- Abnormal urinary stream
- Faecal incontinence or severe constipation
- Palpable bladder
- Spine or buttock abnormality, the latter suggesting sacral agenesis
- Neurological signs or limb abnormalities

Q. What features would raise concern about a structural cause for the urinary incontinence?

A. Antenatal history, e.g. of a duplex kidney

Straining or poor urinary stream suggesting bladder outflow obstruction, e.g. posterior urethral valve or meatal stenosis following circumcision

- Palpable bladder
- Labial adhesions
- Intra-labial mass such as ureterocele
- Bifid clitoris seen in female epispadias

Q. What are the causes of functional urinary incontinence?

A.

- Overactive bladder
- Dysfunctional voiding
- Voiding deferment
- Vaginal reflux
- Constipation
- Giggle incontinence

Q. What is dysfunctional voiding?

A. This describes a specific phenomenon where there is involuntary contraction of the pelvic floor during voiding. Surprisingly, storage symptoms predominate with frequency, urgency and incontinence. Diagnosis can be made with non-invasive bladder assessment (see later discussion). Treatment centres on teaching pelvic floor relaxation, often in the form of biofeedback.

Q. What is vaginal reflux?

A. Characteristically girls who experience this complain of leaking within 10 minutes of voiding and leaving the bathroom. The mechanism is of urine entering the vagina during voiding, and then subsequently dribbling out. It is effectively treated by getting the girl to abduct her legs widely during voiding to separate her labia.

Q. A 7-year-old girl is referred to you because she wets during the day and at night. What history would you ask about her wetting?

A. The history is the most important part of the evaluation of this girl and will set the basis of her management. It is important to establish the incidence, pattern and progression (if any) of the incontinence since birth and establish the type, e.g. urge/stress/continuous/giggle. Therefore, the following points should be clarified:

- *Primary or secondary?* Has she had these symptoms since birth (primary) or have they developed after being continent (secondary)?

  Therefore primary incontinence refers to the group in which there has never been a prolonged dry spell, whereas in secondary incontinence the child has previously been dry for at least 6 months. The former has a higher chance of a significant organic aetiology.

- *The pattern of the incontinence.* Is the incontinence associated with urgency? Is the incontinence continuous, which might be related to an ectopic ureter? In a girl, being wet shortly after voiding may indicate vaginal reflux. A specific entity is 'giggle incontinence' where the only provoking factor is laughing or giggling.

- *Severity of the symptoms.* How often does the wetting occur? When it does occur, how severe is it: does it just make her underwear damp, or is it so bad that she needs to change her clothes? Does she need pads?

Q. What risk factors for incontinence would you inquire about in this child?

A.

- *Voiding frequency.* How often does the child void? This is better evaluated with a frequency-volume chart. However, useful clues can be gleaned from what the child and her parents tell you. 'She often holds on until the last minute' is useful to know. Similarly the child will often give an idea of how often, if at all, she uses the school toilets during the school day. This gives information about urinary frequency or withholding behaviour (voiding postponement).

- *Voiding behaviour.* 'Curtseying' or sitting with the heel of the foot pushed into the perineum to control sudden episodes of urge may indicate detrusor overactivity. Straining to void and poor stream would indicate bladder outlet obstruction. This is perhaps more important in a boy where it may be a sign of meatal stenosis or more rarely posterior urethral valves.

- *Drinking habits.* Drinks containing additives and caffeine may be associated with voiding problems.

- *Constipation.* This requires asking about how frequently the child opens her bowels and whether she strains to pass hard stool. Again, correction of constipation will often improve urinary symptoms. Rarely the co-existence of poor bowel symptoms can be an indicator of a neuropathic aetiology.

- *Urinary tract infections.* These may be a cause for wetting. Episodes of cystitis-like symptoms are worth asking about. Positive urine cultures may be significant, although this information should be interpreted in the context of the child's symptoms at the time, and exactly how the urine was collected.

- *Age at potty training.* A very young age at potty training seems to be associated with later wetting.

- *Antenatal history.* Congenital urological pathology may have been detected but not followed up.

Q. What would you look for when you examine the child?

A.

- *Abdomen.* A palpable bladder or palpable stool would be significant.

- *Genitals.* A split or bifid clitoris may be the only finding in epispadias; a rare condition where the sphincter mechanism will be severely deficient. Perineal excoriation may give an indication of severe wetting or vaginal reflux. In boys who have been circumcised make sure there is no meatal stenosis.

- *Spine.* Inspect and palpate the spine looking for clues of spinal dysraphism such as pigmented or hairy lesions over the midline. Sacral agenesis is characterised by

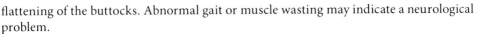

flattening of the buttocks. Abnormal gait or muscle wasting may indicate a neurological problem.

- *General health.* Has the child other medical conditions that may contribute to poor bladder control?

Check blood pressure and perform a urine dipstick at the end of the examination.

Q. The parents have very helpfully brought a frequency-volume chart with them. What instructions would you give to other parents so that they could fill out a frequency-volume chart?

A. Two convenient days are selected. On those days every time the child voids the urine is collected, and the volume and time of each void is recorded. Wetting episodes are also noted. Additional information that should be collected includes time, volume and type of fluid intake. A bladder diary is more exhaustive and would include information about fluid intake and even bowel movements.

Q. What are the things you look at when you interpret a frequency-volume chart?

A. This is most sensibly applied to children over the age of 5 years. According to the International Children's Continence Society normal voiding frequency is four to seven times per day (inclusive). The expected bladder capacity is calculated by adding one to the child's age and then multiplying by 30 to give an answer in millilitres; this formula is useful up to the age of 12 years. This is compared to the Maximum Voided Volume on the chart. The normal range is between 65% and 150% of the expected capacity. The 24-hour urine output can also be calculated in addition to total/type of fluid intake.

Q. Is there any value in a renal ultrasound scan?

A. This will give information about bladder capacity. A post-void residual of more than 20 mL on repeated measurement is significant. A thickened bladder with upper tract dilation may reflect a neuropathic bladder or bladder outflow obstruction. Renal abnormalities, such as a duplex kidney with an abnormal upper moiety may indicate the presence of an ectopic ureter.

Q. What are the general measures that can be taken to help a child with urinary incontinence?

A. This is sometimes called urotherapy. A large part of this is education of the child and parents. An explanation is given of normal bladder function and the cause of their child's incontinence. They are given information about regular voiding habits, normal voiding posture and lifestyle advice about fluid intake and the prevention of constipation. Progress can be monitored with frequency-volume charts and ideally support and encouragement is provided from regular follow-up.

Q. Would you proceed to urodynamics if the child has not responded to urotherapy?

A. Urodynamics are invasive and inappropriate this stage. A non-invasive bladder assessment with a clinical nurse specialist would be more appropriate. This is based on observation of storage and voiding behaviour especially flow rate, flow pattern and residual volume. An alarm can be used additionally to detect incontinence. Recently flow rates are being combined with electromyography (EMG) recordings from pelvic and abdominal floor muscles. This is done noninvasively using skin electrodes. This provides a rich source of information about abdominal wall and pelvic floor contraction during voiding.

Q. Are urodynamics ever performed in children?

A. Videocystometrogram (VCMG) is a test performed under very limited and specific circumstances; most of the required information will have been gathered by the evaluation described above. VCMG is most commonly performed if:

- It has not been possible to achieve a diagnosis by other means
- There has been no response to treatment
- There is a suspicion of a neuropathic bladder

The bladder line may be urethral or suprapubic. Placement of bladder and rectal lines is a significant undertaking and is likely to require sedation or even general anaesthesia.

Nocturnal enuresis

Q. **An 8-year-old boy attends the clinic with his mother. She is very concerned that he always wets the bed during the night. She thinks he is too old to be doing this. You have taken a careful history about continence similar to the one above. He has no daytime urinary symptoms. What is this condition called?**

A. Primary (it has always been present), mono-symptomatic (there are no other urinary symptoms, e.g. urgency) enuresis ('intermittent incontinence while sleeping').

Q. **What is the prevalence of this condition?**

A. Approximately 5%–10% of all 7-year-olds will have this condition. It is more common in boys than in girls and 2%–3% are still wet in their late teens.

Q. **If untreated what is the natural history?**

A. Untreated, 15% will get better every year, although the prognosis may not be so good for children whose symptoms are as severe as this.

Q. **Are there any explanations for the cause of mono-symptomatic nocturnal enuresis?**

A. The normal circadian reduction in urine output during sleep is diminished in at least two-thirds of children with this condition.

Impaired bladder function has been described in children with the moniker of mono-symptomatic nocturnal enuresis, with reduced functional bladder capacity, nocturnal and even daytime detrusor overactivity demonstrated in these children.

It is possible that these children have an abnormal arousal mechanism that prevents the sensation of a full bladder awakening them, as it would in other children. This fits with the observation of many parents of children with this problem who report that their children are very difficult to wake.

Q. **What management strategies could be offered?**

A.

- *Behavioural* – Establish a regular drinking and voiding pattern during the day. Reduce fluid intake in the evening, and void before going to bed. 'Lifting' is where the child is woken and taken to the bathroom, typically at the time his parents are going to bed.
- *Alarm* – An enuresis alarm in the bed is activated when the child wets. This method can often take up to a couple of months before an effect is seen. However, it is associated with the greatest long-term success, with benefit seen in up to two-thirds of children using it.
- *Pharmacology* – Desmopressin will produce results quickly, but these are not sustained once treatment is stopped. Anti-muscarinics may be added as an adjunct to desmopressin. Tricyclic antidepressants have been used to treat this condition but are more frequently associated with side effects.

ANTENATALLY DETECTED HYDRONEPHROSIS – ASSESSMENT

Q. **You are called by a neonatal doctor who is concerned that a newborn has antenatally diagnosed hydronephrosis. Is there useful antenatal history that they can provide you with?**

A. The antenatal history is very useful in giving clues about the possible diagnosis and severity of the condition. It will be well recorded in the mother's notes, which are usually not available when the child is subsequently seen in clinic. The quality of antenatal scans is very high so it would be a shame to lose sight of the information they provide.

Antenatal scans will give information on the kidneys as regards renal cysts, the presence and degree of hydronephrosis (objectively measured by the anterior-posterior [AP] diameter of the renal pelvis), cortical thinning, and echogenicity of the renal parenchyma. Dilated ureters should be noted. The bladder may be thick walled, fail to empty, or never be seen (a sign of bladder exstrophy). Seeing a penis on ultrasound will indicate that the foetus is male. In posterior urethral valves (PUVs) a dilated posterior urethra may be seen. Oligo- or anhydramnios suggests poor urine drainage and is an indicator of poor outcome.

In a newborn, an early USS may not represent the true status of the kidneys, and a follow-up USS ought to be performed in 1–2 weeks' time.

Whereas in a complex renal pathology, e.g. suspected valves, duplex kidney an early USS is helpful to plan further investigations.

Q. **The hydronephrosis affects only one kidney, and arrangements are made for the baby to be seen in your clinic at 6 weeks of age with an up-to-date ultrasound. It is often helpful to have as much of the imaging as possible organised before the child is seen. What would be your indications for a micturating cystourethrogram (MCUG) for this infant?**

A. It depends on what the USSs have suggested as the possible diagnosis:

- To look for VUR. The possibility of this is raised if dilated ureters have been seen on ultrasound. However, dilated ureters may also indicate vesico-ureteric junction (VUJ) obstruction or a mega-ureter.
- If there is a possibility of posterior urethral valves. This is suggested in a boy who has bilateral hydroureteronephrosis, a thick-walled or poorly emptying bladder, a visibly dilated posterior urethra or has had antenatal oligo- or anhydramnios. If the MCUG is being done to look for PUV it should be done postnatally before the child goes home.
- A ureterocele with duplex kidney. It is helpful to know whether this might be obstructing the bladder outlet (as may occur in a large prolapsing ureterocele), or whether there is co-existing vesicoureteric reflux before the ureterocele is treated.

Q. **The paediatric team have been very helpful. They bring you the ultrasound and MCUG images and wonder whether nuclear medicine or functional imaging would help before you see the child and the parents. They are more than happy to organise the test you request, but are not sure whether a dimercapto-succinic acid (^{99m}Tc DMSA) or mercapto-acetyltriglycine (^{99m}Tc MAG3) scan should be organised. How would you help them decide?**

A.

- The ^{99m}Tc MAG3 scan is a dynamic scan. It produces images like a video or cine film. The gamma radiation given off by the tracer can be quantitatively measured to give information like differential function, and washout curves. The images that are then provided to the clinician are similar to a series of still photos taken from the cine film. ^{99m}Tc MAG3 scans are most useful where there is a concern about upper tract obstruction, e.g. pelvi-ureteric junction (PUJ) obstruction or VUJ obstruction. The investigation also approximates differential function.
- A ^{99m}Tc DMSA scan is a static scan and produces only a 'still image'. However the detail and 'resolution' of the image of the kidney produced are much better than that of a ^{99m}Tc MAG3 scan. It will give a good measure of the differential function. It will also provide detail, for example showing cortical defects seen in acute pyelonephritis or with cortical scarring (^{99m}Tc DMSA sensitivity 90% and specificity 100% in detection of renal cortical scarring). It will give good detail in duplex kidneys showing the function of each moiety. A ^{99m}Tc DMSA scan is therefore most useful where detailed information is required about the kidney and there is no concern about obstruction, for example in VUR.

Note:

1. As regards the MAG3 and DMSA nuclear medicine scans, a radio-isotope is bound to both of these carriers. The radio-isotope most commonly used is metastable technetium-99 (^{99m}Tc), which is extracted from a molybdenum-99 generator. The half-life of ^{99m}Tc is 6 hours.

2. Approximately 90% of ^{99m}Tc MAG3 is excreted in the urine by tubular secretion and 10% by glomerular filtration. Furosemide is given to ensure that the kidneys are maximally diuresing. Classically it is given 20 minutes after isotope injection (F+20) or now more commonly 15 minutes before (F−15). The maximal effect of furosemide occurs approximately 18 minutes after injection and thus a F+20 renogram demonstrates obstruction late in the investigation and may give equivocal results in up to 15% of cases. For this reason the F−15 renogram results in maximal stress on the PUJ (in terms of urine flow) earlier in the study and reduces equivocal rates to about 7%. Therefore the F−15 renogram is the investigation of choice. In children it is more practical to give the furosemide at the same time as the isotope injection so the F+0 renogram is usually performed and is acceptable in the majority of cases.

There are three phases of a diuretic ^{99m}Tc MAG3 renogram:

- *Vascular phase (0–10 seconds)* – This reflects renal blood flow (get blush in kidney).
- *Extraction/parenchymal/uptake phase (10 seconds – 5 minutes)* – This reflects renal uptake or parenchymal function, i.e. renal parenchymal uptake and transit of radio-isotope.
- *Excretory phase (5 minutes onwards)* – This occurs with radio-isotope being excreted into the renal pelvis.

After injection of ^{99m}Tc MAG3, images are obtained approximately every 2 seconds for 60 seconds and then every 10–60 seconds for 20–30 minutes. Post-void images are also taken as a full bladder can affect drainage. In a child who is continent and co-operative, indirect ^{99m}Tc MAG3 cytography may be used in the diagnosis/follow-up of vesicoureteric reflux (thus avoiding a micturating cystogram, which is much more invasive and involves significantly more radiation exposure); however, the MAG3 study must be set up to look for reflux, and furosemide is not given.

The diuretic response is proportional to the renal function and thus one should avoid this investigation or interpret results with caution in those patients with a glomerular filtration rate (GFR) of <15 mL/min.

The glomeruli and renal tubules take 3 months to adequately mature after birth and thus isotope renograms should be avoided until this age.

One should be aware of and able to draw the diuresis renogram curves in the viva (sometimes known as 'O'Reilly's' curves, as he pioneered diuresis renography). These are shown in Figure 6.2 (for F+20 renography):

a. A type I curve shows normal renal uptake and drainage.

b. A type II curve demonstrates an obstructed pattern with no response to diuretic.

c.

  i. A type IIIa curve actually represents normal drainage (from a hypotonic renal pelvis). The curve rises initially but falls rapidly on injection of furosemide.

  ii. A type IIIb curve is equivocal and rises initially but neither falls rapidly nor continues to rise following injection of furosemide.

d. A type IV curve, which demonstrates Homsy's sign. The diuretic injection results in a transient response, which seems decompensated at higher urinary flow rates (within 15 minutes of furosemide injection). It is most likely to represent obstruction (although vesicoureteric reflux can result in a similar appearance), i.e. intermittent hydronephrosis. Performing F−15 renography eliminates Homsy's sign and will confirm obstruction in these cases.

3. ^{99m}Tc DMSA is extracted from the peritubular extracellular fluid and deposited in the tubular cells. Static images following the administration of ^{99m}Tc DMSA are obtained 3–4 hours after injection (e.g. planar posterior, left and right posterior oblique, coronal tomographic views).

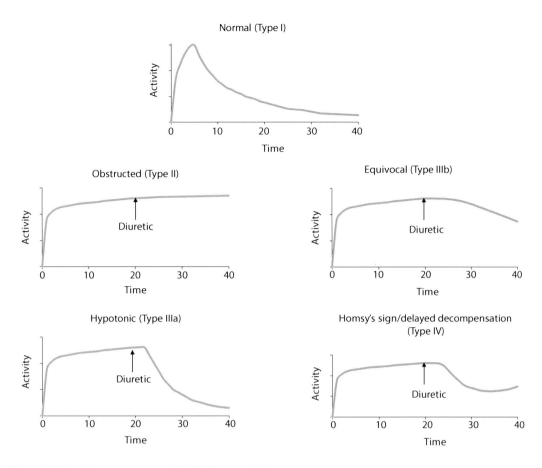

Figure 6.2 Diuresis renogram curves (for F+20 renography).

4. The nuclear medicine studies are usually conducted around 3 months of age, to allow as much renal maturation as possible, yet not delay surgery, but sooner in significant bilateral obstructive pathology, e.g. bilateral significant hydronephrosis suggestive of pelvi-ureteric junction obstruction (PUJO), they may well be conducted sooner to get baseline idea of function due to the need to plan surgery.

Posterior urethral valves

Q. **Concern has been raised from an antenatal scan that a child on the neonatal unit may have posterior urethral valves. The neonatal junior doctor has been reassured by a USS done on the first day of life that looks nearly normal. What is your view of this recent scan result?**

A. In the first few days of life the child is often a little dry, and coupled with immature renal function, urine output is reduced. This would tend to result in a reduction in the degree of hydronephrosis which could be falsely reassuring (the scan needs to be repeated after at least 1 week of age to obtain the correct diameter of the renal pelvis).

Q. **The baby's blood biochemistry has been checked on the first day of life. The neonatal doctors are anxious that the creatinine is elevated at 320 µmols/L. Why should they be worried?**

A. In the uterus the foetus has been dialysed across the placenta. The baby's initial blood chemistry on the first day of life will reflect the mother's blood chemistry. In this case the blood test has detected the mother's poor renal function. It will take a week or so before the baby's blood test reflects his or her own renal function.

Q. **You go and review the child. Antenatal history in this boy includes severe bilateral hydroureteronephrosis, and thickened bladder wall. He has been seen to pass urine only with a poor and dribbling stream. What diagnosis are you concerned about?**

A. The most likely cause is posterior urethral valves. Hydroureteronephrosis may be seen in VUR or VUJ obstruction. A thickened bladder wall may be seen with a neuropathic bladder, or other more rare causes of bladder outlet obstruction.

Q. **He is currently warm, well perfused and well hydrated. Outline the strategy for managing this child during this admission.**

A. Management of posterior urethral valves requires specialist paediatric urology and paediatric nephrology input. The principles are as follows:

Treat possible bladder outlet obstruction with catheter drainage. A 6 Fr feeding tube is suitable as a urethral catheter. Although a suprapubic catheter is sometimes advocated it should be appreciated that these can be difficult to insert into the small and thick-walled bladder that is seen in posterior urethral valves.

Look for and treat post-obstructive diuresis. This will require intravenous fluid and may require help from paediatric nephrologists. Fluid monitoring will include recording urine output, clinical examination, weighing the baby regularly and checking serum biochemistry.

Start prophylactic antibiotics (e.g. trimethoprim 2 mg/kg once a day).

Secure a diagnosis. Although renal tract USS is helpful, the diagnostic test is a MCUG. This should be covered with a short course of treatment dose antibiotics.

Post MCUG, if catheter has been removed, it needs reinsertion, awaiting the cystoscopy.

Resect the valves. Once the baby is stable and well and creatinine levels have reached a nadir value with catheter drainage, the urethral valves can be resected. This is done cystoscopically, under general anaesthesia. A 9.5 Fr resectoscope with a cold blade is a suitable instrument.

The management of any renal impairment should be optimised by paediatric nephrologists before the baby goes home.

Q. **Before he goes home, the medical student on your firm asks you to help him understand the boy's MCUG (Figure 6.3). How has the MCUG been done, and what features do the arrows point to?**

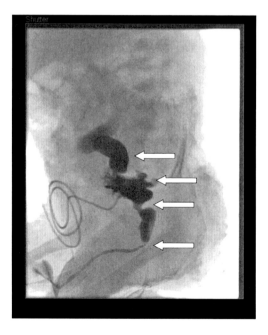

Figure 6.3 Micturating cystourethrogram (MCUG) in an infant with posterior urethral valves.

A. The MCUG (Figure 6.3) has been done by passing contrast down a supra-pubic catheter. From top to bottom, the arrows, respectively, point to:

- VUR into a very dilated ureter, but not entering the pelvicalyceal system on the image seen.
- A very trabeculated bladder.
- A hypertrophied bladder neck.
- The narrowed junction between the dilated posterior urethra, and the narrower anterior urethra. This is the site of the posterior urethral valves.

Q. What are the long-term outcomes for posterior urethral valves?

A. By 20 years of age half will have chronic renal disease, and a third will have end-stage renal disease. Bladder function is also frequently impaired. Potty training may be delayed, and up to half will have day and night incontinence at 5 years of age.

Q. What are the poor prognostic indicators for posterior urethral valves?

A. Rather intuitively, most factors which appear earlier correlate with a worse outcome.

- *Prenatal* – Earlier (<24 weeks) detection, oligohydramnios, high levels of B2 microglobulin (>13 mg/L) in the foetal urine
- *Postnatal* – Presentation under 1 month of age, bilateral VUR
  - *1 year of age* – High nadir creatinine, reduced GFR
  - *5 years of age* – Daytime incontinence and proteinuria
  - *10 years of age* – Urodynamics showing poor compliance or myogenic failure

PUJ OBSTRUCTION AND PYELOPLASTY

Q. In your clinic you see a 3-month-old infant. There was a severe unilateral hydronephrosis detected antenatally. The rest of the renal tract has appeared normal on all the antenatal and postnatal scans. What is the most likely cause of the hydronephrosis?

A. PUJ obstruction.

Q. How does PUJ obstruction present in children?

A.

- Most commonly with antenatal hydronephrosis.
- In older children, PUJ obstruction may present with loin pain. This pain may be exacerbated by drinking large fluid volumes, where the subsequent diuresis exacerbates the stretching of the upper tract. This is referred to as Deitel's crisis.
- PUJ obstruction may be picked up as an incidental finding during the investigation of other complaints.
- More unusually the child may present with a urinary tract infection, a mass or haematuria (a hydronephrotic kidney is more susceptible to trauma).

Q. What is the aetiology of PUJ obstruction in children?

A. Usually the PUJ junction is hypoplastic and aperistaltic in neonates.

A significant proportion of older children, usually after the age of 7 years, who present with PUJ obstruction will have a lower pole anterior accessory vessel crossing the PUJ (these children usually present with intermittent loin pain, which occurs after drinking large amounts; hydronephrosis is only present when patients are symptomatic).

Q. What investigations are useful in children in whom you suspect PUJ obstruction?

A. In children the two most useful tests are ultrasound and dynamic renography. Ultrasound will give information about the degree of hydronephrosis, the AP renal pelvic diameter, degree of calyceal dilation and whether there is renal cortical thinning. It will

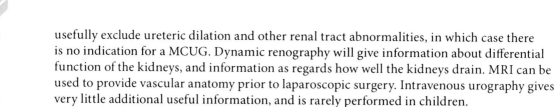

usefully exclude ureteric dilation and other renal tract abnormalities, in which case there is no indication for a MCUG. Dynamic renography will give information about differential function of the kidneys, and information as regards how well the kidneys drain. MRI can be used to provide vascular anatomy prior to laparoscopic surgery. Intravenous urography gives very little additional useful information, and is rarely performed in children.

Note: *If dynamic diuresis renography is equivocal a Whitaker test can be performed, but this is done very rarely, particularly in children. This investigation requires the placement of a nephrostomy in the affected kidney and a catheter in the bladder. With the patient prone a mixture of contrast with saline is infused via the nephrostomy at a rate of 10 mL/min. The pressure difference between the kidney and bladder is measured: if <15 cm H$_2$O the system is not obstructed, and if >22 cm H$_2$O the kidney is obstructed. Results between 15 and 22 cm H$_2$O are equivocal.*

Q. The mother has been told that her baby needs a ^{99m}Tc MAG3 scan. What does MAG3 stand for?
A. Mercapto-acetyltriglycine. It is labelled with metastable technetium-99 (^{99m}Tc).

Q. How is ^{99m}Tc MAG3 handled by the kidney?
A. It undergoes both tubular and glomerular excretion. Dimercapto-succinic acid (DMSA) binds only to the proximal renal tubules. Diethylene-triamine-penta-acetic acid (DTPA) is only filtered by the glomeruli.

Q. She wants to know how it is performed.
A. The study is performed in the nuclear medicine department.

Before the study begins, the mother should ensure that her child has had plenty to drink and is well hydrated. Intravenous access is obtained.

The tracer is injected. Images are acquired, using a gamma camera that records activity over the next 20 minutes or so. Final images are taken after the child has voided, and/or had a change in position. Furosemide may be administered according to a locally agreed protocol. In children, where venous access is often not always easy, the diuretic is often administered at the same time as the tracer.

Q. The mother is very anxious about the dose of radiation. What advice will you give?
A. The radiation dose from a ^{99m}Tc MAG3 test is less than 0.4 mSv (milli Sieverts). For a DMSA scan it is approximately 1 mSV. The higher dose is easier to understand when one considers that ^{99m}Tc MAG3 is excreted by the kidney, whereas ^{99m}Tc DMSA binds to the renal tubule. In both cases the radiation dose is less than for a plain abdominal x-ray.

Q. Please interpret the MAG-3 renogram shown in Figure 6.4.
A. A series of images are shown taken at the intervals marked. 'ROI' indicates the regions of interest that have been drawn around the kidneys; the counts taken from these regions of interest proved the graph shown in the upper right. The differential function is taken by comparing the count from the two kidneys during the early part of the study before the trace has entered the collecting system. 'Eyeballing' the 1–2 minute images and the 2–4 minute images it can be seen that the left kidney carries less function than the right. This is borne out by the measured differential of 39% annotated on the bottom right graph. Tracer moves much more slowly through the left system than the right, with significant tracer remaining in the left kidney at the end of the study. This is reflected in the curves of the top right graph. It would have been advantageous to see how much more drains from the left kidney with voiding. There seems to be some bladder emptying between the 15–20 minute and the 25–30 minute images, but the bladder has not completely emptied. It is not clear from the images whether diuretic has been administered.

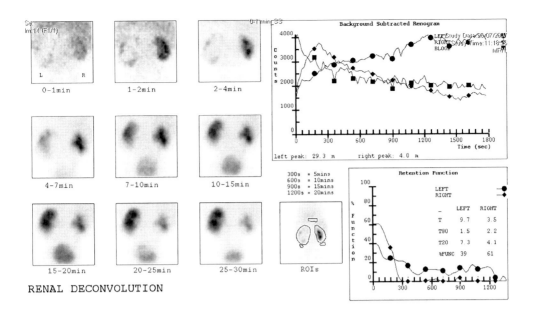

RENAL DECONVOLUTION

Figure 6.4 A ^{99m}Tc MAG-3 renogram.

Q. What are your indications for pyeloplasty in PUJ obstruction?

A.

- Reduced function of the affected kidney. A differential function of less than 40% is significant.
- Symptoms such as pain or urinary tract infection. Older children are able to articulate that they have pain. This is more difficult to establish in infants, and when asked, it is unusual for the mothers of babies with PUJ obstruction to report that they think their child is having pain.
- Deteriorating renal function (a decrease of differential function of more than 10% is significant) or increasing hydronephrosis on follow-up USS.
- Concern that the function of the kidney will decline if left untreated. Based on the 'Natural History' studies by Dhillon [4], gross hydronephrosis, with an AP renal pelvis diameter of more than 50 mm, should be surgically treated. Between 20 and 50 mm things are not so clear cut with an increasing proportion requiring surgery with increased AP renal pelvic diameter as shown in Table 6.1.

Table 6.1 Percent of children requiring surgery for increasing hydronephrosis in PUJ obstruction

AP renal pelvic diameter in transverse plane in PUJ obstruction (mm)[a]	Percent requiring surgery
>50	100
>40	80
>30	55
>20	20
<20	1–3

[a] Those infants with a persistent AP renal pelvic diameter of <10 mm are discharged.

MULTICYSTIC DYSPLASTIC KIDNEY

Q. The paediatrician asks for your advice. He has taken over the care of a 13-month-old girl who had a renal anomaly detected antenatally. USS has a normal kidney on one side, but on the other side there is a 7 cm long kidney composed of large cysts and no normal tissue. A DMSA scan has shown no function in the abnormal kidney. What is the most likely problem affecting this kidney?

A. Multicystic dysplastic kidney (MCDK).

Q. **This is exactly what the paediatrician is concerned about. He would like to know how you would manage the child and your justification for the plan.**

A. Usually these involute, in which case very little further needs to be done. There has been a previous concern about increased risk of hypertension and malignancy in these abnormal kidneys. These problems usually represent episodic case reports rather than a significant risk to the patient. A minority of patients (19%) may have contralateral VUR, but this is rarely associated with scarring. The patient is probably more at risk of reduced renal function and hypertension from having a solitary functioning kidney. Rarely nephrectomy may be necessary if the kidney is causing symptoms from mass effects. So a patient with a MSDK should have follow-up of their renal function, perhaps with checks at 1, 2, 5 and 10 years.

Duplex kidney

Q. **Describe the embryology of a duplex kidney and the Meyer-Weigert rule.**

A. The ureteric bud originates from the lower mesonephric duct, grows cranially and meets the metanephros at 32 days. By *reciprocal induction*, they generate a kidney. Urine production begins at 10 weeks. If an extra ureteric bud is generated it will also head to the metanephros and so develop into a second ureter and a duplex kidney will form. The ureteric bud that meets the more cranial metanephrosis will generate the upper moiety ureter. This ureteric bud will have arisen from a more caudal position on the mesonephric duct than the other ureteric bud. When this part of the mesonephric duct is subsumed into the developing bladder, the more caudal ureteric bud will maintain its lower position.

The resultant relationship with the upper moiety ureter inserting lower and more medially into the bladder is the Meyer-Weigert rule (in comparison the lower renal moiety ureter inserts higher and more laterally into the bladder).

Q. **You see a 3-month-old girl in clinic with her parents. There was a confident prenatal diagnosis of a duplex kidney on one side. What is a duplex kidney and is it common?**

A. It is a kidney with a double collecting system and two separate ureters entering the bladder separately. It is said to occur in 1 in 125 births.

Q. **Where does the ureter of the upper moiety insert relative to the lower moiety ureter?**

A. The upper moiety ureter inserts inferiorly and more medially in comparison to the lower moiety ureter.

Q. **What are the complications associated with a duplex kidney?**

A. In general complications are related to the insertion of the ureter into the bladder.

- The upper moiety ureter may insert into the bladder normally, or its insertion may be related to a ureterocele, or its insertion may be ectopic.

  A ureterocele is a swelling associated with the insertion of the ureter into the bladder. It is usually a cause of obstruction at the VUJ. A ureterocele may be complicated by infection, prolapse and bladder outlet obstruction.

  Ectopic ureter insertion in girls may be into the urethra or vagina, and if below the external sphincter will cause continuous incontinence. The more ectopic the ureter, the more dysplastic the kidney it drains, and the more difficult it can be to spot radiologically. In boys the ectopic insertion may be into the prostate, ejaculatory duct or vas; the insertion of the ectopic ureter is always above the external urethral sphincter in boys so incontinence will not result.

- The lower moiety ureter can insert normally or be associated with vesico-ureteric reflux.

URINARY TRACT INFECTIONS (UTIs) IN CHILDREN

Q. **How common are UTIs in children?**

A. During childhood, UTI occurs in about 3%–5% of girls and 1% of boys. The incidence of UTIs is higher in boys than girls in the first year. Uncircumcised males less than 1 year old are more likely to be affected than circumcised males. After 1 year of age, UTIs in females are more common.

Q. **A 9-month-old boy presents with pyrexia and vomiting. He is very unwell. What microbiology specimens would you like collected?**

A. Airway, breathing, circulation (ABC) and general assessment, including examination of the spine is done. A clean catch urine specimen is the most important. He would also need blood cultures taken.

Note: *A clean catch urine sample means that the urethral meatus should be clean, and if possible urine collected should be from the middle of the stream. For girls, cleaning involves separating the labia and cleaning the area. For circumcised boys, the glans of the penis should be cleaned. For uncircumcised boys the foreskin is gently retracted (where possible) prior to cleaning. After cleaning, the child voids, with the parent 'catching' the urine in a clean specimen container after the first few drops are passed. In those who can void on command, the child can void over the toilet and a clean catch mid-stream voided urine specimen may be easily obtained. Although obtaining clean catch samples can be time consuming and messy, this technique has a high sensitivity and specificity for diagnosing UTIs.*

Q. **The urine of the infant discussed previously shows >500 white cells, CRP is 84. He responds to intravenous (IV) fluids and antibiotics. Is his infection typical?**

A. According to the 2007 National Institute for Health and Care Excellence (NICE) guidelines on the management of UTI [5], an atypical UTI is one where any of the following apply:

- Seriously ill
- Poor urine flow
- Abdominal or bladder mass
- Raised creatinine
- Septicaemia
- Failure to respond to treatment with suitable antibiotics within 48 hours
- Infection with non-*E. coli* organisms

By this definition the infant has an atypical urinary tract infection.

Q. **What imaging is helpful?**

A. A USS of the renal tract.

Q. **The USS shows a large thick-walled bladder. On direct question his mother admits that he has always had a rather 'dribbley' stream. What conditions are you concerned about?**

A. The possibilities are of bladder outlet obstruction (especially posterior urethral valves) or a neuropathic bladder.

Q. **Is any more renal tract imaging appropriate?**

A. According to the NICE guidelines [5], DMSA scan is the only other investigation required in someone who is between 6 months and 3 years of age with an atypical urinary infection. However, in those with a worrying history and an abnormal ultrasound further investigations may also be appropriate. The diagnostic test for PUVs is an MCUG, which must include good views of the urethra during voiding.

The NICE guidelines on radiological imaging in children with UTIs are summarised in Table 6.2.

Table 6.2 Guidelines for imaging in paediatric UTI (adapted from NICE guidelines 2007)

UTI	Age	USS in acute infection	USS in 6/52	DMSA in 4–6/12	MCUG*
Responds well to antibiotics in <48 hours	<6 months		Yes		
Responds well to antibiotics in <48 hours	6 months – 3 years				
Responds well to antibiotics in <48 hours	>3 years				
Atypical UTI	<6 months	Yes		Yes	Yes
Atypical UTI	6 months – 3 years	Yes		Yes	Consider**
Atypical UTI	>3 years	Yes			
Recurrent UTI	<6 months	Yes		Yes	Yes
Recurrent UTI	6 months – 3 years		Yes	Yes	Consider**
Recurrent UTI	>3 years		Yes	Yes	

* Some centres may prefer MAG3 (mercaptoacetyltriglycine) renogram with indirect cystogram in cases suspected to have vesicoureteric reflux.

** Consider MCUG if dilatation on ultrasound, poor urine flow, non-*E. coli* infection, family history of VUR

Q. **A 7-month-old girl presents with pyelonephritis. She is admitted under the paediatricians and responds well to antibiotics. She has a USS before discharge which shows unilateral hydroureteronephrosis. What are the possible causes of unilateral hydroureteronephrosis?**

A. An isolated hydroureteronephrosis raises the possibility of VUR, VUJ obstruction or megaureter.

Q. **An MCUG has been organised by the paediatric team. The mother would like to know a little more about the test before it is performed. What would you tell her?**

A. The test carries a risk of provoking a further UTI, so it should be covered with a short course of treatment dose antibiotics (e.g. trimethoprim).

The test is performed in the radiology department by the radiology doctors and will involve exposure to x-rays. The girl will be catheterised urethrally. Contrast material, 'a special dye that shows on x-ray', is then injected into the bladder and x-rays are taken. At the end of the test the catheter is taken out, and further x-rays taken as she urinates.

The thing that most parents, and patients, dislike about the test is the catheterisation. Above the age of 1 year it becomes much more difficult to catheterise the child as the child will struggle more. An MCUG is not a test that should be requested lightly.

Q. **The mother is very interested by what you say. The girl's aunt has also attended the consultation, but is not as convinced. The aunt, who is an adult, had pyelonephritis last year and objects that no one made all of this fuss with her infection. Why is pyelonephritis in paediatrics taken so seriously?**

A. Investigation of pyelonephritis in the past has had a high yield for detecting problems, with up to 30% of children having a significant underlying renal tract anomaly.

Pyelonephritis in infants is important. During the acute episode it carries its own morbidity. Additionally, following the acute episode, pyelonephritis may result in:

- *Scarring* – Young kidneys are susceptible to damage from the combination of intra-renal reflux and infection. It is unusual for scarring to result in renal impairment unless this is extensive and severe. The importance of scarring is that it carries a significant long-term risk of hypertension.
- *Recurrence* – Up to one-fifth of children with pyelonephritis will have a recurrence within a year.

Note: *There was a concern that a significant proportion of children with end-stage renal disease were thought to have got there because of VUR with associated UTI. It is now thought that this may have been an overestimation, where children, born with poor dysplastic kidneys, were extensively investigated and a bit of VUR identified as the only culprit. It is also being recognised that many children more recently had been overinvestigated with a lower yield of significant pathology. These are perhaps the motivations behind the current NICE guidelines on the investigation of UTI.*

Q. **The MCUG is performed as shown in Figure 6.5. Describe the findings.**

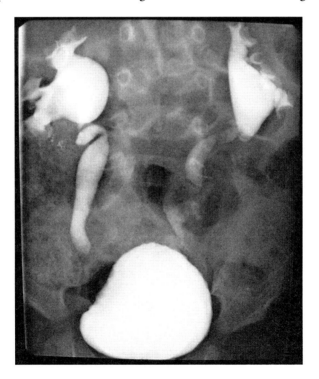

Figure 6.5 Micturating cystourethrogram in infant girl.

A. Bilateral vesico-ureteric reflux with at least moderate ureteric and pelvi-calyceal dilatation.

Q. **What functional imaging would be useful?**

A. A DMSA scan would be very useful. Acutely during the infective episode it will show cortical defects and confirm a diagnosis if it is in doubt; although it is not often used for this indication. After the pyelonephritis has been treated it will show areas of permanent injury or scarring if performed 4–6 months afterwards (in addition to providing relative renal function).

Q. Her DMSA scan is shown in Figure 6.6. What does it show?

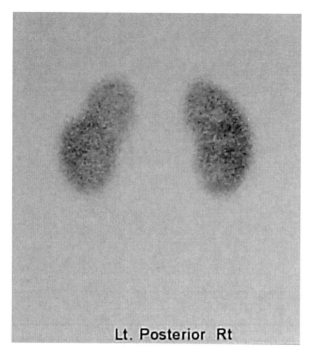

Figure 6.6 A DMSA scan in infant girl.

A. There is a cortical defect in the mid to upper pole of the left kidney. Whether it is a scar depends on whether there has been a sufficient interval since the pyelonephritis; ideally at least 6 months.

Q. What is secondary reflux?

A. It is where the reflux is due to another clearly defined pathology, e.g. posterior urethral valves or neuropathic bladder. In secondary reflux treatment is targeted at the underlying condition.

Q. What is the International Reflux Study Committee grading of primary VUR and the rates of spontaneous resolution?

A. This grading is based upon the extent of retrograde filling and dilatation of the ureter, the renal pelvis and the calyces on a MCUG and is shown in Table 6.3.

Table 6.3 International Reflux Study Committee grading of VUR

Grade of VUR	Characteristics	Rate of spontaneous resolution (%)
Grade 1	Reflux does not reach the renal pelvis; varying degrees of ureteral dilatation	90
Grade 2	Reflux reaches the renal pelvis; no dilatation of the collecting system; normal fornices	80
Grade 3	Mild or moderate dilatation of the ureter, with or without tortuosity; moderate dilatation of the collecting system; normal or minimally deformed fornices	50
Grade 4	Moderate dilatation of the ureter with or without tortuosity; moderate dilatation of the collecting system; blunt fornices, but impressions of the papillae still visible	20
Grade 5	Gross dilatation and tortuosity of the ureter; marked dilatation of the collecting system; papillary impressions no longer visible; intraparenchymal reflux	<10

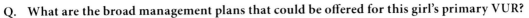

Q. **What are the broad management plans that could be offered for this girl's primary VUR?**

A. Medical or surgical management.

Q. **What are the differences in outcome between surgical and medical management?**

A. Several randomised controlled trials have compared ureteric re-implantation over conservative medical management. On all the most important outcome measures (frequency of UTI, scarring and GFR) there was no difference between the two treatments, except a lower incidence of febrile UTIs in the surgically treated group.

The 2010 Swedish reflux study compared the difference in outcome between surveillance, prophylaxis and endoscopic surgery. Girls on surveillance were more likely to develop UTI than those on prophylaxis or treated surgically. Compared to girls on surveillance, girls on prophylaxis are less likely to scar.

Q. **What are the important elements of conservative/medical management?**

A.

- The most important part of this is educating the parents that if their child has a urinary tract infection, or unexplained pyrexia, that she should be assessed and treated promptly. This requires that urine is sent for culture and sensitivity and then appropriate treatment antibiotics are started. Early treatment of UTI will lessen the chance of longer-term scarring.
- Maintain a good fluid intake.
- Maintain a regular bowel habit and avoid constipation.
- In an older child it is important that the child be encouraged to void frequently. The child should void during each break at school, and parents should encourage the child to void 3 hourly during the day when the child is at home.
- Prophylactic antibiotics have been the mainstay of medical treatment for years. A recent meta-analysis [6] has found that antibiotics do not in fact prevent scars. They do however reduce the risk of pyrexial UTI by about a third, at the cost of an eightfold increase of subsequent breakthrough infections being resistant.

Q. **What are the indications for surgical treatment?**

A. The indications for intervention vary between surgeons. The most common reason for surgery is failure of medical management. This would include breakthrough infections, new renal scarring or difficulty adhering to medical management. Parental preference could be another reason for offering surgery. Sometimes surgery is offered for persisting or high-grade reflux.

Q. **What surgical procedures are available?**

A. *Endoscopic* – Cystoscopy is used to inject a bulking agent around the ureteric orifice. Subtrigonal Teflon (PTFE) injection (STING) has become much less used after Teflon was discovered migrating to distant organs. The most common agent used now is dextranomer/ hyaluronic acid conjugate (Deflux), and success rates of well over 80% are quoted. Although it may require repeat treatments, its advantages are that it can be performed as a day case procedure with minimal morbidity.

Open surgical – There are several methods of re-implanting the ureter.

Intra-vesical re-implantation involves opening the bladder, mobilising the ureter and creating a sub-mucosal tunnel at least five times as long as the diameter of the ureter (Paquin's rule). The easiest is a 'Cohen' cross-trigonal re-implantation (success rate of more than 95%); a 'Leadbetter-Politano' procedure re-implants the ureter into a higher and more medial position in the bladder.

The Lich–Gregoir procedure is an extra-vesical anti-reflux operation and involves burying the ureter in a tunnel of detrusor. The bladder mucosa is not opened in this procedure (and thus a catheter is not necessary post-operatively).

Laparoscopic/vesicoscopic – The previously described open operations are modified in the hands of adept laparoscopic surgeons.

Q. What is the definition of recurrent UTI?

A. Recurrent UTI is defined as (*over a 1-year period or less*):

- Three or more episodes of UTI with cystitis (lower urinary tract infection)
- Two or more episodes of UTI with acute pyelonephritis (upper urinary tract infection)
- One episode of UTI with acute pyelonephritis plus one or more episodes of UTI with cystitis

Q. You see a 7-year-old girl in your clinic with recurrent episodes of cystitis associated with positive urine cultures. What history will you take?

A. In the absence of pyrexial episodes her problems are a real nuisance to her rather than a threat to her health. A similar assessment is made as for the child with incontinence:

- *Symptoms suggesting significant predisposing pathology* – Straining to void, poor stream, frank haematuria and neurological symptoms indicate more detailed evaluation may be necessary.
- *Voiding history and frequency* – Infrequent voiding is a common exacerbating factor; children do not like going to the bathroom to urinate, and the state of most school toilets adds a further disincentive.
- *Fluid intake* – Adequate fluid intake is necessary (with avoidance of fizzy and coloured drinks).
- *Bowels* – Constipation will make episodes of cystitis more likely.

Q. You examine her abdomen and find no masses, her perineum and genitals are unremarkable and she has a normal spine. Is there anything else worth checking?

A. Urine dipstick: to check for leucocytes and nitrites (assessed in the context of whether she has current UTI symptoms), glucose and protein.

Q. Her voiding history is a little vague. How can you find more information about her voiding?

A. A frequency-volume chart.

Q. Are any further investigations required?

A. A renal tract ultrasound is justifiable. It will show upper tract anomalies, bladder volume and residual urine volume.

Q. Ultrasound scan proves normal. What advice do you give to the parents on how to control her frequent episodes of infection?

A. Set up a good voiding habit. She may need to be prompted to void 'by the clock' every 3 hours when she is awake. This also translates into voiding during each break at school. Treating constipation is often effective.

There is some (although not strong) evidence for taking regular cranberry juice and bioactive yogurt. Prophylactic antibiotics – despite the above measures, if the child continues to have problematic infections, it may be worth considering a course of prophylactic antibiotics. Trimethoprim and nitrofurantoin are excreted in the urine and effective in this role whereas ampicillin and cephalosporins affect commensal bowel flora and so may not be as effective.

Persistence of infection may need a thorough bladder assessment and consideration to rule out reflux even in the absence of upper tract dilatation.

The unwell child

Q. A 2-month-old boy is brought into accident and emergency by his parents. He has had a circumcision in the community. There continues to be bleeding and his parents are concerned. Outline your management.

A. Assessment of whether he needs resuscitation takes priority over history and examination.

Q. How would you assess him?

A. The paediatric early warning score is a useful framework to assess a child. This will be integrated into a children's observation chart. The following should be looked for:

- Increased respiratory rate capillary refill time of more than 2 seconds (press on the sternum or forehead for 5 seconds and then release)
- Tachycardia
- Increased respiratory rate
- Changing behaviour, e.g. drowsy, irritable, lethargy, confusion or reduced response to pain
- Hypotension is late sign of hypovolaemia in a child

Note: *Normal paediatric parameters in Table 6.4.*

Table 6.4 Normal paediatric parameters by age group

Age (years)	Respiratory rate (breaths/min)	Systolic blood pressure (mm Hg)	Pulse (beats/min)
<1	30–40	70–90	110–160
1–2	25–35	80–95	100–150
2–5	25–30	80–100	95–140
5–12	20–25	90–110	80–120
>12	15–20	100–120	60–100

Q. The child is hypovolaemic. How would you treat?

A. This should be done jointly with the paediatric team. Oxygen is given. Intravenous access is secured with large-bore intravenous cannula. This will allow blood samples for full blood count, clotting screen and group and save. Fluid resuscitation is with crystalloid (normal saline) or packed red cells.

Q. What volume of bolus should be given?

A. 10–20 mL/kg.

Q. How would you estimate this child's circulating blood volume?

A. 75–85 mL/kg.

Q. Despite applying pressure and adrenaline soaked gauze the bleeding continues. What's the next step?

A. The circumcision will require surgical exploration. This should be done in a setting with appropriate paediatric anaesthesia and high dependency care support.

Until appropriate surgical help is available, he needs a pressure dressing held together with adhesive tapes; temptation to remove any adherent swabs for repeated examination must be avoided.

Q. Paediatric anaesthesia is not available in your unit. The child will require transfer to another hospital. How should this be done?

A. An infant who has required fluid resuscitation for hypovolaemia will need careful transfer. It may be necessary to discuss the transfer with a paediatric intensive care unit retrieval team to ensure that the baby is safe during the journey.

Q. Later that evening as you are walking through the paediatric ward you are asked to prescribe intravenous maintenance fluids for another child. The child has an ileus, is otherwise well and on examination is normally euvolaemic. Which fluids would you prescribe and why?

A. Children are very vulnerable to hyponatraemia which may cause cerebral oedema, permanent neurological deficit and even death. Children should not be prescribed hypotonic fluid (sodium chloride 0.45% or sodium chloride 0.18%). Dextrose is given for calories, glucose quickly moves into the intracellular space, so dextrose solutions are effectively hypo-osmolar (e.g. 0.45% saline with 5% dextrose risks hyponatraemia). Acceptable fluids are sodium chloride 0.9%, sodium chloride 0.9% with dextrose 5% or Hartmann's solution.

If IV fluid is given for a short duration then potassium is not required. If fluid is given for more than 12 hours then potassium should also be given in ready-made bags, e.g. sodium chloride 0.9% plus dextrose 5% plus potassium 10 mmol/L.

Q. How much fluid should be given?

A. According to the child's weight:

Weight (kg)	Fluid rate
Up to 10 kg	4 mL/kg/h for the first 10 kg
10 to 20 kg	2 mL/kg/h for the next 10 kg
More than 20 kg	1 mL/kg/h for every kilogram over 20 kg

For example for a 25 kg child give 40 + 20 + 5 = 65 mL/h.

Post-operatively and during acute illness with the response to stress, fluid requirement can be reduced to two-thirds of this.

REFERENCES

1. Rickwood AM. Medical indications for circumcision. *BJU Int* 1999; 83, (Suppl 1): 45–51.
2. Gairdner D. The fate of the foreskin, a study of circumcision. *Br Med J* 1949; 2: 1433–1437.
3. Oster J. Further fate of the foreskin. Incidence of preputial adhesions, phimosis, and smegma among Danish schoolboys. *Arch Dis Child* 1968; 43: 200–203.
4. Dhillon HK. Prenatally diagnosed hydronephrosis: The Great Ormond Street experience. *Br J Urol* 1998; 81, (Suppl 2): 39–44.
5. www.nice.org.uk/ clinical guideline 54: Urinary tract infection in children. Accessed 2016.
6. Wang HH et al. Efficacy of antibiotic prophylaxis in children with vesicoureteral reflux: Systematic review and meta-analysis. *J Urol* 2015 Mar; 193(3): 963–969.

FURTHER READING

Thomas DFM, Duffy PG, Rickwood AMK (eds). *Essentials of Paediatric Urology*, 2nd edn. Boca Raton, FL: CRC Press.

CHAPTER 7
UROLOGICAL
EMERGENCIES, PART I

*Acute testicular pain, complications of TURP,
sepsis and penile fracture*

Iqbal S Shergill and Basharat Jameel

Contents

ACUTE TESTICULAR PAIN

Q. **A 15-year-old boy (Figure 7.1) is referred to you with acute onset right testicular pain. What is the differential diagnosis?**

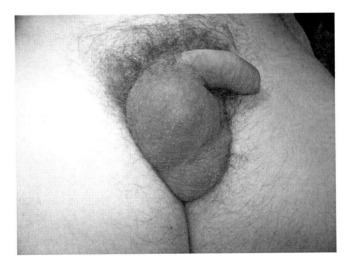

Figure 7.1 Image of a young boy presenting with acute onset right testicular pain.

A. Differential diagnosis includes testicular torsion, epididymo-orchitis, testicular trauma, torted hydatid of Morgagni or mumps orchitis (idiopathic scrotal oedema if under 10 years of age).

Q. How would you assess this patient?

A. I would consider this a urological emergency and see the patient immediately myself, without delay. I would take a history, examine the patient, arrange further investigations (if required) and institute a management plan as appropriate.

Q. What features would be suggestive of testicular torsion?

A. Testicular torsion is a clinical diagnosis. However, even with a high index of suspicion, the definitive diagnosis can only be made at emergency surgical exploration.

Clinical features of testicular torsion are as follows:

- *History*
    - Pain is of acute onset
    - Mainly testicular pain
    - Occasionally radiating to groin, abdomen or thigh
    - History of previous testicular pain (intermittent torsion) may be common
- *Examination*
    - Acutely tender and swollen testicle
    - Horizontal lie (bell-clapper deformity)
    - High riding testis in scrotum (Figure 7.1)
    - Absent cremasteric reflex
    - Mild fever and erythema of the scrotal skin (late signs)
- *Investigations*
    - Urinalysis is usually normal
    - Doppler ultrasound scan (USS) (only in equivocal cases) may show poor or absent blood flow

Q. When does torsion typically occur and what is the difference between intravaginal and extra-vaginal torsion?

A. Testicular torsion can occur at any age but commonly the incidence has a bimodal distribution [1], with the main peak around puberty (12–18 years) and a smaller peak in the first year of life (Figure 7.2).

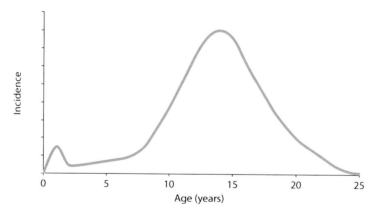

Figure 7.2 The bimodal incidence of testicular torsion.

Intravaginal torsion is the most common form of testicular torsion seen in adolescents and adults and is due to a congenital high investment of the tunica vaginalis on the cord, resulting in a horizontally lying testis, and it produces the 'bell clapper' deformity. This anomaly allows the testis and cord to rotate more readily than a normal testis. The bell clapper deformity is often bilateral, with a significant risk of torsion to the contralateral testis.

Extravaginal torsion is most commonly seen in the first year of life. It can occur both pre- and post-natally. The attachment between the tunica vaginalis and the scrotum is loose, i.e. there is incomplete fixation of the gubernaculum to the scrotal wall, resulting in the entire testis and tunica vaginalis twisting in a vertical axis on the spermatic cord.

Q. **Are there any investigations which can diagnose testicular torsion in certain patients?**

A. Testicular torsion is a clinical diagnosis and the gold standard management for suspected testicular torsion is urgent surgical exploration of the scrotum.

However, in cases where clinical features are equivocal and urgent scrotal exploration is not indicated on clinical grounds, colour Doppler USS may be used to aid diagnosis. Poor arterial blood flow signal in the testicular artery to the testicle suggests a diagnosis of torsion. This technique is operator dependent, with studies demonstrating 85%–90% sensitivity and 75%–95% specificity. Radionuclide imaging has been proposed to be of high sensitivity (87%–98%) and specificity (100%), however it is time consuming and as yet has no place in the clinical assessment of an acute scrotum. The most important point to bear in mind is that the use of radiological investigations must not unnecessarily delay definitive surgical treatment.

The gold standard management for suspected testicular torsion is urgent surgical exploration of the scrotum.

Q. **If you think the patient has testicular torsion, how quickly should you perform the operation?**

A. Salvage rates directly correlate with the number of hours after the onset of pain (Figure 7.3). Hence, I try to operate as soon as is possible.

Figure 7.3 is a graph showing that salvage rates correlate with number of hours after onset of pain.

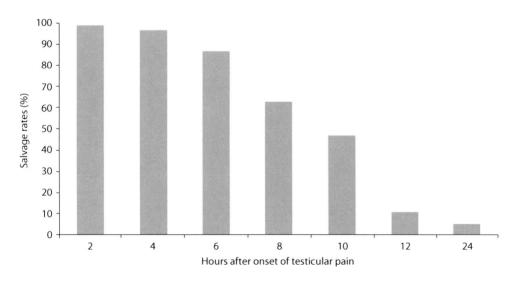

Figure 7.3 Salvage rates according to number of hours after onset of pain.

Q. **The patient appears to have a clinical diagnosis of testicular torsion. What are the key features in the pre-operative consent for emergency scrotal exploration?**

A. The informed consent for emergency scrotal exploration would involve a description of the procedure, discussion of alternative treatments and an explanation of potential complications. The following points would need to be raised [2]:

- Bilateral testicular fixation (orchidopexy) in the case of torsion, where testis is viable
- Orchidectomy in the case of torsion, where testis is not viable, with orchidopexy of contralateral testicle
- No fixation in the case where no torsion is found
- If orchidopexy is performed, non-absorbable sutures may be palpable
- Risk of haematoma, which may require surgical exploration
- Risk of wound infection or orchitis
- Long-term risks of testicular atrophy
- No guarantee of fertility
- Small risk of future torsion despite fixation

Q. What incision do you use? Describe your technique of fixation.

A. At scrotal exploration, although various skin incisions can be employed, including transverse, bilateral vertical and oblique, I use the midline incision through the median raphe.

The layers of the scrotum (skin, dartos, external spermatic fascia, cremasteric fascia, internal spermatic fascia, tunica vaginalis) are divided. The affected testis is delivered and inspected. Testicular torsion occurs inwards and towards the midline and in a case of torsion, the testis is initially untwisted. The testis is then wrapped in a warm saline-soaked swab and the anaesthetist supplies 100% oxygen, via the endotracheal tube.

If the testis is viable, I perform an orchidopexy using the three-point fixation technique. The testis is fixed medially, laterally and infero-anteriorly to the scrotal wall using non-absorbable sutures (typically 3/0 or 4/0 Prolene). If the viability of the testis is questionable, I make a small stab incision through the tunica albuginea to assess for evidence of viability through signs of bleeding. If the testicle is not salvageable, I perform an orchidectomy.

In a case of confirmed testicular torsion, I explore the contralateral testis, through the same incision, and perform a prophylactic three-point orchidopexy, to prevent future torsion on that side. This is supported by reports of contralateral torsion following unilateral orchidopexy and a 40% incidence of anatomical abnormalities predisposing to torsion in the contralateral testis. If an appendix testis is found at operation, I remove it to prevent future torsion of appendix testis mimicking testicular torsion.

Additional procedures have been proposed, namely eversion of the tunica vaginalis at the time of surgical exploration to prevent future re-torsion, as well as the use of a sub-dartos pouch.

In the case where no torsion is found, I do not carry out orchidopexy, due to the potential complications of needle trauma (including breach of the blood-testis barrier). The testis should be replaced intact. In addition, I do not perform contralateral exploration.

Q. Are you aware of any potential complications of testicular torsion?

A. Misdiagnosis, especially as an epididymo-orchitis, is the most common problem. If a patient shows no improvement, despite 48–72 hours of antibiotic therapy, the diagnosis of testicular torsion (dead testis) should be considered. An infarcted testis left in the scrotum, may result in abscess or sinus formation. The potential long-term complication of this event is the formation of antisperm antibodies, causing infertility in the contralateral testis. Other long-term complications include future torsion in a testis that has undergone previous inadequate prophylactic fixation. This risk may be minimised by performing orchidopexy in the contralateral testis when torsion is found. In the case where orchidectomy is carried out, a testicular prosthesis insertion may be considered, in the future, to improve cosmetic outcome and psychological recovery. In my practice, I do not insert the prosthesis at the time of emergency exploration, through the scrotal route, due to the significant risk of erosion.

MANAGEMENT OF COMPLICATIONS OF TRANSURETHRAL RESECTION OF THE PROSTATE

Q. **A fit 75-year-old man presents for transurethral resection of the prostate (TURP). Pre-operative assessment revealed good effort tolerance, no symptoms of cardiac failure and all investigations were normal. He undergoes spinal anaesthetic after a preload of 500 mL saline, and is given oxygen via Hudson mask. Surgery begins after the block was confirmed at the T8 level. At 60 minutes into the procedure, the patient complains of nausea and was given ondansetron. HR: 106 bpm, BP: normal. Then, 15 minutes later, he becomes anxious, pulls off the oxygen mask off and tries to get off the operating table. What is the probable diagnosis and how does it occur?**

A. I would strongly suspect the diagnosis is likely to be transurethral resection (TUR) syndrome.

TUR syndrome is a multifactorial syndrome, which arises from absorption of large volumes of irrigation fluid (1.5% glycine), typically during TURP. Although it is commonly thought to be due to dilutional hyponatraemia exclusively, fluid overload and effects of glycine toxicity contribute significantly to the pathophysiology of this condition.

Q. **What is the incidence of TUR syndrome?**

A. Classical studies quote an incidence of 0.5%–2.0% following TURP [3,4]. Recent contemporary studies suggest an even lower incidence, based on technological evolution. Interestingly, TUR syndrome may also be associated with transurethral resection of bladder tumour (TURBT) and percutaneous nephrolithotomy (PCNL).

Q. **What concentration of glycine is used in resection, and what is its osmolality?**

A. Typically, 1.5% glycine is used. It is an inhibitory amino acid, and a non-electrolyte solution, with an osmolality of 200 mOsomol/L – hence, it is hypotonic, with respect to plasma.

Q. **How is glycine handled in the body?**

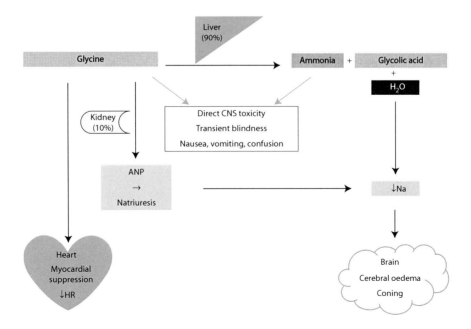

Figure 7.4 Handling and toxic effects of glycine.

A. Figure 7.4 shows handling and toxic effects of glycine. In a typical TURP, there is approximately 20 mL/min fluid absorption and thus during a 60 minute resection one would anticipate 1.2 L of glycine solution being absorbed. Absorption of 1.5% glycine solution occurs directly (and thus immediately) into the periprostatic venous plexus, as well as indirectly (resulting in delayed absorption) from the perivesical and retroperitoneal spaces. This amount of absorbed hypotonic fluid is relatively easily dealt with in a normal individual, with 90% of glycine being metabolised to ammonia, glycolic acid and water, by the liver, and the remaining 10% being metabolised by the kidney.

Q. Can you explain the symptoms of TUR syndrome?

A. TUR syndrome is a multifactorial syndrome, which arises from absorption of large volumes of 1.5% glycine solution, resulting in dilutional hyponatraemia, fluid overload and effects of glycine toxicity. Knowledge of these three factors allows an understanding of the clinical symptoms of TUR syndrome (Figure 7.4).

The dilutional hyponatraemia results in osmotic shift of water from plasma into the brain. Symptoms are generally dependent on sodium concentration, resulting in cerebral herniation and death, if left untreated (Table 7.1).

Furthermore, glycine induces an osmotic diuresis, which results in absolute losses of sodium from the body, and this can be further exacerbated by the release of atrial natriuretic peptide, which promotes natriuresis (Figure 7.4).

Table 7.1 Symptoms associated with dilutional hyponatraemia

Na concentration (mmol/L)	Symptoms
130–135	Asymptomatic
120–130	Restlessness Confusion
115–120	Nausea
<115	Seizures Coma

With fluid overload patients initially develop hypertension, shortness of breath, chest pain and cyanosis, from resultant pulmonary oedema and cardiac failure. Later clinical features include bradycardia and a marked decrease in systolic arterial pressure.

Glycine is an inhibitory neurotransmitter in the retina, present at a concentration of 400 mol/L in humans. An excess amount slows down the transmission of impulses from the retina to the cerebral cortex, with prolongation of visual evoked potentials and deterioration of vision occurring after absorption of as little as a few hundred millilitres of glycine. Thus, clinically, if the patient is under spinal anaesthesia, he may report seeing flashing lights. Prickling sensations and facial warmth are also early signs of glycine absorption. At higher concentrations, glycine results in bradycardia due to direct and indirect cardiotoxic effects. Late clinical features include hypotension and coma.

Q. How would you manage TUR syndrome?

A. I conveniently divide the management of TUR syndrome into prevention, recognition and definitive treatment.

Prevention – Initially, I diagnose and treat any pre-existing hyponatraemia, before considering the patient for TURP. Second, I identify putative risk factors for TUR syndrome. In the American Urological Association (AUA) co-operative study, of immediate and postoperative complications of almost 4,000 patients from 13 institutions, Mebust et al. [3] identified significant differences in TUR syndrome when time of resection and size of gland were assessed. Among patients with a resection time of >90 minutes, the incidence of TUR syndrome was 2.0% compared to 0.7% where there was a shorter resection time ($p < .01$) [3]. Similarly, a statistically significant difference was noted in patients with glands >45 g (incidence 1.5%) as opposed to <45 g (incidence 0.8%) [3]. It would therefore, at first glance, seem logical to suggest standard TURP be avoided if the operative time would exceed 90 minutes or if the prostate gland size was larger than 45 g. However, in my practice, and in contemporary practice in the United Kingdom, an operative time of 60 minutes is usually standard, and open prostatectomy is only usually performed for gland sizes >100 g.

Other potential risk factors, such as height of irrigation fluid and intravesical pressure, race and age have also been suggested, but the evidence for these is less robust. Despite this, in my practice, I use the Iglesias continuous flow resectoscope, avoid aggressive resection near the capsule and try to complete the TURP as soon as the capsule is breached. In addition, if a prolonged procedure is inevitable, I request the anaesthetist to administer furosemide prophylactically, to off-load the excess fluid that may be absorbed. More recently, other preventative strategies have included the use of bipolar or laser resection with normal saline irrigation, as well as the use of 5% glucose as an irrigation solution in a randomised, prospective trial.

Recognition – I aim to perform TURP with the patient awake, under spinal anaesthesia, as several of the clinical factors described above will become apparent if TUR syndrome develops. With general anaesthetic, however, hypertension, from fluid overload, may be the only early warning sign, often detected by the anaesthetist. Arrhythmias, hypotension and decreased oxygen saturation are usually late features. Although not universally used, I am aware that 1% ethanol in the irrigant can be a useful strategy for detection, as it allows breath alcohol levels to be checked by a breathalyser, allowing an estimate of the volume of excess fluid that has been absorbed. Furthermore, the use of weighing machines being added to the ordinary operating table has also been reported as a technique for measuring fluid overload.

Definitive Treatment – In mild cases of established TUR syndrome, supportive management along with a period of watchful waiting is often sufficient. In my practice, the serum sodium and electrolytes are checked, but the result is not awaited prior to commencing medical treatment, in the form of the loop diuretic furosemide. (This drug results in relative loss of more water than sodium thus decreasing fluid overload and also increasing serum sodium levels.) Typically, a dose of 40 mg is given intravenously. More diuretic may be warranted depending on the serum sodium levels, as slower absorption from the retroperitoneal or perivesical space occurs (an alternative to furosemide given by many is mannitol). Concurrently, I ensure that I quickly control any haemorrhage and finish the operation as soon as possible. In addition, I think it is essential to have early input from the intensive care team, in all cases of TUR syndrome.

Severe cases occur due to lack of recognition or inadequate early treatment of mild cases. In these cases it is extremely vital that the high-dependency unit/intensive therapy unit (HDU/ITU) team are called early. Using this multidisciplinary approach, a central line and invasive arterial monitoring are usually performed as well as transferring the patient to HDU/ITU, when stable. Clearly, in extreme cases the patient may need to be intubated and ventilated. Furthermore, the intensive care environment is useful for the small minority of patients who have a dangerously low serum sodium, which requires correction with hypertonic saline solution. A correction of 1 mmol/l per hour is recommended to avoid the devastating complication of rapid correction of hyponatraemia, resulting in central pontine myelinolysis.

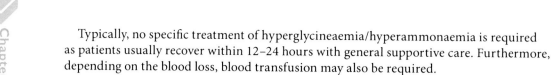

Typically, no specific treatment of hyperglycineaemia/hyperammonaemia is required as patients usually recover within 12–24 hours with general supportive care. Furthermore, depending on the blood loss, blood transfusion may also be required.

Q. **A 65-year-old man with recurrent acute urinary retention undergoes TURP. Prostate volume was 70 mL and during the procedure, it was noted that the prostate was extremely vascular. A large perforation of the surgical capsule was made on the left side, but otherwise the procedure was performed uneventfully. Post-operatively, in the recovery room, you are called because the catheter is draining dark red urine and the patient is pale, drowsy and looking unwell. HR is noted to be 120/min and BP = 80/55 mm Hg. How will you manage this patient?**

A. I would consider this a urological emergency and see the patient immediately, myself, without delay, as I suspect that he may have uncontrolled haemorrhage after TURP.

Normally 2%–5% of patients require blood transfusion after TURP and although venous ooze usually settles with conservative management, arterial bleeding may be present and necessitate early return to theatre. Importantly, several manoeuvres described below often need to be performed in quick succession or simultaneously and early help should be enlisted from HDU/ITU.

Initially, using basic principles of Advanced Trauma and Life Support (ATLS), I would resuscitate this patient, with the close involvement of my HDU/ITU anaesthetic colleagues. I would administer 100% high flow oxygen and give good analgesia. In addition, I would draw blood to check the full blood count (FBC) (Hb), clotting, urea and electrolytes (U+E) (Creatinine) and cross-match four units of blood.

Urologically, I would first check to see if the catheter is blocked and that the irrigation is running adequately. If clot retention is present, I would immediately perform a bladder washout, to remove all clots. If this does not improve the situation, or clot retention is not present, I would inflate the catheter balloon to 50 mL and maintain in-line traction with the irrigation running on maximum flow. There is no recognised time limit for traction on the catheter, although clearly, the longer this is applied, in some cases many hours, the higher is the risk of future contracture due to bladder neck ischaemia. I usually apply traction for 20–30 minutes and release for 5 minutes. Traction can then be reapplied at a later stage if further bleeding occurs.

In the meantime, I would give blood transfusion and correct any clotting abnormalities, as required. If the traction does not stabilise the situation and if there is ongoing bleeding, persistent hypotension, persistent clot retention or excessive blood transfusion requirement, the patient needs urgent return to theatre, which I will organise.

In theatre, initially, clot evacuation, endoscopic washout and careful diathermy to bleeding points is performed. In my practice, I perform a thorough washout with a resectoscope (26 or 28 Fr) and Ellick evacuator, using the diathermy loop to dislodge any organised clot (without current). Use of a bladder syringe attached to the end of the resectoscope can aid the evacuation of clot resistant to washout with the Ellick evacuator. If arterial bleeding is present, it can be difficult to detect in the presence of hypotension. Careful observation with low pressure irrigation can sometimes help.

If there is ongoing bleeding despite this, then the patient needs open surgical exploration and packing of the prostatic fossa.

Alternatively, if facilities are available, super-selective internal iliac artery embolisation may be performed. The procedure can be performed under local anaesthesia and may be a safer option in frail elderly patients.

Q. **How do you perform open surgical exploration of the prostatic fossa?**
A. In my practice, I perform a Pfannenstiel incision and the bladder is opened to pack the prostatic fossa (around the urethral catheter) with swabs through a transvesical approach.

The packs are left in place for 48 hours to tamponade any bleeding points and subsequently removed in theatre, with the definitive closure of the anterior abdominal wall.

SEPSIS FOLLOWING TRANSRECTAL ULTRASOUND (TRUS) BIOPSY

Q. **A fit and healthy 65-year-old man has TRUS-guided prostate biopsy (TRUS-Bx) for a raised prostate-specific antigen (PSA). He had been given prophylactic 120 mg gentamicin (IV) and 500 mg metronidazole (PR), and subsequently started a 5-day course of 500 mg bd ciprofloxacin (PO). Then 36 hours later, the urology clinical nurse specialist is contacted by the patient's wife, as he has developed severe flu-like symptoms. What advice do you give the urology clinical nurse specialist?**

A. I would consider this a urological emergency and advise the urology clinical nurse specialist that I will contact the patient immediately, myself, without delay, advising him to attend accident and emergency urgently, where I would arrange to see him personally. I would strongly suspect that this patient has developed sepsis following TRUS-Bx.

Q. **What is systemic inflammatory response syndrome – SIRS?**

A. Response of the body to a variety of infectious (sepsis) or non-infectious (burns, pancreatitis) stimuli. Two of the criteria listed in Table 7.2 are required.

Table 7.2 Criteria for diagnosis of systemic inflammatory response syndrome

Temperature	>38°C or <36°C
HR	>90/min
RR	>20/min or p_aCO_2 <32 mm Hg (<4.3 kPa) or need for mechanical ventilation
WCC	<4 or >12

Q. **How do you define sepsis, severe sepsis, septic shock and refractory septic shock?**

A. The definitions are stated in Table 7.3.

Table 7.3 Definitions of sepsis, severe sepsis, septic shock and refractory septic shock

Term	Definition
Sepsis	Proven infection causing SIRS.
Severe sepsis	Sepsis associated with organ dysfunction, hypoperfusion or hypotension. Hypoperfusion and perfusion abnormalities may include but are not limited to lactic acidosis, oliguria or an acute alteration of mental status.
Septic shock	Sepsis with hypotension despite fluid resuscitation along with the presence of perfusion abnormalities that may include, but are not limited to lactic acidosis, oliguria, or an acute alteration in mental status.
Refractory septic shock	Septic shock lasting >1 hour, resistant to fluid resuscitation or pharmacological intervention.

Q. **How would you initially manage this patient?**

A. I would consider this a urological emergency and see the patient myself, without delay. Based on international guidelines for surviving sepsis, on arrival, I would resuscitate the patient according to the sepsis 6 care bundle protocol used in my hospital (Table 7.4).

Table 7.4 Components of the sepsis 6 care bundle protocol

Component	Notes
100% oxygen	I would give 15 L/min via facemask with reservoir bag unless oxygen restriction necessary (e.g. in chronic CO_2 retention aim for an SaO_2 of 88%–92%).
IV fluid bolus	I would give a 500–1000 mL bolus of Hartmann's through a large bore Venflon. Larger bolus may be required, e.g. if systolic BP less than 90 or lactate greater than 4, consider 1500–2000 mL.
Blood cultures	I would take blood cultures as per hospital guidelines.
IV antibiotics	I would administer as per hospital guidelines, in my practice to include gentamicin (3–5 mg/kg), metronidazole and a third-generation cephalosporin.
Lactate + bloods	I would take lactate on arterial or venous sample. I would also request FBC, U&E, LFT, clotting (INR and APTT) and glucose if not yet done. I would also consider blood transfusion if Hb less than 7 (or above this with co-morbidities).
Monitor urine output	Consider catheter. Monitor output hourly. Dip urine and send midstream specimen of urine (MSU)/catheter specimen urine (CSU).

In addition to sepsis 6 care bundle protocol, I would contact my HDU/ITU anaesthetic colleagues and involve them early in the multidisciplinary management of this patient, as I am conscious of the high morbidity and mortality risk from this condition. If he is very unwell, he may need invasive monitoring or pharmacological support in the HDU/ITU setting.

Q. What are the most common organisms?

A. The most likely organisms would include gram-negative and anaerobic organisms, such as *Escherichia coli, Klebsiella, Pseudomonas, Enterococci* and *Bacteroides*.

PENILE FRACTURE

Q. A 34-year-old man presents with acute penile pain and swelling following sexual intercourse. He says he heard a 'cracking' sound during coitus and there was immediate detumescence. What is the likely diagnosis?

A. Penile fracture.

Q. Anatomically, what actually gets 'fractured' in this condition?

A. A penile fracture involves a full-thickness tear of the tunica albuginea of the penis. However, it may also involve the urethra in approximately 10% of cases. During erection, the thickness of the tunica albuginea typically reduces from 2 to 0.25 mm, predisposing the penis to injury, either from bending or buckling. The ventral tunica albuginea is the thinnest area and penile fractures are commonly located in this area.

Q. How do you diagnose this condition?

A. It is actually a clinical diagnosis based on the history and examination findings. However, I am aware that additional investigations can help with confirming the diagnosis and locating the site of the fracture which helps with surgical planning:

- Penile ultrasound is non-invasive and easily available. Ultrasonography can detect the site of the tunical tear and overlying haematoma.
- Magnetic resonance imaging (MRI) is an accurate pre-operative investigation and can detect even small tears of the tunica albuginea. Although difficult to perform in the emergency setting, it can be used when there is diagnostic doubt.
- Cavernosography is an invasive procedure rarely used and has potential side effects including reaction to contrast, priapism and risk of corporal fibrosis from extravasated contrast material.

Q. How do you exclude a urethral injury?

A. Clinical features suggesting urethral injury include blood at urethral meatus, haematuria and an inability to pass urine, following the injury. An on-table retrograde urethrogram should be performed if urethral injury cannot be excluded.

Q. What is the management of penile fracture?

A. I would consider penile fracture as a urological emergency and see the patient myself, without delay. Early surgical exploration and repair of the tunica albuginea is considered the treatment of choice. Conservative treatment is associated with high incidence of penile fibrosis, erectile dysfunction and penile curvature.

Q. Outline the principles of surgical repair.

A. The surgical approach depends on the site of the fracture and the experience of the surgeon. Surgical exploration can be performed by degloving the penis using a circum-coronal incision together with a circumcision.

Alternatively a longitudinal peno-scrotal incision avoids the need for degloving and circumcision and provides exposure to the urethra and corpus cavernosum. Once the haematoma overlying the fracture has been evacuated and the defect in the tunica albuginea identified, the defect should be repaired using interrupted absorbable sutures, either 0 PDS or 2/0 PDS. If there is a concomitant urethral injury, then 4/0 absorbable sutures are used to repair the defect over a urethral catheter. Depending on the size of the urethral disruption, a pericatheter urethrogram can be performed before removing the catheter.

REFERENCES

1. Li CY, Zaman F, Minhas S. Testicular torsion and acute testicular pain. In: *Urological Emergencies in Hospital Medicine* (eds. Shergill IS, Arya, M, Patel HR, Gill IS), pp. 1–9. London: Quay Books; 2007.
2. https://www.baus.org.uk/_userfiles/pages/files/Patients/Leaflets/Torsion%20of%20testis.pdf
3. Mebust WK et al. Transurethral prostatectomy: Immediate and postoperative complications. A cooperative study of 13 participating institutions evaluating 3,885 patients. *J Urol* 1989; 141: 243–247.
4. Pickard R et al. The management of men with acute urinary retention. National Prostatectomy Audit Steering Group. *BJU* 1998; 81: 712–720.

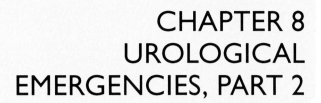

CHAPTER 8
UROLOGICAL
EMERGENCIES, PART 2

Genitourinary trauma and urethral stricture

Davendra M Sharma, Iqbal S Shergill and Manit Arya

Contents

RENAL TRAUMA

Q. **A 26-year-old motorcyclist, travelling at 20 mph, collides with a car. The motorcyclist is thrown from his bike. You are called to accident and emergency (A&E) because he complains of left flank pain. His pulse is 90 beats/minute, blood pressure (BP) 120/80 mm Hg, respiratory rate (RR) 16, oxygen saturation 99%. How would you assess this patient?**

A. As with all trauma cases, advanced trauma life support (ATLS) principles are strictly followed. It is important to have a multidisciplinary approach, consulting with emergency, orthopaedic, general surgical and any other speciality doctors if necessary (standard answer to trauma question).

Traumatic injuries remain an important cause of mortality and morbidity in the civilian population. Trauma may be generally classified as due to blunt or penetrating injury. Blunt trauma, which is much more common in the United Kingdom, may result in significant genitourinary injury. Urologists are expected to understand the principles of trauma management and safely manage these patients.

Q. **Your colleagues have 'cleared' this patient of other major injuries. What specific information would you like to have to assess him urologically?**

A. I would take a focussed history and relevant examination (standard answer). It is important to elucidate the following points from the history:

1. The mechanism of injury
2. Whether there is any previous urological or renal history
3. Whether the patient has noticed any blood in the urine

Q. What examination findings are important?

A.

- Extent and location of any bruising and tenderness.
- Haematuria (macroscopic in adults or dipstick/macroscopic in children) – particularly in first sample following accident. *I am aware that microscopic analysis (at least five red blood cells per high power field) is more reliable in assessing the extent of haemorrhage than dipstick testing. However, this is very rarely used in daily clinical practice.*
- Blood pressure (BP) – has there been a significant drop in BP, i.e. systolic <90 mm Hg, at any time since the accident?

Q. This patient has dipstick haematuria. What would you do?

A. If the patient has had a measured (even single) drop in his systolic BP (<90 mm Hg), then an urgent contrast spiral computed tomography (CT) scan is arranged. If there is no significant drop in BP recorded, the patient is admitted for analgesia, 24 hours of observation and repeat full blood count (FBC).

Q. In a stable adult patient with dipstick haematuria, are there any factors that would lower your threshold for imaging, and why?

A. Yes. If the mechanism of injury is that of a rapid deceleration injury or a fall from a significant height, imaging is recommended. These patients may have a pelviureteric junction (PUJ) disruption or vascular injury which may not result in haematuria or a fall in BP. In fact haematuria (microscopic and macroscopic) may be absent in up to 40% of renal injuries and 25% of pedicle injuries.

Q. What are the indications for imaging (CT with contrast) in a *stable* patient following renal trauma as suggested by the European Association of Urology (EAU)?

A.

- Penetrating trauma
- Deceleration injuries (or other 'significant' mechanism of injury, e.g. fall from a considerable height)
- Blunt trauma in adults associated with a systolic BP <90 mm Hg at any time following the injury
- Blunt trauma in adults associated with frank haematuria (thus blunt trauma associated with dipstick/microscopic haematuria in adults is not an indication for imaging providing it is not a deceleration injury and BP has been stable)
- Blunt trauma in children associated with dipstick/microscopic or frank haematuria – in children, a lower threshold for imaging (ideally spiral CT with contrast) is required as hypotension is a late manifestation of hypovolaemia

Q. What are the objectives of radiographic imaging in renal trauma and which modality best delivers these objectives?

A.

1. Accurately stage the injury
2. Document contralateral renal function
3. Recognise pre-existing renal pathology
4. Identify injuries to other organs

A contrast spiral CT scan is superior to all other forms of imaging in trauma. As well as delivering the objectives above, it is quick and now familiar to most surgeons. Ultrasound resolution is inferior to CT but it may be useful in the follow-up of renal injury.

Q. How is the CT scan performed and why?

A. Spiral CT scan with contrast:

1. *Arterial and/or portal venous phase* – Demonstrates vascular and parenchymal injury as well as haematoma
2. *Delayed images (10–20 minutes)* – PUJ or collecting system injury. May be omitted if, on the early phase scan, the kidneys are normal, and there is no perinephric, retroperitoneal, pelvic or perivesical fluid present.

Q. **What do Figures 8.1 and 8.2 show? How would you stage the injury and what are the different grades? What are the essential components of the staging system?**

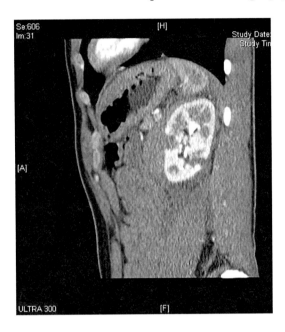

Figure 8.1 Sagittal contrast CT demonstrating grade 3 renal trauma.

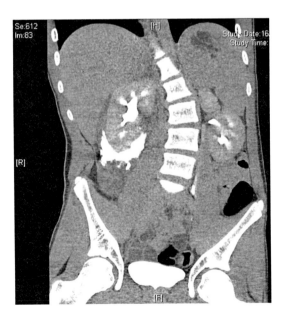

Figure 8.2 Coronal contrast CT demonstrating grade 4 renal trauma.

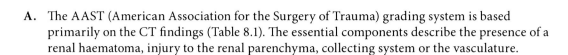

A. The AAST (American Association for the Surgery of Trauma) grading system is based primarily on the CT findings (Table 8.1). The essential components describe the presence of a renal haematoma, injury to the renal parenchyma, collecting system or the vasculature.

Table 8.1 The American Association for the Surgery of Trauma (AAST) renal trauma severity scale

Grade (AAST)	Type	Description
I	Contusion	
	Haematoma	Subcapsular, not expanding with no parenchymal laceration
II	Haematoma	Not expanding perirenal haematoma confined to renal retroperitoneum
	Laceration	<1 cm parenchymal depth of renal cortex with no urinary extravasation
III	Laceration	>1 cm parenchymal depth of renal cortex with no urinary extravasation
IV	Laceration	Parenchymal laceration through corticomedullary junction extending into collecting system
	Vascular	Segmental renal artery or vein injury with contained haematoma, or partial vessel laceration, or vessel thrombosis
V	Laceration	Completely shattered kidney
	Vascular	Avulsion of renal pedicle or hilum which devascularises kidney

Q. What proportion of renal trauma is due to blunt trauma?

A. In the United Kingdom the majority (over 95%) of injuries are due to blunt trauma. In South Africa and territories affected by violent conflict, the incidence of penetrating trauma is much higher.

Q. You are called to theatre later that night by the on-call trauma team. Another blunt trauma patient was taken to the emergency theatre as he was not able to maintain his BP despite fluid boluses. No imaging was performed prior to laparotomy, which reveals normal viscera and no intraperitoneal blood. There is, however, a large left retroperitoneal haematoma. What is your next step?

A. Arrange a one-shot on-table intravenous urography (IVU).

Q. Why do a one-shot IVU and how would this be performed?

A. Most importantly, it shows whether there are two functioning kidneys. Delayed contrast excretion or extravasation may also be detected. A normal film may obviate the need for renal exploration.

A one-shot IVU depends on a rapid bolus administration of 2 mL/kg contrast (e.g. Omnipaque). A single portable plain abdominal x-ray is performed at 10 minutes. Fluoroscopy (C-arm) results in poor images and should be avoided.

Q. What are the absolute indications for exploring the kidney in trauma?

A.

1. Persistent life-threatening blood loss believed to stem from renal injury
2. Renal pedicle avulsion (grade 5 injury) which is suspected clinically, by imaging or by the observation of an expanding pulsatile retroperitoneal haematoma at laparotomy
3. Penetrating renal trauma (most cases)

Q. What are the principles to exploring a kidney in trauma?

A.

- A midline generous laparotomy incision from sternum to pubis.
- The small bowel is lifted out of the peritoneal cavity in order to expose the retroperitoneum.
- Incise peritoneum over aorta above the inferior mesenteric artery and dissect alongside it superiorly up to the left renal vein (if a large perirenal haematoma obscures the site for

this incision then make incision medial to inferior mesenteric vein). The left and right renal arteries are then easily identified. Vessel loops can then be placed around the renal artery and vein thus establishing early vascular control.

- The colon can now be reflected thus exposing the kidney (or haematoma).
- If nephrectomy is avoided then renal tissue is preserved by controlling bleeding and debriding all non-viable tissue.

Q. How would you deal with a non-expanding, non-pulsatile haematoma at laparotomy?
A. In this situation haematoma should be left alone. This is so as exploration increases the probability of loss of the kidney because of bleeding, which can be controlled only by nephrectomy.

Q. What proportion of patients suffering blunt trauma to the kidneys require surgical intervention?
A. Less than 5%.

Q. What is the role of angioembolisation?
A. Selective renal artery angioembolisation is increasingly used to successfully manage stable patients with haemorrhage following blunt and penetrating trauma.

Q. What are the potential complications of conservatively managed renal trauma and how are they managed?
A. *Early*:

- Secondary haemorrhage requiring radiological or surgical intervention.
- Urinary extravasation leading to urinoma (or if superimposed infection to perinephric abscess formation). Radiological drainage with or without internal stenting may be necessary.
- Infection, e.g. perinephric abscess or systemic sepsis.
- Vascular complications including arterio-venous fistula (AVF) or pseudoaneurysm formation.

Late:

- *Hypertension* – Re-evaluate to look for renal artery thrombosis, subcapsular haematoma, extensive fibrosis (Page kidney is hypertension due to scar formation) or AVF.
- *Renal insufficiency* – Follow-up DMSA scan to look for significant functional loss.
- Calculus formation and chronic pyelonephritis.

It is recommended that higher-grade renal injuries (4 and 5) are imaged by CT 48–72 hours after injury to look for complications such as secondary haemorrhage or urinoma formation.

Q. How are renovascular injuries managed?
A.

- *Arterial* – Irreversible damage ensues after 2–6 hours so most kidneys will not function following arterial injury. Reconstruction should be attempted in solitary kidneys, bilateral renal injury or if diagnosed very quickly. Incomplete injury, e.g. intimal flaps, can be managed conservatively. Segmental arterial injuries are managed with angioembolisation. Endovascular techniques are also described for main artery and branch injuries and may take the primary role in the future.

    Hypertension develops in a small subset of patients with major arterial injury – elective nephrectomy may be necessary in these cases.
- *Venous injuries are rare and difficult to identify* – Avulsion from the inferior vena cava (IVC) following blunt trauma requires urgent laparotomy, IVC repair and nephrectomy. The left renal vein may be tied leaving the kidney to drain from the gonadal and adrenal veins. Penetrating injuries should be repaired.

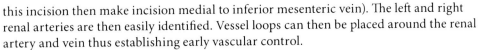

Q. **What does the image show in Figure 8.3?**

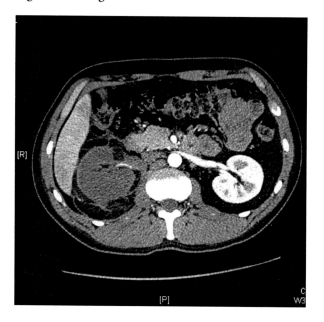

Figure 8.3

A. Figure 8.3 is a contrast CT scan (arterial phase) showing right arterial injury with absence of right nephrogram.

Q. **Figure 8.4 is an investigation of this previously discussed patient 3 months later. What does this demonstrate?**

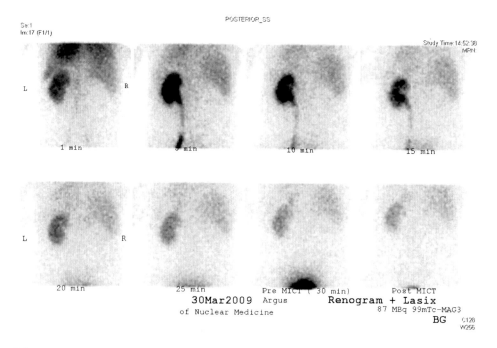

Figure 8.4

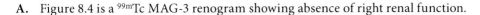

A. Figure 8.4 is a ^{99m}Tc MAG-3 renogram showing absence of right renal function.

Q. **Can you summarise the management of blunt renal trauma?**
A. I use the management algorithm in Figure 8.5, which is based on the EAU guidelines, for managing blunt renal trauma.

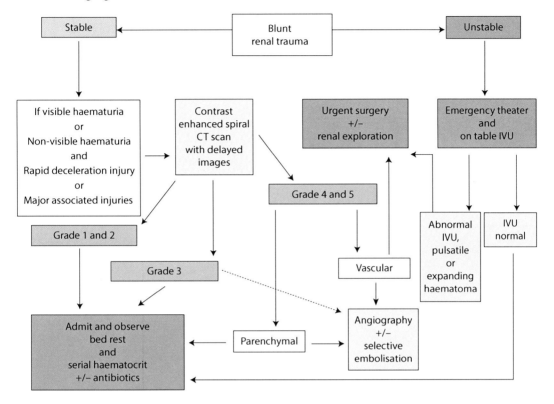

Figure 8.5 Management of blunt renal trauma in adults (EAU guidelines).

Q. **Can you summarise the management of penetrating renal trauma?**
A. I use the management algorithm in Figure 8.6, which is based on the EAU guidelines, for managing penetrating renal trauma.

URETERIC INJURY

Q. **You are called by the Gynaecology SpR on call. She is concerned about a patient who had an abdominal hysterectomy 2 days ago. The patient is unwell and complaining of left flank pain and a urological injury is suspected by the gynaecology team. What would you do initially?**
A. One must consider this a urological emergency and review the patient without delay. Bear in mind that a urological complication of gynaecological surgery may have occurred, and hence may have future medicolegal implications. On arrival, carefully review all the medical notes, especially the operation note, and speak personally to the gynaecological surgeon who performed the procedure, to establish

  - Indication for surgery (cancer versus benign aetiology)
  - Difficulties encountered at time of surgery (prolonged procedure, untoward bleeding, presence of adhesions)

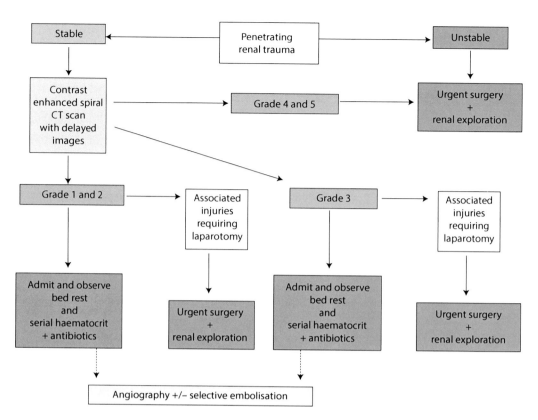

Figure 8.6 Management of penetrating renal trauma in adults (EAU guidelines).

- Past medical history, for endometriosis, previous abdominal surgeries and previous radiotherapy treatment

  Then take a focussed history, perform a physical examination and carry out necessary investigations.

Q. What features in the history and examination are you interested in?

A. First, characterise the pain (type, location, etc.) and note any previous urological history and the patient's co-morbidity.

An abdominal examination is necessary looking for scars, full bladder and loin tenderness/mass. Perform a bimanual vaginal examination with a chaperone if the patient can bear it (to look for a vesico-vaginal fistula).

The presence of a pyrexia and tachycardia should be noted as should the patient's BP. If a drain is present, what is it draining and how much? Is a catheter present? If so, what colour is the urine and how much is the urine output?

Q. Assessment reveals a stable but pyrexial patient with left loin tenderness and excess clear fluid from the drain. What investigations are necessary?

A.
- *Blood tests* – FBC, urea and electrolytes, C-reactive protein and Group & Save (G&S).
- Urine dipstick and midstream specimen of urine for culture (or catheter specimen urine (CSU) if catheter present).
- *Drain fluid* – Send for biochemical analysis (particularly urea and creatinine – creatinine levels >300 µmol/L will be urine if serum creatinine is normal).
- *Urgent CT-IVU* – To identify the injury and look for *another* concomitant injury.

A retrograde ureteropyelogram is very sensitive for detecting ureteric injury but may be

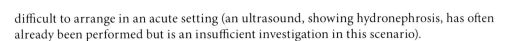

difficult to arrange in an acute setting (an ultrasound, showing hydronephrosis, has often already been performed but is an insufficient investigation in this scenario).

If a urological injury is suspected the patient should be transferred immediately to a urology ward.

Q. What potential injuries may have occurred?

A. Ureteric (unilateral or bilateral) or bladder or a combination of both.

Q. What does Figure 8.7 show?

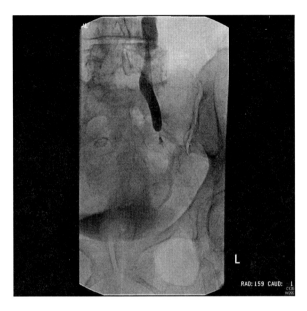

Figure 8.7

A. Figure 8.7 is an antegrade nephrostogram demonstrating a left ureteric stricture as a result of iatrogenic injury following gynaecological surgery.

Q. What are the management options? Are you aware of any staging systems for ureteric injury?

A. Management depends on the stage, location and timing of the injury, and the patient's general condition (Tables 8.2 and 8.3).

Table 8.2 Staging system and management options for ureteric injury

Grade of ureteric injury (AAST)	Injury	Management
I	Haematoma only	Conservative ± stent
II	Laceration <50% circumference	Stent ± suture
III	Laceration >50% circumference	Stent ± suture Ureteroureterostomy + stent
IV	Complete tear <2 cm of devascularisation	Ureteric reconstruction
V	Complete tear >2 cm of devascularisation	Ureteric reconstruction

Ideally, this patient should be taken back to theatre as soon as possible for cystoscopy (excludes associated bladder injury), bilateral retrograde studies (excludes injury to the contralateral ureter), an attempt at retrograde stenting or alternatively formal repair or reconstruction if necessary.

Table 8.3 Options for ureteric reconstruction

Location of injury	Reconstructive option
Upper ureter	Ureteroureterostomy Ureterocalycostomy Transureteroureterostomy
Mid ureter	Ureteroureterostomy Boari flap Transureteroureterostomy
Lower ureter	Ureteroureterostomy Direct reimplantation Psoas hitch Boari flap
Complete injury (e.g. avulsion)	Ileal interposition Renal autotransplantation

Traditionally, it has been suggested that if ureteric injury was diagnosed within a few days then, if open repair/reconstruction is needed, this should ideally be performed immediately. However, if the injury was discovered after approximately 7–14 days, then, if open repair/reconstruction is necessary, this should be delayed for at least 3 months (as this is generally thought to be the time of maximal oedema and inflammation). Currently, it is believed that an earlier repair can still give good results and that the time of diagnosis of the ureteric trauma is not so important.

Delayed repair is certainly essential if the patient is unwell or there are any contraindications for re-operation, e.g. infected urinoma at site of injury. In these cases, nephrostomy drainage should be arranged. A careful attempt at antegrade stenting can be tried in expert centres (Figure 8.8).

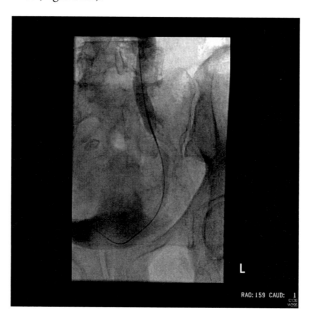

Figure 8.8 Antegrade guidewire prior to stenting across iatrogenic ureteric stricture.

Q. What basic principles govern ureteric reconstruction?
A.

1. Mobilization of the ureter preserving the adventitia
2. Debridement of non-viable tissue

3. Spatulation
4. Tension-free mucosa to mucosa anastomosis with fine absorbable sutures (5 or 6 O)
5. An internal ureteric stent and separate drain placed near site of anastomosis

Omental interposition to separate the repair from associated intra-abdominal injuries or suture lines is recommended.

A bladder catheter should be inserted to limit stent reflux.

Q. How would you manage the patient post-operatively?
A. Remove the bladder catheter 2 days post-operatively. The drain can also be removed at day 2 if output is minimal. The ureteric stent is removed at 6 weeks. A dynamic renogram and IVU are arranged at 3 months (or earlier if the patient has worrying symptoms).

Q. How do missed ureteric injuries present?
A. Missed ureteric injuries are relatively common. They may present with ureteric obstruction (stricturing), urinoma, abscess formation, or fistulation. Ureteric obstruction can result in nephron loss, stones, infection and pain.

Q. What is the likely outcome of ureteric injuries?
A. The outcome of ureteric reconstruction is usually favourable if the principles outlined above are adhered to. Ureteric reflux may result from reconstruction but this is not felt to be an important problem in the adult patient.

Q. What is the role of the interventional radiologist in ureteric injury and reconstruction?
A. The interventional radiologist has several key roles:

- Relieving renal obstruction by percutaneous nephrostomy.
- Performing nephrostoureterograms which are essential in planning definitive management.
- Antegrade stenting with or without retrograde assistance ('rendezvous procedure') may be definitive in partial or short ureteric defects although this requires careful follow-up to look for ureteric stricturing.
- Balloon dilatation of ureteric strictures may be successful in 50% of cases.

Q. What is the role of ureteroscopy in managing ureteric strictures?
A. Short ureteric strictures can be managed by incision $\pm$ balloon dilatation and stenting. Success rates have been quoted at 75%. Endoscopic treatment of strictures of 2 cm or greater have high failure rates. Longer-term stents are being evaluated and may become established as an option in the future in well-selected patients.

Q. Is there a role for laparoscopy in ureteric reconstruction?
A. Yes, experienced laparoscopists have successfully reconstructed ureteric injuries and this may in the future be the surgical approach of choice.

BLADDER TRAUMA

Q. A 36-year-old male presents to A&E with acute lower abdominal pain. He was punched in the abdomen having had several pints of beer. He is stable but has been referred to you because of pain and difficulty voiding. What findings make you suspicious of urological injury?
A. The classic triad of lower abdominal pain, inability to void, and frank haematuria with a history of direct trauma to a full bladder suggest a bladder perforation.

(Note that in spinal cord injury/spina bifida patients who have augmented bladders spontaneous bladder rupture can occur without significant pain; the presenting features may be those of sepsis or vague symptoms of non-specific illness.)

Q. What are the common causes of bladder injury?
A. Pelvic fractures, blunt or penetrating trauma to a distended bladder, and iatrogenic causes (associated with lower abdominal and pelvic and endoscopic surgery).

Q. What percentage of pelvic fractures is associated with a bladder injury?
A. Approximately 5%–6%. However around 80% of bladder injuries are due to pelvic fractures.

Q. How would you assess this patient?
A. As with all trauma cases, ATLS principles guide management. It is important to have a multidisciplinary approach, consulting with emergency and general surgical colleagues if necessary.

Q. What specific investigation would you request?
A. In a stable patient, I would request a stress (retrograde) cystogram.

Q. Is there any other investigation that could be requested and might yield more information?
A. Yes, a CT stress (retrograde) cystogram.

Q. How is a stress (retrograde) cystogram performed?
A. In the absence of urethral trauma, the bladder is catheterised and filled to capacity by gravity with diluted (50:50) water-soluble contrast. At least 300 mL must be infused in adults in order to distend the bladder and adequately diagnose a perforation (otherwise blood clot or small bowel/omentum may fill the perforation and prevent extravasation of contrast). Anterior-posterior and post-drainage films are obtained. The post-drainage films are particularly important for diagnosing a posterior bladder perforation, which may be obscured by a bladder filled with contrast.

Q. Why not do an IVU and wait for the cystographic phase?
A. The bladder is a low-pressure highly compliant organ. Intravesical pressure has to be raised by adequate bladder distension (at least 300 mL in adults) or the injury may easily be missed.

Q. What classification do you use for bladder injuries?
A.

- Bladder contusion
- Intraperitoneal rupture (30%–40%)
- Extraperitoneal rupture (50%–60%)
- Combined intra- and extraperitoneal ruptures (5%–10%)

Q. What does the (CT retrograde) cystogram in Figure 8.9 show and how would you manage it?

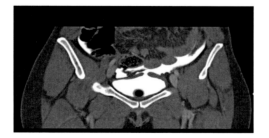

Figure 8.9

A. Figure 8.9 is a CT (retrograde) cystogram showing an intraperitoneal bladder perforation. Contrast is seen leaking into the peritoneal cavity (note that in *extraperitoneal* bladder perforation contrast only extravasates into the surrounding perivesical space).

The patient should be resuscitated and put on broad-spectrum antibiotics. *Intraperitoneal perforations require surgical repair* and thus a lower midline laparotomy is performed to inspect the viscera and close the bladder rupture with absorbable sutures. A urethral catheter (±suprapubic catheter) and intra-abdominal drain should be placed.

Q. How would you manage extraperitoneal ruptures?

A. *Generally, extraperitoneal ruptures do not require surgical repair.* They are managed with a urethral catheter on free drainage for 10–14 days and antibiotics. A stress (retrograde) cystogram is then performed to ensure healing has occurred.

Q. Are there any indications to proceed with surgical repair in *extraperitoneal* ruptures?

A. Yes.

1. Failure of catheter to drain – e.g. clot obstruction
2. Persistent extravasation
3. Bladder neck injury
4. Patients undergoing internal fixation for pelvic fracture or laparotomy for other viscus repair (e.g. bowel, rectum, vagina) can have concurrent bladder repair
5. Bone spike puncturing bladder on imaging

Q. What complications may be seen after missed bladder perforation injury?

A. Intraperitoneal urinary extravasation can result in urinary ascites, peritonitis, ileus and systemic sepsis.

Injuries involving the bladder neck can result in incontinence or stricture. Recto-/ colovesical fistulae and vesicovaginal fistulae may also occur.

Q. How would you manage a penetrating injury to the bladder?

A. Operative exploration, closure, bladder drainage and antibiotics. Careful attention should be paid to the posterior bladder wall, the ureters and neighbouring viscera.

URETHRAL TRAUMA

Q. What constitutes the anterior and posterior urethra and how are they most commonly injured?

A.

- Anterior urethra (bulbar and penile and navicular) – straddle/fall astride mechanism is the most common cause of injury, which usually results in bulbar urethral damage. Penile fracture, obviously affecting the penile urethra, is another cause.
- Posterior urethra (prostatic and membranous) – pelvic fracture (due to road traffic accidents or fall from heights) is the cause of injury in virtually all cases (of blunt trauma). Complete injury occurs due to the shearing effects of bone disruption. Thus the prostate, attached to the puboprostatic ligaments, moves in one direction and the membranous urethra, fixed in the urogenital diaphragm, moves in another. Partial injury results from ligamentous avulsion.

Q. What is the AAST classification of urethral injuries?

A. The AAST classification is demonstrated in Table 8.4.

Table 8.4 The American Association for the Surgery of Trauma (AAST) urethral trauma severity scale

Group	Type	Description
I	Contusion	Blood at urethral meatus; normal urethrogram
2	Stretch injury	Elongation of the urethra without extravasation on urethrography
3	Partial disruption	Extravasation of contrast at injury site with contrast visualised in the bladder
4	Complete disruption	Extravasation of contrast at injury site without visualisation in the bladder; <2 cm urethral separation
5	Complete disruption	Complete transaction with >2 cm urethral separation, or extension into the prostate or vagina

Q. What is the 'butterfly' pattern of perineal bruising following anterior urethral injury?

A. In order to explain this one must understand the fascial layers of the scrotum and anterior abdominal wall.

In the anterior abdominal wall the subcutaneous fatty layer is known as Camper's fascia. Scarpa's fascia lies deep to this. Scarpa's fascia is attached to the coracoclavicular ligaments superiorly. Inferiorly, it fuses with the deep fascia of the thigh (fascia lata) 1 cm below the inguinal ligament. Medially, Scarpa's fascia is continuous with Colles' fascia in the perineum. Colles' fascia attaches to the posterior edge of the urogenital diaphragm and perineal body and the inferior ischiopubic rami. Colles' fascia is continuous with the dartos fascia of the penis and scrotum.

In the penis, Buck's fascia lies beneath the dartos fascia (which as already mentioned is continuous with Colles' fascia). Buck's fascia is attached distally to the base of glans (coronal sulcus) and laterally to pubic rami, ischial spines and tuberosities.

If the anterior urethra has ruptured but Buck's fascia is intact, e.g. as may occur in a penile fracture, then urine and haematoma are confined in a sleeve-like or tubular configuration along the length of the penis.

If, however, Buck's fascia is breached or ruptured or the bulbar urethra is injured, e.g. as may occur in a straddle injury to the bulbar urethra, blood and urine extravasation are limited by the attachments of Colles' fascia, i.e. their spread is limited by the fusions of Colles' fascia to the ischiopubic rami laterally and to the posterior edge of the urogenital diaphragm and perineal body posteriorly – the subsequent bruising is therefore butterfly shaped. Bruising and urine can also travel up the anterior abdominal wall beneath Scarpa's fascia to the clavicles (coracoclavicular ligaments) but extravasation will not extend down the leg or into the buttock.

A posterior urethral injury will only be associated with a butterfly distribution of bruising if the pelvic fracture has resulted in urethral disruption with the tear extending below the urogenital diaphragm into the bulbar urethra.

Q. A 40-year-old farmer is brought into A&E after being run over by a tractor. He is resuscitated by the trauma team and is now stable. He has a pelvic fracture. What urological injuries could this patient have and how might they present?

A.

- Bladder injury characterised by suprapubic pain, inability to void, frank haematuria
- Urethral injury characterised by blood at external meatus (present in 37%–93% of patients with posterior urethral injury and at least 75% of those with anterior urethral injury), pain or inability to void, palpable bladder (latter two suggest urethral disruption)

Q. How would you assess the patient?

A. As with all trauma cases, ATLS principles guide management. It is important to have a multidisciplinary approach, consulting with emergency, orthopaedic and general surgical colleagues if necessary. The patient should be questioned about previous urological problems.

Positive examination findings include

- Blood at the penile meatus.
- Bruising in the perineum.
- Distended bladder on palpation.
- Digital rectal examination (DRE) may demonstrate a pelvic haematoma (soft and boggy swelling) or blood on the glove (latter suggests a rectal injury, which is associated in 5% of cases of pelvic fracture). The classically described 'high riding prostate' (which occurs as a result of prostate-membranous urethral disruption with the subsequent haematoma pushing up the prostate) can be difficult to feel due to the associated pelvic haematoma.

Q. The previously discussed patient with a pelvic fracture has blood at the meatus, perineal bruising and a large pelvic haematoma on rectal examination. There is no blood on the glove after DRE. What is the likely diagnosis?

A. This is typical of a posterior urethral distraction injury (pelvic fracture urethral distraction defect [PFUDD]) usually occurring between the prostatic and membranous urethra. As mentioned earlier, the injury occurs due to the severe shearing effects of bone disruption. Thus the prostate, attached to the puboprostatic ligaments, moves in one direction and the membranous urethra, fixed in the urogenital diaphragm, moves in another.

Q. How commonly are pelvic fractures associated with urethral injury?

A. Approximately 3%–25% of pelvic fractures are associated with urethral injury. The incidence of double injuries involving the urethra and bladder is 10%–20%.

Q. What investigation would you do?

A. Immediate retrograde urethrogram.

Note: *In an unstable patient, one careful attempt can be made to pass a urethral catheter. If there is any resistance a suprapubic catheter is inserted (either via ultrasound scan [USS] guidance or via a formal open approach) and a retrograde urethrogram performed later. It is extremely unlikely that gentle passage of a urethral catheter would convert a partial injury into a complete injury.*

Q. How is the urethrogram performed?

A.

- I am aware that in a normal situation, the patient should be positioned in a 30% oblique position with bottom leg flexed at hip and knee, but in this pelvic trauma case, as the hips and knees may not be able to be flexed, I would perform supine with anterior-posterior views, with an option to use the C-arm obliquely, to make sure that extravasation from the bulbar urethra is not masked. This is because in the AP views, the bulbar urethra is superimposed upon itself.
- A 12F catheter is placed in the fossa navicularis and the balloon inflated with 2 mL water to create a seal preventing leakage of contrast.
- Then 20–30 mL of full-strength water-soluble contrast is injected slowly into the urethra using fluoroscopic guidance. If fluoroscopy is not available, then a series of plain x-rays using 10 mL aliquots each time gives sufficient information.

Q. How would you treat a partial urethral injury?

A. Partial urethral injuries can be managed with a suprapubic catheter (SPC) or urethral catheter for 4 weeks. If an SPC is *in situ*, voiding cystourethrography is then performed. If there is neither contrast extravasation nor stricturing, the SPC can be safely removed and normal voiding can be re-established.

If a urethral catheter is *in situ* a urethrogram can be performed via a 6 Fr nasogastric (NG) tube inserted alongside the urethral catheter. Contrast can then be passed down the NG tube to exclude extravasation (*one uses the same method to perform a retrograde urethrogram following urethroplasty when the urethral catheter is* in situ).

Q. **What does the antegrade urethrogram in Figure 8.10 show?**

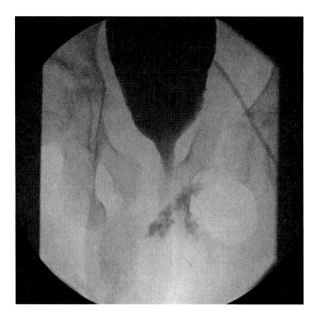

Figure 8.10

A. Figure 8.10 shows an antegrade urethrogram demonstrating complete disruption of the posterior urethra with extravasation of contrast due to a pelvic fracture urethral distraction injury. This occurs in 65% of urethral injuries. Partial injuries make up the remaining 35%.

Q. **How would you manage the above patient initially?**
A. SPC drainage of the bladder to minimise urinary extravasation and broad-spectrum antibiotics.

Q. **What difficulties might be anticipated in performing the suprapubic puncture?**
A. The bladder may not be palpable. The pelvic haematoma can cause significant distortion of the anatomy and difficulty identifying the normal tissue planes. Thus one must never insert an SPC blindly in this situation. Ultrasound can be used to guide the puncture, otherwise open cystotomy is recommended.

Q. **On inserting the SPC into the bladder via USS guidance, the urine is found to be blood stained. What do you suspect and how will you manage this?**
A. A combined urethral and bladder injury. A cystogram should be performed via the SPC and the bladder injury dealt with accordingly.

Q. **What is the next step in the management of the PFUDD following an antegrade urethrogram?**
A. *A more detailed urethrogram* – the up-and-downogram (i.e. simultaneous retrograde and antegrade urethrogram) – is performed to assess the site, severity and length of the urethral defect.

   Definitive reconstruction is performed between 3 and 6 months post-injury (deferred treatment).

Q. **Why wait prior the reconstruction?**
A.
   1. To allow the patient to recover from major trauma.

2. To allow the pelvic haematoma and any urinary extravasation to resolve. This reduces the length of the defect, and allows the tissue planes to return to normal.

Q. What operation is used to re-establish urethral continuity (following the above PFUDD) and what steps can be used to bridge the urethral defect?

A. Bulbo-prostatic anastomotic (BPA) urethroplasty via a perineal approach. It is sometimes necessary to use a combined abdominal and perineal approach.

The steps used to deal with the defect include bulbar urethral mobilisation and if necessary, midline separation of the corporal bodies, inferior pubectomy, and supracorporal urethral rerouting. Defects up to 7 cm can be dealt with using these manoeuvres in sequence.

Q. What are the approximate success rates for deferred treatment and how is the outcome of urethral reconstruction following pelvic fracture judged?

A. The success rate of deferred BPA approaches 95%. The outcome is judged by observing restricture rates (<10%), incontinence (5%) and erectile dysfunction (ED) (20%).

Q. Is there a role of 'early' urethral realignment following PFUDD?

A. Early realignment is performed either by open or endoscopic surgery. Immediate open repair is associated with a high incidence of strictures (70%), incontinence (20%) and ED (44%).

Although the incidence of incontinence and ED is reported to be less with endoscopic realignment, there are high restricture rates requiring multiple follow-up procedures. This is an acceptable initial treatment if carried out expeditiously.

Due to the relatively poor outcomes of early surgical realignment, deferred repair is preferred in specialist centres in the United Kingdom.

The only indications for early realignment are concomitant bladder neck or rectal injury. These injuries require immediate open exploration and repair. Bladder neck injury combined with PFUDD will result in incontinence in most cases so repair is essential. Early realignment is recommended in these cases.

Q. How are fall astride injuries managed?

A. The principles are similar to the management of PFUDDs. However, the injury differs in that it is due to a crushing force on the bulbar (anterior) urethra which results in an obliterative stricture and loss of normal urethral length. Deferred treatment is again recommended with initial suprapubic diversion to minimise extravasation, antibiotics to minimise infection and abscess formation, and time to allow bruising and haematoma to resolve. After 3 months stricture excision and primary anastomosis can be performed.

GENITAL TRAUMA

Q. A 21-year-old university student is kicked in the groin during an intercollegiate football match. He is brought to hospital because he has a swollen painful scrotum. He is otherwise well. How would you assess this patient and what injuries may have been sustained?

A. He should have a focussed history and examination. It is important to rule out the possibility of other major injuries prior to concentrating on the genitalia. The possible injuries include scrotal bruising with localised haematoma formation, haematocele, testicular, epididymal and spermatic cord injury (including torsion).

Q. How may testicular injuries be classified?

A. Tunica albuginea disruption (testicular rupture) or contained intratesticular haematoma or testicular dislocation.

Q. Is there any role for imaging?

A. Yes. An adequate physical examination is often difficult due to the presence of bruising, swelling, haematoma and pain. Scrotal ultrasound is the imaging method of choice for detecting intrascrotal injury – the primary goal being to assess the integrity (intact tunica albuginea) and vascularity of the testis. It has a specificity of 75% and a sensitivity of 64% in detecting testis rupture (although the sensitivity may be higher in more experienced hands). A combination of clinical and ultrasound findings will guide management.

Q. What may be seen on ultrasound of an injured testis?

A. Disruption of the tunica albuginea may be detected. However, more commonly the diagnosis is made by a combination of findings including the presence of a haematocele, a contour abnormality of the testis indicating disruption of the tunica albuginea and heterogenous echotexture of the testis (the latter suggestive of associated parenchymal bleeding).

Q. What does this intraoperative scrotal image in Figure 8.11 show?

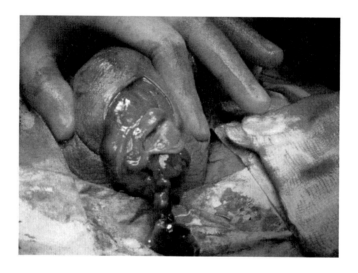

Figure 8.11

A. Figure 8.11 shows testicular rupture.

Q. How would you manage this patient?

A. This patient should be counselled for urgent scrotal exploration. Extruded or necrotic seminiferous tubules should be debrided and the tunica albuginea closed with fine (4-0) absorbable sutures. A small drain may be left to drain dependently and the patient put on broad-spectrum antibiotics for 7 days. For reproductive, endocrine and psychological reasons, every effort should be made to preserve the testis but in the presence of gross injury, orchidectomy should be performed.

Q. Is there a role for delayed (>48 hours) scrotal exploration?

A. Studies have shown that testicular salvage after blunt trauma decreased from 80% to 30% if exploration was delayed by more than 3 days.

Q. **How would you manage a haematocele?**

A. Prompt drainage is recommended for large haematoceles to prevent infection, testicular ischaemia, and prolonged pain. Scrotal haematomas, bruising and smaller haematoceles can be treated conservatively with ice, rest and elevation.

Q. **How does the management of bilateral testicular injury differ?**

A. The consequences include loss of fertility, hypogonadism and significant psychosexual issues. Sperm banking should be considered in the early post-injury phase and testosterone levels monitored.

URETHRAL STRICTURE

Q. **What is the blood supply of the urethra?**

A. The blood supply to the urethra is derived from the internal pudendal branch of the internal iliac artery. It enters the perineum via the pudendal canal (of Alcock) and terminates in the common penile artery which provides three branches that supply the structures of the penis. The urethra gets a generous blood supply from the bulbourethral and dorsal penile branches which arborise in the glans penis.

Q. **A previously well 24-year-old man is referred to you with a history of slow urinary stream. He has recently been treated for a urinary tract infection but is otherwise well. What is the most likely cause of this patient's problems?**

A. A urethral stricture. The differential diagnosis includes bladder neck obstruction, neuropathic bladder and late presentation of posterior urethral valves.

Q. **What is the aetiology of urethral strictures?**

A.

1. Posterior urethral strictures (prostatic and membranous urethra) are due to a fibrotic process that narrows the lumen and most commonly these are due to trauma such as a PFUDD or surgery, e.g. radical prostatectomy, TURP, cryotherapy, laser use.

2. Anterior urethral strictures (bulbar, penile and navicular urethra) are a result of scar formation in the spongy erectile tissue of the corpus spongiosum. This scarring may be subsequent to

   a. *Inflammatory processes* – Gonococcal urethritis, balanitis xerotica obliterans (BXO).
   b. *Trauma* – Direct blow or straddle/fall astride injury (usually affects bulbar urethra).
   c. *Iatrogenic* – Traumatic catheterisation, instrumentation, post-hypospadias repair/urethral surgery.
   d. *Idiopathic/congenital* – May be the result of a previous straddle injury, which may have gone unnoticed. However, there is a distinct group of young men in whom strictures occur between the proximal and middle thirds of the urethra, which contain a high content of smooth muscle on biopsy and are termed 'congenital' (form between point of fusion of the urethra from its two different embryological origins).

Q. **What would you look for on examination?**

A. In patients with urethral strictures, there are often no external signs of the disease process. However, it is important to inspect for BXO, meatal stricturing, hypospadias and evidence of prior surgery. Palpation may reveal spongiofibrosis adjacent to the stricture.

Q. **What does the flow curve in Figure 8.12 show? What other investigations are important?**

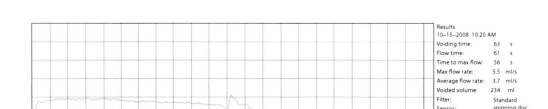

Results		
10–15–2008 10:20 AM		
Voiding time:	63	s
Flow time:	61	s
Time to max flow:	56	s
Max flow rate:	5.5	ml/s
Average flow rate:	3.7	ml/s
Voided volume:	234	ml
Filter:	Standard	
Sensor:	spinning disc	

Figure 8.12

A. Figure 8.12 demonstrates a prolonged slow flow classical of a urethral stricture. This is typically termed a 'plateau'-shaped trace with little change in flow rate.

Further investigations would include the following:

- *Flexible urethroscopy* – Direct inspection of the urethral lumen is probably the most common first line of investigation in the United Kingdom.
- *Urethrography* – Ascending and descending studies. In specialist centres, urethrography is performed in place of urethroscopy as it provides the most detailed information about the urethra. A diagnosis and management plan can be formulated and the patient counselled appropriately.

Additionally USS may show a thickened bladder wall and residual urine. If hydroureteronephrosis is present then estimation of renal function should be performed. Urinalysis will exclude concurrent urinary tract infection (UTI).

Q. What does this antegrade urethrogram in Figure 8.13 show?

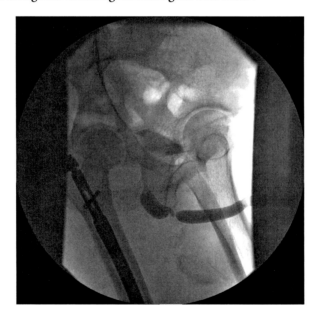

Figure 8.13

A. Figure 8.13 is an antegrade urethrogram illustrating a short narrowing of the bulbar urethra consistent with a stricture. Ascending, descending and dynamic images should be reviewed.

Q. How would you manage this patient and why?

A. I would counsel this patient for an optical urethrotomy. The alternative is a urethral dilatation or a combination of urethrotomy and dilatation. There is no advantage in terms of outcome but the optical urethrotomy is done under direct vision so may be considered safer. Approximately 50% of urethral strictures require no further treatment following optical urethrotomy urethral dilatation. These are typically short (<1.5 cm), located in the bulbar urethra, associated with minimal spongiofibrosis and have had no previous interventions.

A urethral catheter should be left *in situ* for 3 days following an optical urethrotomy and the patient should be taught intermittent self-catheterisation/dilatation, which should be continued for 6 months (reduces restructuring rates).

Q. How would you manage a patient whose short bulbar stricture recurs following an optical urethrotomy?

A. If the patient is fit for anaesthesia, and the stricture <2 cm in length I would counsel the patient for an anastomotic bulbar urethroplasty which is curative in approximately 90% of cases at 10 years' follow-up. Any anastomotic repair must be spatulated, tension free and 'stented' (catheterised in this case).

Note: *The alternative option is palliative (if this is preferable to the patient) repeat urethral dilatation/optical urethrotomy followed by long-term self-dilatation. Older age should not be considered a contraindication to urethroplasty.*

Q. What are the indications for anastomotic urethroplasty?

A. This procedure is used in two situations:

- Short strictures of the bulbar urethra no more than 2 cm in length.
- A pelvic fracture–related injury of the membranous urethra or bulbo-membranous junction. This is not so much a stricture but a distraction defect with no continuity of the urethra and obliteration of the lumen by fibrous tissue, which separates the ends of the urethra.

Note: *The membranous urethral strictures following TURP, sometimes known as 'sphincter strictures' because they are due to fibrosis within the external sphincter mechanism, are best treated by urethral dilatation in order to avoid incontinence.*

Q. Which manoeuvres can be used to bridge the defect during anastomotic urethroplasty (in order to bring the two ends of the urethra together) if bulbar urethral mobilisation alone is not adequate?

A. If the elasticity of the urethra and mobilisation are not sufficient to bridge the defect then the principle is to straighten out the natural curve of the bulbar urethra so that its course from the penoscrotal junction to the prostatic apex is a straight line (rather than a semicircle). The manoeuvres used to do this are

- Separation of the crura at the base of the penis
- Wedge pubectomy of the inferior pubic arch
- Re-routing of the urethra around the shaft of the penis

Defects up to 7 cm can be bridged using these steps in sequence.

Q. What specific complications can occur post bulbar anastomotic urethroplasty?

A. Bleeding, wound infection, post-micturition dribbling (due to division of the bulbospongiosus muscle) and stricture recurrence.

Q. What operative options are available for longer bulbar strictures?

A. Substitution urethroplasty: this is used for bulbar strictures too long for anastomotic repair and in strictures of the penile urethra where anastomotic urethroplasty is not

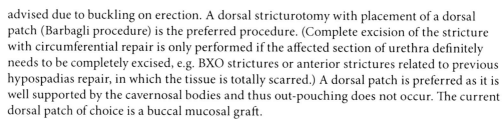

advised due to buckling on erection. A dorsal stricturotomy with placement of a dorsal patch (Barbagli procedure) is the preferred procedure. (Complete excision of the stricture with circumferential repair is only performed if the affected section of urethra definitely needs to be completely excised, e.g. BXO strictures or anterior strictures related to previous hypospadias repair, in which the tissue is totally scarred.) A dorsal patch is preferred as it is well supported by the cavernosal bodies and thus out-pouching does not occur. The current dorsal patch of choice is a buccal mucosal graft.

Other options include an augmented anastomotic urethroplasty, which is not commonly performed and a perineal urethrostomy, which is generally used only when reconstructive surgery fails.

Q. For complex strictures such as those related to radiotherapy should one use a graft?

A. No. In the presence of diseased tissue, e.g. following radiotherapy, grafts will not take. Thus any tissue transfer needs to have its own blood supply and a genital skin flap is used pedicled on the vascular dartos layer of the penis.

Q. What are the success rates of anastomotic and substitution urethroplasty?

A. Anastomotic urethroplasty is associated with an approximately 90% success rate at 10 years. Substitution urethroplasty success rates are worse with 85% patency rates at 1–3 years and deteriorating at 3%–5% per year so that by 10–15 years approximately half the patients have developed recurrent strictures.

Q. What options are available for the management of penile urethral strictures?

A. The management of penile strictures is complex. Aetiology, length, location and the condition of the surrounding tissues are important. Urethral dilatation or optical urethrotomy will inevitably fail in penile strictures and anastomotic urethroplasty should not be performed for penile strictures as this will result in unacceptable penile deformity on erection. More proximal simple penile urethral strictures (i.e. those not caused by BXO or failed hypospadias repair) can be managed with a stricturotomy and penile skin flap (Orandi flap). Distal strictures, usually related to previous hypospadias repair or BXO, can be managed with excision of the affected segment followed by a circumferential repair involving a two-stage urethroplasty using buccal mucosal graft (for BXO genital skin cannot be used as the disease will recur in this tissue).

Q. Why has buccal mucosa become the graft of choice?

A. Several reasons including

- Ready availability in sufficient quantities
- Minimal morbidity to the donor site
- Tough, easy to handle
- Behaves like a full-thickness graft, so little or no contraction and rich sub-dermal plexus (much more vascular than skin) and thus takes well
- Accustomed to a wet environment
- Appears to have antibacterial properties
- Resistant to skin diseases

Q. What specific donor site complications can occur after harvesting of a buccal mucosal graft?

A. Discomfort, bleeding, donor site infection, injury to parotid duct (Stenson's), numbness in oral cavity, persistent difficulty with mouth opening and change in salivary function.

FURTHER READING

1. Santucci RA et al. Evaluation and management of renal injuries: Consensus statement of the renal trauma subcommittee. *BJU Int* 2004; 93: 937–954.
2. European Association of Urology. http://uroweb.org/guideline/urological-trauma
3. McAninch JW, Ed. Genitourinary trauma. *Urol Clin North Am* 2006; 33: 1–132.
4. Andrich DE et al. Urethral strictures and their surgical treatment. *BJU Int* 2000; 86: 571–580.
5. Gommersall L, Kapasi F, Potluri B. Diagnosis and management of renal trauma. Chapter 7 In: Shergill IS, Arya M, Patel HR, and Gill IS, Eds. *Urological Emergencies in Hospital Medicine*, London: Quay Books, 2007, pp. 61–70.
6. European Association of Urology. http://uroweb.org/guideline/urological-trauma

CHAPTER 9
URINARY TRACT INFECTIONS

Vibhash Mishra and Jas S Kalsi

Contents

DEFINITIONS

Q. What is the definition of *urinary tract infection*?

A. Urinary tract infection (UTI) is the inflammatory response of urothelium to micro-organism invasion (commonly bacterial), usually associated with bacteriuria and pyuria.

Q. What is the definition of *bacteriuria*?

A. Bacteriuria is the presence of bacteria in urine.

Q. What is the definition of *pyuria*?

A. Pyuria is the presence of white blood cells (WBCs) in urine.

Q. What is the definition of *sterile pyuria* and what is the differential diagnosis?

A. Sterile pyuria is pyuria, without bacteriuria. Possible causes include tuberculosis, carcinoma *in situ* of bladder, schistosomiasis, urinary tract stones, partly treated UTI and other inflammatory bladder conditions (interstitial cystitis or leucoplakia).

Q. What is the definition of *cystitis*?

A. Cystitis is a clinical syndrome of dysuria, frequency and urgency with or without suprapubic pain.

Q. What is the definition of *acute* and *chronic pyelonephritis*?

A. Acute pyelonephritis is a syndrome comprising flank pain, nausea and vomiting, fever (>38°C) or costovertebral angle tenderness. Chronic pyelonephritis is a radiological diagnosis describing a scarred, shrunken kidney, which may or may not have resulted from recurrent infections.

Q. What is the definition of an *isolated UTI*?

A. An isolated UTI is one which occurs at least 6 months after the previous UTI.

Q. What is the definition of *recurrent UTI*?

A. Recurrent UTI is an episode of UTI after documented, successful resolution of an earlier episode and occurring at a frequency of at least twice in the last 6 months, or three times in the last 12 months. Recurrent UTI can be sub-classified as 'persistent' or 're-infection':

- **What is the definition of persistence?**
  Persistence refers to recurrent UTI caused by the same organisms. It indicates a possible focus of infection in the urinary tract such as stones (commonly struvite), chronic prostatitis, bladder diverticulum, urethral diverticulum and colo-vesical fistula.

- **What is the definition of re-infection?**
  Re-infection refers to recurrent episodes of UTI caused by different organisms. It usually indicates an increased susceptibility to UTI (including genetic), and is associated with poor hygiene, sexual intercourse, post-menopause. More than 95% of all recurrent UTIs in females are due to re-infection.

Q. What is the definition of *unresolved infection*?

A. An unresolved infection is one that has not responded to treatment. Possible causes include natural or acquired bacterial resistance to antimicrobial therapy, development of resistance in a previously susceptible organism, simultaneous infection with multiple organisms, rapid reinfection, an overwhelming size of bacterial inoculums or antimicrobial level below the minimum inhibitory concentration.

Q. What is the definition of a *complicated UTI*?

A. A complicated UTI indicates infection in the presence of a structurally or functionally abnormal urinary tract, or UTI in the presence of underlying disease which is known to increase the risk of acquiring infection, or failing therapy.

   Factors suggesting complicated UTI include male gender, being elderly and pregnancy, The presence of an indwelling catheter, stent (urethral, ureteral, renal) or the use of intermittent bladder catheterization, indwelling catheter/stent, recent urinary tract instrumentation, immunosuppression, diabetes, symptoms for >7 days at presentation, hospital-acquired infection, recent antimicrobial use, functional (vesicoureteric reflux) or anatomical abnormality of the urinary tract (ileal loop or pouch, post-void residual urine of >100 mL, an obstructive uropathy of any aetiology (upper and lower urinary tracts), e.g. bladder outlet obstruction (including neurogenic urinary bladder), stones and tumour, or chemical or radiation injuries of the uroepithelium [1].

Q. What is the definition of an *uncomplicated UTI*?

A. An uncomplicated UTI indicates infection in the presence of a structurally or functionally normal urinary tract, or UTI in the absence of any underlying disease that increases the risk of acquiring infection, or failing therapy.

RECURRENT UTIs

Q. A 45-year-old woman has been referred by the GP with a history of recurrent UTIs. How will you approach this case?

A. I would first take a thorough history. In my history I would try to establish whether this is a case of an isolated or recurrent UTI, cystitis or pyelonephritis and whether there are any features which make this a complicated infection. I would also like to exclude symptoms which may be attributable to a sexually transmitted infection such as itching, vaginal discharge or any symptoms in the partner. I would make sure that all the midstream specimen of urine (MSU) results from GP are available so that it is possible to ascertain which organism caused the infection or whether there is a non-infective process, i.e. interstitial cystitis, stones, Carcinoma in situ (CIS). The MSU results would also allow me to differentiate re-infection from persistence and the number of confirmed UTIs in 1 year.

I would then ask about their past medical history (diabetes, stones, constipation, neurological illness or previous UTIs as a child). This would help differentiation between a complicated and uncomplicated UTI. It is important to establish whether there is a family history of UTIs (UTIs associated with ABO blood group antigen non-secretors, Lewis non-secretor or P blood group secretors). The pregnancy status of the patient should always be established and whether they are on an oral contraceptive pill (possible interactions with antibiotics).

Q. What will you look for on clinical examination?

A. On physical examination (with a chaperone), I would aim to identify any underlying anatomical predisposing factors such as a palpable kidney or a palpable bladder (incomplete emptying) and whether there is any loin tenderness. On vaginal examination (PV) (again with a chaperone) I would ascertain the state of tissue oestrogenisation, the presence or absence of genital prolapse (cystocele) and/or urethral diverticulum. I would also perform a focussed neurological examination.

Q. Which investigations will you request in this case?

A. I would in general request urine dipstick followed by an MSU for urine microscopy and C and S, an x-ray kidney, ureter and bladder (KUB) and a renal tract ultrasound (USS) with a post-void residual (PVR) measurement.

Q. What findings on urinalysis suggest the presence of an infection?

A. The presence of blood, leucocytes and nitrites. I would also note the urinary pH.

Q. Can you explain how urinary dipstick analysis works?

A. *Blood*: The chromogen indicator on the dipstick, orthotolidine, is a peroxidase substrate. When haemoglobin, which contains peroxidase activity, comes in contact with orthotolidine, an oxidation reaction takes place resulting in colour change (blue colour) of the indicator. False-positives (oxidising agents) can result from exercise, dehydration, menstrual blood, povidone iodine and hypochlorite solutions (bleach). False-negatives (reducing agents) can be due to vitamin C, gentisic acid and poorly mixed urine. Dipstick positive but microscopy negative indicates dilute urine (low specific gravity).

Leucocytes: Neutrophils (present in infected urine) produce the enzyme leucocyte esterase. This enzyme causes hydrolysis of an indoxyl carbonic acid ester (substrate on dipstick) to indoxyl, which in turn oxidizes a diazonium salt chromogen on dipstick to produce the colour change. False-positives are contamination from vaginal discharge and presence of formalin. False-negatives include high specific gravity of urine, dehydration, glycosuria, presence of urobilinogen, ingestion of large amounts of vitamin C and also if the test is read too soon (<2 min) or the sample has been left standing for too long (lysis of WBCs).

However, not all patients with bacteria in their urine (bacteriuria) have significant pyuria. The sensitivity of this dipstick test for the detection of infection is 70%–95%, meaning 5%–30% of patients with an infection will have a dipstick negative for leucocyte esterase.

Nitrites: Most gram-negative bacteria, the most common uropathogens, convert nitrates (present in urine) to nitrites (not normally present in the urine). Nitrites then react with the aromatic amine reagent on the dipstick, to form a diazonium salt. Then the diazonium salt interacts with hydroxybenzoquinolone to form a pink-coloured azo dye (Griess reaction). It usually takes 4 hours to make the Griess reaction. False-positives occur due to contamination. False-negatives include non-nitrite converting bacteria (gram-positive organisms and Pseudomonas), urine present in the bladder <4 hours, absent dietary nitrates, ascorbic acid and dilute urine (low specific gravity).

The sensitivity of nitrite dipstick detection is 35%–85% while the specificity is 92%–100%. This means that if the nitrite test is positive the patient is likely to have a UTI but a negative test often occurs although an infection is present. The combination of the nitrite test with leukocyte esterase with a positive result on either is more specific but less sensitive than either test alone (sensitivity 75%–84%, specificity 82%–98%).

Q. Why is the urinary pH important?

A. The average urine pH varies between 5.5 and 6.5. A consistently alkaline pH >7.5 in the presence of a UTI suggests the possibility of stones. Certain organisms (*Proteus, Klebsiella, Staphylococcus, Pseudomonas, Providencia, Serratia*) produce the enzyme urease, which catalyses hydrolysis of urea into carbon dioxide and ammonia. Ammonia raises the pH of urine causing precipitation of calcium magnesium ammonium phosphate to form staghorn stones.

Q. How would you ask a patient to take a urine sample which is to be sent for microscopy and culture?

A. In female patients, I would ask for an MSU sample to be collected by asking them to spread the labia, wash and cleanse the periurethral area with a moist gauze from front to back, void the first 100–150 mL of urine in the toilet and then place a wide-mouthed sterile container to collect the next 10–15 mL.

In circumcised men, no special preparation is required. I would ask uncircumcised men to retract their foreskin, wash their glans penis with soap and rinse with water, keep the foreskin retracted and then collect 10–15 mL of midstream urine as previously described.

The collected sample should be cultured within a couple of hours and if that is not possible, refrigerated immediately and then cultured within 24 hours.

For microscopy, sediment is obtained by centrifuging 5–10 mL of the sample for 5 minutes at 2000 rpm and this is then examined for the presence of bacteria and white blood cells.

For culture, 0.1 mL of urine is delivered onto each half of a split-agar plate, which contains blood agar on one half for gram-positive organisms and eosin-methylene blue (EMB) on the other half for gram-negative organisms. The number of colonies is then estimated after an overnight incubation.

Q. How is Gram staining performed?

A. Gram staining is performed in the following manner: The bacterial smear is stained on a slide with crystal violet for 1–2 minutes. This is then poured off and Gram's iodine is added for 1–2 minutes. After this time, the iodine is poured off and the stain is then decolourised by washing the slide with acetone for 2–3 seconds. The slide is washed with water and safranin counterstain added for 2 minutes. Finally, the slide is washed with water and dried.

Q. **What is the basis behind the Gram stain?**

A. The cell wall of Gram-positive bacteria retains the purple colour of crystal violet, whereas that of Gram-negative bacteria takes up the pink safranin counterstain.

Q. **What is the microbiological definition of significant bacteriuria?**

A. Kass was the first person to introduce the concept of quantitative microbiology in the diagnosis of urinary infections. In the context of pyelonephritis in pregnant women, he proposed 10^5 cfu/mL pure growth as a cut-off for significant bacteriuria [2]. This remained an essential criterion for the diagnosis of a UTI for many years. However, it is now known that 20%–40% of women with symptomatic UTIs present with bacteria counts of 10^2–10^4 cfu/mL of urine (pure growth) [3]. The following bacterial counts are currently considered significant in the relevant groups of patients (all pure growth) [1]:

- $\geq 10^3$ cfu/mL of MSU in acute uncomplicated cystitis in women
- $\geq 10^4$ cfu/mL of MSU in acute uncomplicated pyelonephritis in women
- $\geq 10^4$ cfu/mL of straight catheter urine sample in a complicated UTI in women
- $\geq 10^4$ cfu/mL of MSU in men (all UTIs considered complicated in men)
- $\geq 10^5$ cfu/mL of MSU in a complicated UTI in women

Q. **Despite your investigations, no causes for the infections have been identified. Can you please explain to the patient why she may be getting UTIs?**

A. I would explain to the patient that in the absence of an identifiable cause, recurrent UTIs are a function of the individual's susceptibility, the virulence of the organism and the host defence mechanisms.

Q. **What is meant by susceptibility to infections?**

A. Studies have demonstrated that women who suffer with recurrent UTIs may be inherently more susceptible due to their increased epithelial cell receptivity for uropathogens. Pathogenic bacteria adhere more readily to the vaginal, urethral and buccal epithelial cells of susceptible women due to the presence of an increased number of receptor sites. This trait (of increased susceptibility to UTI) is associated with HLA-A3 phenotype, Lewis blood group status Le(a−b-) and Le(a+b-), P blood group secretors and ABO blood group antigen non-secretors.

Q. **What is pathogenicity?**

A. It is defined as the ability of an organism to cause disease.

Q. **What is virulence?**

A. It is the degree of pathogenicity.

Q. **What are bacterial virulence factors?**

A. They are the characteristics of uropathogens which allow them to colonise and flourish within the host. They can be divided into factors directed against external agents or those against the host.

1. Factors which are directed against external agents, e.g. antimicrobial resistance, can be inherited chromosomally (Proteus' intrinsic resistance to nitrofurantoin), acquired chromosomally (mutations) or extra-chromosomally mediated (via plasmids).
2. Factors which are directed against the host include:
   a. Toxin production, e.g. haemolysin.
   b. Enzyme production, e.g. urease.
   c. Production of antihumoral substances, e.g. IgA inactivating protein by gonorrhoea and proteus.

d.   General mechanisms, e.g. penetration of host by *Schistosoma* spine, phage variation by organisms to change from a fimbriated to a non-fimbriated form to evade phagocytosis.

    e.   *Adherence mechanisms* – Bacterial adherence to vaginal and urothelial epithelium is a pre-requisite for the initiation of a UTI. To facilitate this process, certain uropathogens express a number of antigenically and functionally active proteins called *adhesins* on their cell surface. These adhesins may take the form of fimbriae or pili or may be afimbrial. The most well-known afimbrial adhesin is the Dr adhesin, associated with UTIs in children and pregnant women. The most well-described pili, found on *Escherichia coli*, are as follows:

        i.   *Type 1* – Associated with *E. coli* causing cystitis. Also known as mannose sensitive pili, as the haemagglutination of guinea pig erythrocytes mediated by these pili is inhibited by mannose.

        ii.   *p pili* – Found strains of *E. coli* causing pyelonephritis. Also called mannose resistant pili, as the haemagglutination reaction is not inhibited by mannose.

        iii.   *s pili* – Associated with both bladder and kidney infection.

Q. What are the normal host defence mechanisms against UTIs?

A. A number of host defence mechanisms exist to reduce the incidence and propensity to acquire and develop urinary tract infections. These defences normally work in parallel and include:

1. The normal commensal flora of the vaginal introitus and periurethral area, e.g. lactobacilli reduce the ability of uropathogens to colonise by lowering the vaginal pH by converting glycogen to lactic acid.

2. The normal antegrade flow of urine.

3. The vaginal environment related to oestrogen and cervical IgA.

4. The physical and chemical characteristics of urine (osmolality, pH, urea and organic acid concentration).

5. The normal exfoliation of urothelial cells.

6. Tamm-Horsfall protein (secreted by cells of ascending limb of loop of Henle) – binds the type 1 pili of *E. coli* and thus prevents adherence.

7. The presence of an intact GAG layer.

Q. Are you aware of any risk factors for the development of recurrent UTIs?

A. There are certain factors which increase the propensity to develop recurrent urinary tract infections. These may be divided into general and specific factors.

    The general factors are applicable to all patient groups and include the following:

1. Factors that reduce the normal antegrade flow of urine such as bladder outflow obstruction, low fluid intake and a neurogenic bladder

2. Factors that promote bacterial colonisation such as sexual intercourse, the use of spermicides and vaginal oestrogen depletion

3. Factors that facilitate the retrograde ascent of pathogens such as female gender, the presence of an indwelling catheter, urinary/faecal incontinence and incomplete bladder emptying with ischaemia of the bladder wall

4. Factors that reduce the ability of the immune system to fight infection such as diabetes mellitus, steroid use or HIV positivity

Certain specific factors are applicable to females of different age groups such as:

1. Premenopausal women

    a.   Sexual intercourse

    b.   Use of spermicide

    c.   A new sexual partner
    d.   Previous UTIs
    e.   Age at first UTI
    f.   Maternal history of UTI
2. Pregnant women
    a.   UTI in non-pregnant state
    b.   Asymptomatic bacteriuria
    c.   Length of gravidity (maximum between weeks 9–17)
3. Menopausal women
    a.   History of UTI before menopause
    b.   Urinary incontinence
    c.   Atrophic vaginitis due to oestrogen deficiency
    d.   Cystocele
    e.   Increased post-void urine volume
    f.   Blood group antigen secretory status
    g.   Urine catheterisation and functional status
    h.   Deterioration in elderly institutionalised women

Q. What are opportunistic infections?

A. They are infections caused by non-pathogens (e.g. commensals) due to a weakened host defence mechanisms.

Q. You have found no cause for infections in this woman. How will you manage her?

A. As the investigations have revealed no reversible factors, it is unfortunately not possible to ensure her recurrent UTIs will not re-occur. I would explain to the patient that the aim of her management in her case would be to first control her symptoms and second to reduce the frequency of infections. To this effect, I would first give her general advice such as to:

1. Ensure a high fluid intake.
2. Void before and after sexual intercourse.
3. Avoid detergents in her bath.
4. Avoid spermicidal contraceptives as spermicides promote colonisation of pathogens by destroying the commensal bacterial flora.
5. Try to keep her urine acidic if possible.
6. Consider applying lactobacilli topically to the vaginal area (bioyoghurt).
7. Apply topical oestrogen to the vagina (if there is evidence of vaginal atrophy) to eliminate pathogenic colonisation by restoring normal vaginal environment and recolonisation with lactobacilli.
8. Encourage a regular daily intake of cranberry juice or cranberry tablets. It is known that the active ingredient proanthocyanidins block bacterial adherence to urothelium and reduce frequency of infections by up to 12%–20%.

    More specifically, I would then counsel the patient regarding the potential use of antimicrobial therapy. Three regimes are available depending upon the frequency of UTIs, relationship with intercourse and preference and acceptability of the patient:

1. Self-start intermittent therapy usually involves a 3-day course of a quinolone, trimethoprim or nitrofurantoin at full therapeutic dose. These may be initiated by the patient upon the onset of symptoms. The patient is asked to take an MSU sample before starting treatment and keep it in the fridge. If the antibiotics are successful then the MSU sample does not necessarily need to be cultured. However if the symptoms do not resolve then the sample can be used to assess bacterial sensitivities. The literature suggests that 3-day courses are superior to single-dose therapy and equivalent to longer courses with

fewer side effects [4]. However, 7-day courses are recommended for men and for women with symptoms for ≥1 week or with complicating factors.

2. Post-intercourse prophylaxis involves a single dose of a quinolone, trimethoprim, cephalexin or nitrofurantoin to be taken immediately after intercourse if UTIs are closely related to sexual activity [5].

3. Low-dose long-term antibiotic prophylaxis works by eliminating the introital and enteric reservoirs of pathogenic bacteria and does not seem to cause reinfections with resistant organisms. It is prescribed in the form of one tablet every night of trimethoprim (100 mg), cephalexin (250 mg), nitrofurantoin (50 mg) or a quinolone (e.g. ciprofloxacin 250 mg) for 6–12 months [6]. In general, breakthrough infections should be treated by therapeutic courses of a different antibiotic chosen on the basis of sensitivities (if available) and prophylaxis resumed after treatment. Recurrences may be reduced by up to 95%. However, prophylaxis does not alter the long-term baseline infection rate and ~60% women start getting infections again a few months after stopping the regime [1].

Q. **You find out she is now pregnant. How common are UTIs in pregnancy?**

A. Urinary infections are not uncommon in pregnancy. Approximately 4%–7% of pregnant females have asymptomatic bacteriuria (same percentage as that of normal population). However, of these, 20%–40% will develop pyelonephritis during pregnancy (usually in the third trimester). Hence, pregnancy is one condition where asymptomatic bacteriuria should be treated.

Q. **Which antibiotics may be used safely in pregnancy and what other precautions are required?**

A. The safe antibiotics during pregnancy are penicillins and cephalosporins. Nitrofurantoin may be used in the first and second trimesters only. The antibiotics to avoid during pregnancy are as follows:

Tetracyclines	All trimesters
Quinolones	All trimesters
Trimethoprim	First trimester
Aminoglycosides	Second and third trimesters
Chloramphenicol	Third trimester
Sulphonamide	Third trimester
Nitrofurantoin	Third trimester

It is very important that once the treatment has been completed a negative urinary culture is performed to confirm eradication of the bacteria. This is in contrast to simple uncomplicated UTIs where this is not necessary.

Q. **How would you treat recurrent UTIs in pregnancy?**

A. In case of recurrent UTIs in pregnancy a low dose of cephalexin, 125–250 mg daily, is usually safe and effective.

Q. **Can you describe the mode of action/side effects of the common antibiotics?**

A. The mode of action and the side effects of the most common antibiotics are listed in Table 9.1.

Table 9.1 The mode of action and the side effects of the most common antibiotics used in treatment of UTI

Agent	Action	Mode of action	Common side effects and cautions	Relevance in pregnancy
Penicillins	Bactericidal	Interference with bacterial cell wall synthesis	Hypersensitivity, diarrhoea	Safe
Cephalosporins	Bactericidal	Interference with bacterial cell wall synthesis	Hypersensitivity, diarrhoea	Safe
Macrolides (erythromycin, etc.)	Bacteriostatic	Inhibition of ribosomal protein synthesis		Safe
Quinolones (ciprofloxacin, etc.)	Bacteriostatic	Prevent DNA replication by inhibiting DNA gyrase	Tendon damage (higher risk when given with steroids), diarrhoea, contraindicated in epileptics, interaction with warfarin	Unsafe
Tetracyclines	Bacteriostatic	Inhibition of ribosomal protein synthesis	Hepatotoxicity, deposition in growing bones and teeth	Unsafe
Trimethoprim	Bacteriostatic	Prevents DNA replication by inhibiting dihydrofolate reductase		Unsafe in first trimester
Aminoglycosides (gentamicin)	Bactericidal	Inhibition of ribosomal protein synthesis	Nephrotoxicity, ototoxicity, impairs neuromuscular transmission, caution in elderly and those with renal impairment	Unsafe in second and third trimesters
Nitrofurantoin	Bactericidal	Damages bacterial DNA by inhibiting multiple enzyme systems	Acute and chronic lung toxicity, hepatotoxicity, allergic reactions, inadequate urine concentration at GFR <50	Unsafe in third trimester

Q. How do you administer therapeutic doses of gentamicin?

A. I use gentamicin at a single daily dose of 3–7 mg/kg body weight based on the Hartford protocol as long as there are no contraindications. The advantages of this regime include convenience for the patients and staff, need to check levels less frequently and lower risk of nephrotoxicity as too many peak serum levels are avoided and a more steady level is achieved. The treatment outcome is better as the ratio of peak serum concentration to minimum inhibitory concentration is higher. Subsequent interval adjustments are made by using a single concentration in serum and hospitals use their own protocols for monitoring of once-daily therapy.

An example of one such protocol is as follows:

- Give the first dose when indicated
- Give the second and subsequent doses at 1700 hours the next day
- Check gentamicin levels after the third dose at 1200 hours

Give the next dose based on the levels:

- <1 mg/L – Same dose
- 1–2 mg/L – Reduce dose by 25% and re-check levels before next dose
- >2 mg/L – Omit that day's dose, re-check levels next day

URINARY TRACT TUBERCULOSIS

Q. **A 53-year-old Bangladeshi woman has been referred to you with a few months history of frequency, nocturia and malaise. Urine cultures with the GP have been negative. How will you investigate this patient?**

A. I would first take a general and focused urological history. However, given the ethnic background, the chronicity of the symptoms and the associated malaise I am concerned that there may be an underlying history of urinary tuberculosis (TB). However, recurrent UTI, stones and interstitial cystitis should be considered in the differential.

  I would specifically ask about previous exposure to TB, loss of appetite, fever, night sweats, loin pain, haematuria and suprapubic pain. I would then ask about a past history of pulmonary TB and renal stones. I would want to exclude any underlying conditions which may result in an immunocompromised state such as diabetes mellitus, steroid use and HIV status.

  In the examination, I would specifically record the temperature and the presence or absence of any lymphadenopathy. A general examination of the chest and abdomen is mandatory as well as a specific examination of the genitalia. I would then perform a dipstick urinalysis and send the urine off for formal microscopy and culture and sensitivities (C&S) if required. I would also request baseline blood tests (including full blood count [FBC], urea and electrolytes [U&Es], erythrocyte sedimentation rate [ESR], liver function tests [LFTs]). I would then ask for radiological tests including a chest x-ray, a plain x-ray KUB, and then a renal tract USS with a formal post-void residual.

Q. **The dipstick urinalysis shows blood and WBCs, but no nitrites. What would be your next step in the investigation process?**

A. I would send the urine for cytology and arrange for three early morning urine (EMU) samples to be sent for acid-fast staining and TB culture.

Q. **Why would you send three samples and why early morning?**

A. The organism causing TB is excreted only intermittently in the urine and therefore, sending multiple samples of urine that has been standing in the bladder overnight gives us the best chance of a positive yield.

Q. **How are EMU samples processed? Why is Gram stain not used?**

A. The smear made of the urine sample is stained using the Ziehl-Neelsen stain to look for acid-fast bacilli and the specimen is also cultured using the Lowenstein-Jensen culture medium. The causative organism of TB, *Mycobacterium tuberculosis* (an obligate aerobic rod, is not suitable for Gram staining due to high lipid content of the cell wall), is a slow growing organism and cultures may take 6–8 weeks to grow.

Q. **How is acid-fast staining performed? What is the basis behind this stain?**

A. Acid-fast staining may be performed in the following way. First, a fixed smear of the bacteria is covered on a slide with a piece of blotting paper. This is then stained with carbol fuchsin for 2 minutes. The blotting paper is then removed and the stain is decolourised with a mixture of HCl and ethanol for 10–15 seconds and rinsed. The stain is then restained with crystal violet for 1 minute and rinsed again.

  When viewed under oil immersion, acid-fast cells appear pink, whereas non-acid-fast cells appear purple.

Q. **Are there any other investigations to potentially confirm the presence of TB?**

A. Yes, a molecular biologic technique called polymerase chain reaction (PCR) using pooled urine samples to amplify *M. tuberculosis* species-specific DNA by *in vitro* enzymatic replication is also available.

Q. **Does the tuberculin test have a role in the diagnosis of urinary TB?**

A. This is a skin test involving an intradermal injection of a purified protein derivative of *M. tuberculosis*. A positive result suggests an exposure to TB, not necessarily an active infection. The importance is that in a patient with suspected TB, a positive tuberculin test is consistent with the diagnosis, a negative test excludes it.

Q. **How is TB acquired?**

A. Primary TB is usually acquired in childhood by inhalation of infected droplets causing deposition of bacilli in the lungs. In immunocompetent individuals, this primary infection is self-limiting or subclinical. Clinical features may later develop as post-primary manifestations at times of reduced immunity. The spread of infection from lungs to the urinary system is haematogenous and starts in the kidney, from where it spreads by direct extension to the ureters and bladder. In the genital tract, the primary site of involvement by haematogenous spread is the epididymis in males and fallopian tubes in females, from where it may spread by direct extension to adjacent organs such as the testes, prostate, and uterus.

Q. **What are the pathological manifestations of urinary TB?**

A. The pathognomonic lesion of TB is a caseating granuloma, which comprises Langhans giant cells surrounded by lymphocytes and fibroblasts. The healing of these lesions results in fibrosis and calcification. That is the reason for the scarring, calcification and parenchymal destruction and distortion seen with healed TB. The kidney classically becomes small, shrunken and distorted, resulting, in extreme cases, in 'autonephrectomy'. The calyceal necks as well as the ureters may develop strictures most commonly in the region of vesico-uretric junction (VUJ). There may be distortion of ureteric orifices (golf-hole appearance) leading to reflux (VUR). In the bladder, active lesions show bullous oedema, ulceration and haemorrhage. Chronic lesions in the bladder may take the form of discrete stellate appearance or the whole bladder may become small and fibrotic (thimble bladder).

Q. **What is this investigation in Figure 9.1 and what does it show?**

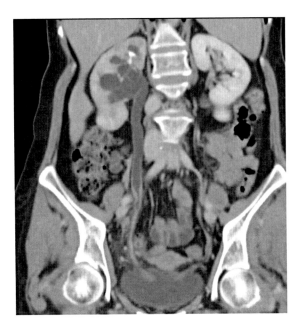

Figure 9.1 Coronal CT scan of the abdomen.

A. Figure 9.1 is a coronal reconstruction of a computed tomography (CT) scan of the abdomen showing right renal upper pole cortical atrophy, linear calcification in the upper pole calyx with infundibular stenosis, lower pole hydronephrosis and dilated proximal ureter with a long distal ureteric stricture.

Q. **What is your radiological investigation of choice?**

A. I would ideally request a CT urogram or an intravenous urography (IVU) to assess the anatomy, the presence of calcification, parenchymal destruction or areas of narrowing.

Q. **How would you manage this patient?**

A. In my experience, genito-urinary TB is still rare and may be complicated. In accordance with National Institute for Health and Care Excellence (NICE) TB guidelines (2016), the clinician responsible for care should refer the person with TB to a clinician with training in, and experience of, the specialised care of people with TB. Thus I believe the patient is best managed in a multidisciplinary team setting involving shared care between urologists, microbiologists and respiratory physicians. The mainstay of management is usually medical treatment with multidrug antituberculous therapy with isoniazid (with pyridoxine), rifampicin, pyrazinamide and ethambutol for 2 months then isoniazid (with pyridoxine) and rifampicin for a further 4 months.

Q. **Why is TB treated with three or four drugs?**

A. Multidrug anti-TB regimens are used to achieve prompt bacterial eradication, to decrease the duration of therapy and to decrease the likelihood of development of drug-resistant organisms.

Q. **Can you describe the names, dosages and common side effects of anti-tuberculous drugs?**

A. The names, dosages and common side effects of anti-tuberculous drugs are listed in Table 9.2.

Table 9.2 Names, dosages and common side effects of anti-TB medication

Drug	Dose (mg/kg)	Associated side effects
Isoniazid (INH)	5	Hepatotoxicity, peripheral neuropathy
Rifampicin	10	Hepatotoxicity, orange discoloration of urine
Pyrazinamide	20	Hepatotoxicity, arthralgia
Ethambutol	20	Retrobulbar neuritis, reduced visual acuity, altered colour vision with reduced red-green discrimination

Q. **Is there a role for the use of steroids n the management of urinary TB?**

A. Steroids are indicated in cases of ureteric stricture not responding to anti-tuberculous therapy alone in 4–6 weeks on serial IVU or CT urogram.

Q. **Which patients are high risk for multi-drug-resistant TB and what should you do?**

A. Patients with a history of previous TB drug treatment, especially with a known poor adherence to treatment, contact with a known case of multi-drug-resistant TB and birth or residence in a country in which the World Health Organization (WHO) reports that a high proportion (5% or more) of new TB cases are multidrug resistant.

For people with clinically suspected multi-drug-resistant TB, a TB specialist should request rapid diagnostic nucleic acid amplification tests for rifampicin resistance on primary specimens.

Q. **What are the radiological manifestations of genito-urinary TB?**

A. Radiologically the following may be seen: small shrunken kidneys, calyceal distortion, infundibular stenosis, cavitation, calcification, ureteric dilatation proximal to a VUJ stricture, multiple ureteric strictures or a contracted and calcified bladder. There may be the presence of pelvic calcification secondary to calcification of vas, seminal vesicle or prostate.

Q. What is the radiological investigation of choice?
A. I would ideally request a CT urogram or an IVU.

PYELONEPHRITIS

Q. A 47-year-old man is in the accident and emergency (A&E) with high fever and severe right loin pain. How will you manage this case?
A. This is a urological emergency and I would see the patient myself, in A&E without delay. On arrival, I would resuscitate him using basic principles of advanced life support. I would administer 100% high-flow oxygen, insert two large-bore Venflons, taking blood for FBC, U&Es, C-reactive protein (CRP), clotting and blood cultures. In addition, I would ensure that he is catheterised and a catheter specimen of urine (or a prior MSU) is sent for urine dipstick and subsequent microscopy and C and S. The patient should be provided with adequate analgesia.

I would then take a general and focused urological history asking specifically for a history of dysuria, haematuria, recent urological intervention or a prior history of stones. I would also ask questions pertaining to a non-urological cause (gastrointestinal or respiratory symptoms). It is important to establish the patient's immune status (diabetes, steroid use, HIV).

Upon examination, I would record the patient's mental state, pulse, blood pressure (BP), temperature, respiration and O_2 saturation. A full and thorough examination is then required to look for a septic focus including chest, abdomen, loins, genitalia and rectal examination (prostatic tenderness).

After ensuring that he is appropriately resuscitated with IV fluids, I would commence the patient on broad-spectrum IV antibiotics. In my practice, I initially give gentamicin (3–7 mg/kg) together with a second-generation cephalosporin. Subsequent antibiotic treatment is reviewed according to culture results, microbiology advice and the clinical situation. Clearly, these patients are admitted for inpatient parenteral antibiotic treatment and observation. In my practice, I seek the early assistance of the microbiologist and if necessary high-dependency unit/intensive therapy unit (HDU/ITU) anaesthetic colleagues, to help in the multidisciplinary management of these patients.

Q. What is systemic inflammatory response syndrome (SIRS)?
A. Response to a variety of infectious (sepsis) or non-infectious (burns, pancreatitis) stimuli. Two of the criteria listed in Table 9.3 are required.

Table 9.3 Criteria for diagnosis of systemic inflammatory response syndrome

T°	>38° or <36°
HR	>90/min
RR	>20/min or p_aCO_2 <32 mm Hg (<4.3 kPa) or need for mechanical ventilation
WCC	<4000 or >12,000 cells/mm³

Q. What is the definition of *sepsis*?
A. Sepsis is defined as proven infection causing SIRS.

Q. What is the definition of *severe sepsis*?
A. Severe sepsis is defined as sepsis with evidence of organ dysfunction, e.g. confusion, lactic acidosis and oliguria.

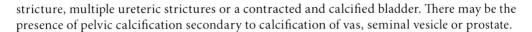

Q. What is the definition of *septic shock*?

A. Septic shock is defined as sepsis-induced hypotension (systolic BP <90 mm Hg) persisting despite adequate fluid resuscitation.

Q. What is the definition of *refractory septic shock*?

A. Refractory septic shock is defined as septic shock lasting for >1 hour and not responding to fluid administration or pharmacological intervention.

Q. What is your understanding of the pathogenesis of sepsis?

A. The major pathogenesis of sepsis is secondary to the presence of endotoxins released by Gram-negative bacteria in the circulation. This in turn results in a cascade of events resulting in release of mediators such as TNFα, interleukins (IL-2, IL-6, IL-8) from target cells (e.g. neutrophils, macrophages, lymphocytes and plasma cells) and activation of the kinin, complement and fibrinolytic systems. These events result in widespread microvascular injury, tissue ischaemia and clinical manifestations of sepsis.

Q. Unfortunately, in spite of your initial management the patient's BP is falling. What would you now do?

A. I would acknowledge that this patient is very unwell. In order to manage this patient effectively, the further treatment of this patient should take place in an ITU setting and will include consideration of vasopressors, inotropes, steroids and recombinant human activated protein C. Once the patient is more haemodynamically stable, radiological investigations should be organised to identify the source of sepsis and steps taken to eradicate it.

Q. What imaging would you like to arrange?

A. I would initially request an ultrasound scan of the renal tract.

Q. Ultrasound shows strong focal echoes in the right renal parenchyma without acoustic shadowing. What would you do now?

A. This is not diagnostic, although hydronephrosis (infected obstructed kidney) has been excluded, I would therefore organise a CT scan of the abdomen with contrast, providing there are no contraindications (such as renal failure).

Q. This is the CT scan (Figure 9.2). Can you describe this? What is the likely diagnosis?

A. Figure 9.2 is a CT scan of abdomen showing air fluid level and debris in the right renal pelvis suggestive of an emphysematous pyelonephritis (EPN).

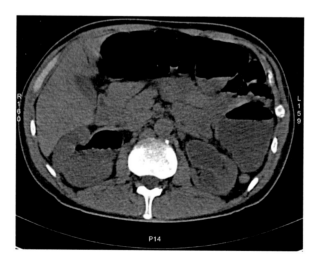

Figure 9.2 Sagittal CT scan of the abdomen.

Q. **What is EPN?**

A. It is an acute necrotizing parenchymal and perirenal infection caused by gas-forming organisms. It commonly occurs in diabetics. Other associated conditions may be urinary tract obstruction, stones and impaired immunity.

Q. **What is this condition commonly caused by?**

A. The most common organisms isolated include *E. coli* and *Klebsiella*. However, it may also be associated with *Proteus, Pseudomonas* and *Streptococcus* infection.

Q. **What is the pathogenesis of EPN?**

A. Unfortunately, this is a poorly understood process. The possible mechanisms leading to accumulation of gas include a mixed acid fermentation of glucose by bacteria and an overwhelming local inflammation coupled with slow transport of the end products due to diabetic microangiopathy. The analysis of accumulated gas has shown to include nitrogen, hydrogen, carbon dioxide and oxygen.

Q. **Are you aware of any different types of EPN and what is the significance?**

A. EPN may be classified on the basis of the CT appearance into type I and type II. Type I is classically characterised by gross parenchymal destruction with either absence of fluid collection or presence of streaky or mottled gas radiating from the medulla to the cortex. Type II EPN is associated with a confined, bubbly or loculated intrarenal gas pattern, presence of renal or perirenal fluid or gas within the collecting system. The differentiation is important as type I EPN is associated with a higher mortality rate of up to 60% versus around 20% for type II.

Q. **Four days after treatment in the ITU, the patient is still not better. What can you do next?**

A. In this patient, the CT does not show any evidence of obstruction or a large perirenal fluid collection; therefore, the next step would be a nephrectomy. The functional status of the contralateral kidney will determine the involvement of nephrologists. In the presence of obstruction or perirenal fluid collection, percutaneous drainage may stabilize the patient, allowing complete urological workup and deferred nephrectomy.

Q. **Figure 9.3 is a CT scan from a different patient whose symptoms have not resolved with conservative treatment. What does it show?**

A. This is a CT scan with contrast showing a large right-sided collection in and around the kidney. The collection distorts and enlarges the renal contour, infiltrates perinephric fat and

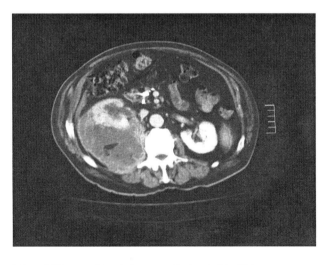

Figure 9.3 Cross sectional slice of CT scan of the abdomen at the level of the kidneys.

extends into the psoas muscle. The normal renal collecting system fat has been obliterated by the process. This is highly indicative of a perinephric abscess.

Q. What is your management plan?

A. Surgical drainage, or nephrectomy if the kidney is non-functioning or severely infected, is the classic treatment. However, more recently renal ultrasound and CT make percutaneous aspiration and drainage of small perirenal collections possible. In this case, I would consider percutaneous drainage to be contraindicated as it is a large abscess cavity which is likely to be filled with thick, purulent fluid. Moreover, percutaneous drainage may be more appropriate if this was a single kidney or single functioning kidney.

Q. How would you differentiate a case of acute pyelonephritis clinically from a perinephric abscess?

A. The literature suggests that most patients with uncomplicated pyelonephritis are symptomatic for less than 5 days before hospitalization, whereas most with perinephric abscesses are symptomatic for longer than 5 days. Moreover, patients with acute pyelonephritis do not usually remain febrile for longer than 4 days once appropriate antimicrobial agents are started. In contrast, patients with a perinephric abscess often have fevers for on average 7 days. Therefore, a perinephric abscess should be suspected in patients with abdominal pain or a flank mass with a persistent fever after 4 days of antimicrobial therapy.

Q. What is a perinephric abscess caused by?

A. The most common causes of a perinephric abscess are secondary to the rupture of an acute cortical abscess into the perinephric space or from haematogenous spread from other sites of infection (e.g. skin). When patients develop an obstructed infected kidney (pyonephrosis) secondary to an obstructing stone, they are at high risk of developing a perinephric abscess if the obstruction is not relived early. This is especially true in patients with immunosuppression and diabetes mellitus (30% of patients). Rarer causes include secondary infection of a perirenal haematoma or infection from nearby structures (bowel perforation, Crohn's disease, osteomyelitis from the thoracolumbar spine).

Q. Figure 9.4 is a CT scan from a different patient with a history of fever, rigors and right flank pain. Can you describe the findings and what is the likely diagnosis?

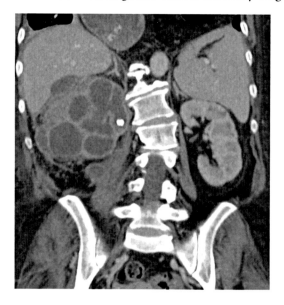

Figure 9.4 Sagittal CT scan of the abdomen demonstrating the renal tract.

A. This demonstrates a coronal reconstruction of a CT scan of the abdomen showing an expanded non-enhancing right kidney invading into the surrounding tissues and a stone within it suggesting a xanthogranulomatous pyelonephritis (XGP).

Q. **What is XGP?**
A. It is a severe chronic renal infection resulting in diffuse parenchymal destruction and an enlarged non-functioning kidney usually associated with calculi.

Q. **What are the common organisms?**
A. XGP is most commonly associated with infection with either *E. coli* or *Proteus* species. However, *Pseudomonas* and *Klebsiella* infection is also frequently demonstrated.

Q. **What is the pathology?**
A. Under the microscope, the pathology seen in cases of XGP is described as diffuse infiltration of inflammatory cells, e.g. lymphocytes, giant cells and plasma cells within the kidney. The characteristic finding is the presence of xanthoma cells, which are lipid-laden foamy macrophages.

Q. **What is the usual course of events in this condition?**
A. If a patient is systemically unwell, the patient is usually admitted to the HDU/ITU and requires intensive treatment for sepsis. On subsequent imaging, the distinction from cancer may be difficult and a nephrectomy is usually performed. If nuclear medicine function scans such as dimercapto-succinic acid are performed these often demonstrate that the kidney is associated with very poor or no function. Moreover, the formal diagnosis is often delayed until the post-operative histology is available.

Q. **How will you perform a nephrectomy in this patient?**
A. Performing a nephrectomy in a patient with XGP is usually technically very challenging as there is usually extension of the inflammatory process into the retroperitoneum. Furthermore, the inflammation results in tissue planes being very stuck and difficult to dissect. As a result, I believe that an open nephrectomy is more suitable than a laparoscopic approach as there is a high risk of injury to the blood vessels, bowel and other neighbouring organs due to the difficult tissue planes.

CHRONIC PELVIC PAIN SYNDROME (CPPS)

Q. **A 52-year-old man is referred with recurrent UTIs. What questions are important in the history?**
A. It is known that recurrent UTIs are very uncommon in male patients. Therefore, in the history I would ask specifically about the presence of any lower urinary tract symptoms (LUTS), particularly a reduced or prolonged flow and a feeling of incomplete emptying to exclude a urethral stricture or a large post-void residue. I would also enquire about a past or present history of renal stone disease. Other important questions in the history include the possible presence of pneumaturia, a previous history of diverticular disease, recurrent diarrhoea, or rectal bleeding which may indicate the possibility of a colo-vesical fistula. I would also ask about the presence of dysuria, storage-type LUTS symptoms, perineal/suprapubic discomfort and ejaculatory problems. These may indicate underlying CPPS [7]. In general, recurrent UTIs can be either due to re-infection or bacterial persistence. As re-infections are very uncommon in men, it is important to try to elicit symptoms which may suggest a persistent focus of infection.

Q. He has been having frequency, urgency, dysuria, perineal discomfort and painful ejaculation intermittently for a few years. What do you think this suggests?

A. On the basis of these symptoms, the most likely diagnosis at this stage would be chronic pelvic pain (CPP), however, that is quite often a diagnosis of exclusion and it is important to exclude other conditions.

Q. What is CPPS?

A. Chronic pelvic pain is chronic or persistent pain perceived in structures related to the pelvis of either men or women. It is often associated with negative cognitive, behavioural, sexual and emotional consequences as well as with symptoms suggestive of lower urinary tract, sexual, bowel, pelvic floor or gynaecological dysfunction. CPPS is the occurrence of CPP when there is no proven infection or other obvious local pathology that may account for the pain.

Q. What do you want to do next for this patient?

A. I would want to ascertain more details from the history about the duration of his symptoms, what his most bothersome symptoms are and how badly these symptoms are impinging on his quality of life. Furthermore, I would like to know if he has previously had any medical or surgical treatments for the condition. To be able to effectively measure the severity of the condition and the possible effect of any treatments I would use the National Institutes of Health Chronic Prostatitis Symptom Index (NIH-CPSI) questionnaire as a baseline.

After obtaining all the necessary information in the history, I would then perform a focussed physical examination of the kidneys, suprapubic region, external genitalia and prostate. This would be followed up by some basic investigations in the form of dipstick urinalysis, MSU for microscopy and C and S, x-ray KUB, renal US, flow rates and PVR.

Q. What is NIH-CPSI?

A. NIH-CPSI stands for National Institutes of Health Chronic Prostatitis Symptom Index. It is a validated questionnaire initially produced by the NIH/NIDDK workshop on chronic prostatitis (CP). It is recommended for use in both clinical practice as well as research. It is a nine-item questionnaire with three main domains (pain, urinary symptoms and quality of life). It is used to establish the patients' baseline bother which can be used to assess the need for any treatment. It can also be used to stratify patients on the basis of their predominant symptoms and to monitor the response to treatment [8].

Q. How do you establish a diagnosis of prostate pain syndrome (PPS)?

A. In PPS, whereas the VB-2 specimen is sterile, EPS and VB3 show <10,000 cfu of uropathogenic bacteria in expressed prostatic secretions and insignificant numbers of leucocytes or bacterial growth in ejaculates. However, this test is impractical in the standard clinical setting. Hence, diagnostic efficiency may be enhanced cost-effectively by using PPMT (described later) [9]. It must be emphasised, however, that these tests help only a little in the diagnosis of PPS, because 8% of patients with suggested PPS have been found to have positive prostatic localisation cultures, similar to the percentage of asymptomatic men [10].

Q. What is bladder pain syndrome (BPS) and how would you establish the diagnosis?

A. The European Society for the Study of IC/PBS (ESSIC) has proposed to use the name *bladder pain syndrome* (BPS), followed by a type indication. Other terms that have been used include 'interstitial cystitis', 'painful bladder syndrome', and 'PBS/IC' or 'BPS/IC'. These terms are no longer recommended.

In general, BPS is a diagnosis of exclusion and therefore it is important to exclude conditions such as benign prostatic hyperplasia (BPH), urethral stricture or UTI which may cause similar symptoms.

Bladder pain syndrome (BPS) is defined as the presence of persistent or recurrent pain perceived in the urinary bladder region (>6 months) and accompanied by at least one other symptom, such as pain worsening with bladder filling and daytime and/or nighttime urinary frequency [11]. Specifically, there should be no proven infection or other obvious bladder pathology. BPS is often associated with negative cognitive, behavioural, sexual or emotional consequences, as well as with symptoms suggestive of lower urinary tract and sexual dysfunction [7].

In 2008–2009, ESSIC suggested a standardised scheme of sub-classifications [11] to acknowledge differences and make it easier to compare various studies (Table 9.4).

Table 9.4 ESSIC classification of BPS types according to results of cystoscopy with hydrodistension and biopsies

Biopsy	Cystoscopy with hydrodistension			
	Not done	Normal	Glomerulations[a]	Hunner's lesion[b]
Not done	XX	IX	2X	3X
Normal	XA	IA	2A	3A
Inconclusive	XB	IB	2B	3B
Positive[c]	XC	IC	2C	3C

[a] Cystoscopy: glomerulations grade 2–3.

[b] Lesion per Fall's definition with/without glomerulations.

[c] Histology showing inflammatory infiltrates and/or detrusor mastocytosis and/or granulation tissue and/or intrafascicular fibrosis.

In Table 9.4 the first symbol (1, 2 or 3) relates to cystoscopy with hydrodistension and the second symbol (A, B or C) to biopsy:

- 1, 2 or 3 represent increasing grade of severity at cystoscopy with hydrodistension
- A, B or C represent increasing grade of severity of biopsy findings
- X indicates not done for both

After excluding these conditions, BPS is diagnosed on symptoms and localisation of organisms and/or leucocytes in segmented urogenital specimens. The gold standard is the four-glass test described by Meares and Stamey. It involves microscopy and culture of urine and expressed prostatic secretion (EPS) [12].

Q. How do you perform the four-glass test?

A. In my practice, I perform this test in a standardised manner as follows:
1. I ask and confirm that the patient has drunk 400 mL of water 30 min before the test.
2. I make sure that four sterile specimen containers are marked VB_1, VB_2, EPS and VB_3 and their lids are removed.
3. The glans penis is exposed and the foreskin kept retracted throughout the test.
4. I cleanse the glans penis with a soap solution and the soap removed with sterile gauze.
5. I make sure the first 10–15 mL of urine is collected in the container marked VB_1.
6. I then ask the patient to pass the next 100–200 mL of urine into the toilet and then collect the subsequent 10–15 mL in the container marked VB_2.
7. I then ask the patient to bend forwards holding the container marked EPS near their urethral meatus.
8. I then massage the prostate until a few drops of prostatic secretion are collected in the EPS container.

9. Immediately after the prostatic massage, I ask the patient to again urinate and collect the first 10–15 mL of urine in the container marked VB_3.

Q. How are the results of the four-glass test interpreted?

A. I ensure that all four specimens are set off for formal microscopy and culture. A positive VB_1 or VB_2 indicates urethritis and cystitis, respectively. A diagnosis of CP is made in the presence of organism(s) and/or leucocytes in the EPS or VB_3 specimen.

Q. Are you aware of any alternative methods of diagnosis to the four-glass test?

A. An alternative method is the pre- and post-massage test (PPMT) proposed by Nickel. It is less tedious, time-consuming and expensive, but an equally effective modification of the four-glass test. This test involves microscopy and culture of a pre- and post-prostatic massage urine sample with a positive post-massage sample indicating the possibility of CP.

Q. The four-glass test in this man shows leucocytes in EPS, but no organisms. What does that mean?

A. This result is consistent with a diagnosis of type IIIA prostatitis.

Q. What types of prostatitis are you aware of?

A. The contemporary classification of prostatitis is the NIH classification (1995). It divides prostatitis into the following categories:
- *Type I* – Acute bacterial prostatitis (acute bacterial infection)
- *Type II* – Chronic bacterial prostatitis (recurrent bacterial infection)
- *Type III* – Chronic non-bacterial prostatitis/CPPS (no demonstrable infection)
  - *Type IIIA – Inflammatory* – WBC in semen/EPS/post-prostatic massage urine
  - *Type IIIB – Non-inflammatory* – No WBC in semen/EPS/post-prostatic massage urine
- *Type IV* – Asymptomatic inflammatory prostatitis

Q. How is CPPS caused?

A. The aetiology of CPPS is poorly understood. It is likely that there are multiple factors operating not only in different patients, but also within an individual patient. The proposed aetiological factors include infection, chemical irritation, dysfunctional high pressure voiding, intraductal reflux, neuromuscular disturbances and altered immunity. Even when the triggering factors are not known, the resultant inflammatory process causes tissue oedema and intraprostatic pressure leading to local hypoxia and varied mediator-induced tissue damage. It is proposed that this in turn leads to altered neurotransmission in sensory nerve fibres resulting in pain and other symptoms associated with the condition.

Q. How would you manage this patient?

A. I would manage this patient according to what his predominant symptoms were and their impact on his quality of life. It is imperative to have a long, frank discussion with the patient to provide reassurance about the benign nature of the condition and explanation about the lack of unequivocal evidence in favour of any treatment. The goal should be symptom control rather than eradication and the management should be multimodal, of an appropriate duration and incremental in nature.

The European Association of Urology (EAU) chronic pelvic pain guidelines have suggested a diagnostic and phenotyping (classification) of CPPS for both sexes (Figures 9.5 and 9.6) [7].

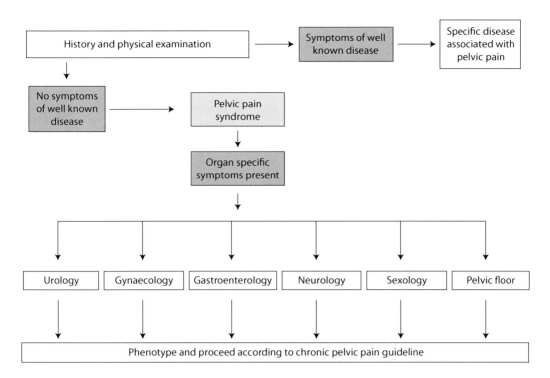

Figure 9.5 Diagnosing chronic pelvic pain. (Adapted from EAU guidelines, http://uroweb.org/guideline/urological-infections/.)

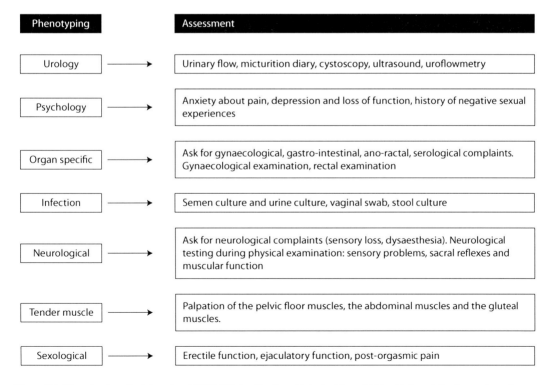

Figure 9.6 Phenotyping of pelvic pain – UPOINTS classification. (Adapted from EAU guidelines, http://uroweb.org/guideline/urological-infections/.)

The cornerstones of management are antibiotics, anti-inflammatories and alpha-blockers.

For non-steroidal anti-inflammatory drugs (NSAIDs), a trial has reported that the pain, quality of life, and total NIH-CPSI scores were in favour of the treatment, but effects were limited to the duration of therapy [10]. Two recent meta-analyses concluded that anti-inflammatory drugs were 80% more likely to have a favourable response than placebo [13,14].

With regards to the use of alpha- blockers, a recent systematic review and network meta-analyses have shown significant improvement in total symptoms, pain, voiding and quality of life scores [15].

I would start him on a combination of antibiotics and an NSAID and if there is an improvement in 2 weeks, I will continue these agents for 6 weeks.

Q. Which antibiotics are particularly suitable for PPS and why?

A. I regularly use either quinolones, tetracyclines, azythromycin, trimethoprim or amoxycillin. Quinolones and tetracyclines are particularly useful as they show good penetration and bioavailability into the prostate with oral as well as parenteral administration and are likely to be effective against the usual pathogens.

Empirical antibiotic therapy is widely used currently and patients responding to antibiotics should be maintained on medication for 4–6 weeks or even longer [7]. Unfortunately none of the biochemical or microbiological tests predict antibiotic response in patients with PPS [16]. A meta-analysis of randomised controlled trials using quinolones (ciprofloxacin and levofloxacin) and tetracycline hydrochloride has been published. Although direct meta-analysis has not shown significant differences in outcome measures, network meta-analysis has suggested significant effects in decreasing total symptoms, pain, voiding and quality of life scores compared with placebo. The network meta-analysis also shows combination therapy of antibiotics with alpha-blockers has shown even better outcomes in network meta-analysis [17].

Based on the evidence, the EAU guidelines currently do not recommend 5-alpha-reductase inhibitors for use in PPS in general, but symptom scores may be reduced in a restricted group of older men with an elevated prostate-specific antigen [18].

Q. Is there any evidence that using antibiotics in a patient when there is no evidence of infection is helpful?

A. There is a lack of strong evidence that antibiotics are of any benefit. The treatment strategies used in the management of this condition are based on expert opinion panels. It is generally believed that even in culture-negative cases, there may be an underlying sub-clinical infection with chlamydia, ureaplasma and other fastidious organisms. Thus a trial of an agent such as a tetracycline seems sensible.

Q. There is no response to these agents in 2 weeks. What will you do next?

A. I will continue the NSAID for a total of 6 weeks and also consider adding in an alpha-blocker, which I will advise for at least 3 months.

Q. Unfortunately, the symptoms are only partly relieved. Are you aware of any other options?

A. The NSAID can be replaced with a muscle-relaxant such as diazepam or baclofen, or a tricyclic antidepressant and I would counsel the patient with respect to considering regular prostatic massage on a bi- or tri-weekly basis for 6–12 weeks, depending on the response.

Q. How is prostatic massage supposed to work?

A. The benefits of prostatic massage are believed to be derived from a combination of several factors including expression of inspissated prostatic secretions, relief of pelvic muscle spasm, physical disruption of any protective biofilm (see following discussion), improved circulation and thus penetration of antibiotics.

Q. **In your clinical experience, do you believe it works?**

A. The results of prostatic massage in my experience are variable. Unfortunately, the benefit has not been shown in the setting of a randomised controlled trial, but there are case series and anecdotal reports suggesting some symptomatic relief in a quarter to a third of patients.

Q. **What is a biofilm?**

A. A biofilm is a complex aggregation of organisms on a solid substrate, protected by an extracellular mucopolysaccharide matrix in an aqueous environment.

EPIDIDYMO-ORCHITIS

Q. **You have been called to A&E to review a 30-year-old man presenting with a few hours history of pain in the scrotum. What is important in the history?**

A. I will see this patient without delay as this is a urological emergency. The main differentials in this situation are trauma, testicular torsion and epididymo-orchitis. I would ask about a history of trauma, similar self-limiting episodes in the past, mode of onset, exact duration of symptoms and any other associated symptoms such as fever, dysuria, urethral discharge and urinary symptoms. I would also take a thorough past sexual history including any recent unprotected casual sexual contact.

Q. **The patient is sexually active and has no long-term lower urinary symptoms. The pain started yesterday with some chills and dysuria. What is important in the examination of this patient?**

A. The history is consistent with epididymo-orchitis. I would perform a general survey to exclude features of sepsis such as high-grade fever, tachycardia, tachypnoea and mental confusion and then proceed to a local examination of the genitalia to elicit signs of inflammation and exclude a missed torsion and abscess formation.

Q. **How would you distinguish between torsion and epididymo-orchitis?**

A. It is sometimes difficult to distinguish epididymo-orchitis from torsion clinically and I have a low threshold for exploring a patient unless there are obvious features to suggest an infection. The history of a sudden onset of pain and an absence of urinary symptoms points more towards a torsion. Similarly, demonstration of redness and raised local temperature, at least early in the course of the illness, is more likely in epididymo-orchitis. A urethral discharge is suggestive of epididymo-orchitis. In early torsion, actual twists in the spermatic cord may be palpable and elevation of the affected side of the scrotum relieves the pain in epididymo-orchitis, but aggravates it in torsion. However, if there is any doubt, one must surgically explore the patient.

Q. **Elevation of the affected side of the scrotum relieves the pain. What is this finding called and how reliable is it?**

A. It is called Prehn's sign. It is not hugely reliable and I do not base my decision to explore or otherwise purely on this finding.

Q. **Your history and examination do indeed point towards epididymo-orchitis. What is the likely cause in this man?**

A. A sexually acquired chlamydial or gonococcal infection singly or in combination. Gonococcal infection is more common in homosexual men.

Q. How will you manage him?

A. I would investigate him with urinalysis, urine culture and Gram staining and culture of any urethral discharge. I would also send off baseline blood tests including a FBC, U&Es and CRP. I will then manage him with bed rest, scrotal support, analgesics and antibiotics.

Q. What might you see on Gram staining of the urethral discharge in gonococcal infection?

A. Gram-negative intracellular diplococci.

Q. On investigation, how may chlamydial infection be diagnosed in the absence of a urethral discharge?

A. Detection of DNA of *Chlamydia trachomatis* is now possible by performing polymerase chain reaction on a first-void urine sample.

Q. Which antibiotic would you use?

A. I usually treat epididymo-orchitis in a young man with ciprofloxacin (500 mg bd) and doxycycline (100 mg bd) for at least 2 weeks.

Doxycycline covers chlamydial infection and ciprofloxacin covers gonococcal infection.

However, it should be noted that there is increasing resistance of gonococcal infection to ciprofloxacin, penicillins and tetracyclines. Thus current first-line treatment in those with a confirmed infection with *Neisseria gonorrhoeae* is a stat dose of oral cefixime 400 mg (also if chlamydial/gonococcal infection, sexual contacts must be traced and treated).

Q. This patient is unfortunately allergic to doxycycline. What antibiotic can you give him as an alternative for chlamydial infection?

A. As he is allergic to doxycycline, I would use a stat dose of 1 g of azithromycin instead of doxycycline.

Q. If this man was 67 instead of 30 years old, would your approach be any different?

A. Yes, in that age group the likely cause of epididymo-orchitis is an ascending urinary infection as a result of bladder outflow obstruction and the likely organism is *E. coli* (i.e. Gram-negative enteric organisms are the most common cause of epididymo-orchitis in this age group). I would therefore treat him with a course of ciprofloxacin without doxycycline. I would ask specifically about any preceeding lower urinary tract symptoms and their impact on the patient's quality of life. After the infection has settled I would investigate his lower urinary tract with uroflowmetry and post-void residual ultrasound of the bladder. I could then address any abnormalities that may be seen and therefore attempt to prevent any recurrence of the infection.

Q. Four days after the initiation of treatment, the patient is not getting better, in fact the pain is getting worse. What will you do?

A. I would check the patient's compliance with medication, chase the culture result and modify the antibiotic regime if indicated. I would also arrange a scrotal ultrasound to exclude an abscess.

Q. What does the ultrasound show in Figure 9.7?

A. The ultrasound demonstrates a small hydrocele surrounding a relatively normal looking testis and a thick expanded epididymal head with fluid levels suggestive of an epididymal abscess.

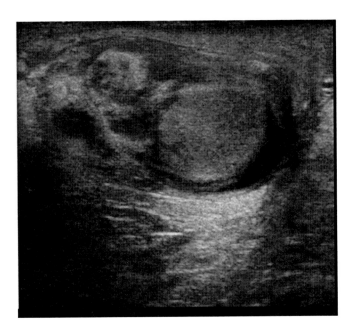

Figure 9.7 Scrotal ultrasound scan of patient.

Q. What would you do now?

A. I would advise the patient that the infection has unfortunately gotten worse and now developed into an abscess. After appropriate counselling and consent, I would organise for the patient to undergo incision and drainage of the abscess under a general anaesthetic. It is important to explain that despite the drainage, the infective process may continue or may indeed need an orchidectomy at the time of drainage if there is severe infection that has spread into the testicle itself. It may also be necessary to leave the wound open with or without a drain.

REFERENCES

1. Bonkat G et al. EAU Guidelines on Urological Infections 2017. http://uroweb.org/guideline/urological-infections/
2. Kass EH. Bacteriuria and pyelonephritis of pregnancy. *Arch Intern Med* 1960; 105: 194–198.
3. Stamm WE et al. Management of urinary tract infections in adults. *N Engl J Med* 1993; 329: 1328–1334.
4. Warren JW et al. Guidelines for antimicrobial treatment of uncomplicated acute bacterial cystitis and acute pyelonephritis in women. Infectious Diseases Society of America (IDSA). *Clin Infect Dis* 1999; 29: 745–758.
5. Melekos MD et al. Post-intercourse versus daily ciprofloxacin prophylaxis for recurrent urinary tract infections in premenopausal women. *J Urol* 1997; 157: 935–939.
6. Harding GK et al. Long-term antimicrobial prophylaxis for recurrent urinary tract infection in women. *Rev Infect Dis* 1982; 4: 438–443.
7. European Association of Urology. http://uroweb.org/guideline/urological-infections/
8. Litwin MS et al. The National Institutes of Health chronic prostatitis symptom index: Development and validation of a new outcome measure. Chronic Prostatitis Collaborative Research Network. *J Urol* 1999; 162: 369–375.

9. Nickel JC et al. How does the pre-massage and post-massage 2-glass test compare to the Meares-Stamey 4-glass test in men with chronic prostatitis/chronic pelvic pain syndrome? *J Urol* 2006; 176: 119.

10. Nickel JC et al. A randomized, placebo controlled, multicenter study to evaluate the safety and efficacy of rofecoxib in the treatment of chronic nonbacterial prostatitis. *J Urol* 2003; 169: 1401.

11. European Society for the Study of IC/PBS. http://www.essic.eu/pdf/ESSICconsensus2007.pdf

12. Meares EM et al. Bacteriologic localization patterns in bacterial prostatitis and urethritis. *Invest Urol* 1968; 5: 492–518.

13. Zhao WP et al. Celecoxib reduces symptoms in men with difficult chronic pelvic pain syndrome (Category IIIA). *Braz J Med Biol Res* 2009; 42: 963.

14. Bates SM et al. A prospective, randomized, double-blind trial to evaluate the role of a short reducing course of oral corticosteroid therapy in the treatment of chronic prostatitis/chronic pelvic pain syndrome. *BJU Int* 2007; 99: 355.

15. Anothaisintawee T et al. Management of chronic prostatitis/chronic pelvic pain syndrome: A systematic review and network meta-analysis. *JAMA* 2011; 305: 78.

16. Nickel JC et al. Predictors of patient response to antibiotic therapy for the chronic prostatitis/chronic pelvic pain syndrome: A prospective multicenter clinical trial. *J Urol* 2001; 165: 1539.

17. Thakkinstian A et al. Alpha-blockers, antibiotics and anti-inflammatories have a role in the management of chronic prostatitis/chronic pelvic pain syndrome. *BJU Int* 2012; 110: 1014.

18. Nickel JC et al. Dutasteride reduces prostatitis symptoms compared with placebo in men enrolled in the REDUCE study. *J Urol* 2011; 186: 1313.

FURTHER READING

European Association of Urology. http://uroweb.org/guideline/urological-infections/

CHAPTER 10
URINARY TRACT STONES

Thomas Johnston, Mark Rochester and Oliver Wiseman

Contents

STAGHORN STONES

Q. **A 44-year-old woman presents with a 6-month history of recurrent urinary tract infections (UTIs) and occasional left loin ache. A recent midstream urine culture grew *Proteus mirabilis* 10^5 cfu/mL with >200 leucocytes. Her GP has requested an ultrasound of the renal tract and plain kidney, ureter and bladder (KUB) x-ray. What does the KUB x-ray in Figure 10.1 show?**

A. Figure 10.1 shows a large left staghorn calculus and upper third right ureteric calculus.

Q. **What further investigations are required?**

A. This woman should have urine sent for culture and sensitivity in the first instance and blood for full blood count (FBC), urea and electrolytes (U+Es), calcium and urate and a urine spot test for cystine. Imaging to define the stone burden and calyceal anatomy, and also split renal function is then required prior to planning definitive treatment.

Q. **Which imaging modalities would you use and why?**

A. The choice of imaging to determine burden and anatomy is a non-contrast computed tomography of kidneys, ureters and bladder (CT-KUB) scan. Some endourologists would state that a contrast phase to look at the anatomy of the collecting system would be helpful to plan treatment, but this is not standard.

The function of the affected kidney is determined by renography, typically a ^{99m}Tc DMSA (^{99m}Tc dimercapto-succinic acid) renogram. DMSA is a protein which is actively extracted and bound by functioning renal tubules with very little filtered. It is the drug of choice for high-quality cortical imaging. The standard dose is 100 MBq. Images are taken 2–3 hours

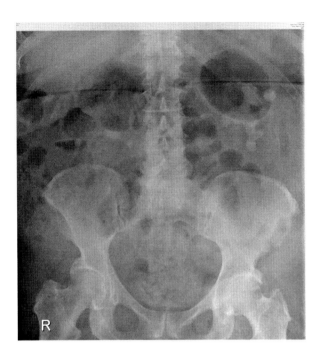

Figure 10.1

later with a gamma camera, or after a longer interval in the presence of renal failure. Posterior and posterior oblique views are taken.

Q. Should the left staghorn renal calculus be treated or be left alone? Justify your answer.

A. The case for a more aggressive approach to staghorn calculi was outlined in a paper by Blandy and Singh [1]. This paper was in three parts:

Part 1

The first part of this paper was a post-mortem study. The authors retrospectively studied 8,996 consecutive post-mortems. Only nine staghorns were discovered. Five of these had caused severe symptoms and were thought to have contributed to the death of the patients. The authors concluded that 'the notion of an incidentally discovered silent staghorn is false.

Part 2

The second part of this paper concerned the conservatively managed staghorn calculus. Sixty staghorns were identified retrospectively over the period 1955–1975, in patients where stones were not removed. Twenty had early nephrectomy. Of 40 observed 16 went on to develop pyonephrosis and had drainage and difficult nephrectomies with a high mortality. Overall 17/60 (28%) died during follow-up (mostly from renal failure). All others were said to have had pain and infection.

Part 3

The final section of this paper described a case series of surgical removal of staghorn calculi. In this retrospective series 152 staghorns were found in 125 patients. The authors described stone 'clearance' in 80%, and 'dust' only remaining in a further 5%. The mortality was 7% during follow-up.

The authors concluded that there is no such clinical entity as a 'silent staghorn' based on the post-mortem study. Furthermore, they stated that long-term survival is better in those treated surgically (mortality 7%) than in those managed conservatively (mortality 28%).

Critical analysis of this paper allows the following points to be raised. It is a simple message which has been supported by subsequent data. Good data concerning the fate of residual fragments is presented. However, it could be criticised for its retrospective design, and no statistical analysis was performed. Case selection error is likely, and autopsy data may be incomplete. For example, five symptomatic staghorns are referred to in part 1, but 24 deaths in parts 2 and 3. Furthermore, almost half the staghorns found in the autopsy series were asymptomatic, perhaps not supporting the authors' first conclusion. Complications of surgery were probably underestimated due to the retrospective design, and questions could be raised as to the method of assessment of renal function, which is not described.

Further guidance on the management of staghorn calculi can be taken from Teichman et al. [2], who analysed retrospectively 177 consecutive staghorn calculus patients to determine risk factors for ultimate renal deterioration and renal cause–specific death. Over a mean follow-up of 7.7 years, the overall rate of renal deterioration was 28%. This was associated more frequently with solitary kidneys (77% versus 21%), previous stone disease (39% versus 14%), hypertension, complete staghorn calculi and neurogenic bladder as well as those who refused treatment (100% versus 28%). With respect to mortality, no patient with complete clearance of fragments died of renal-related causes versus 3% of those without clearance of fragments and 67% of those who refused treatment, comparing favourably with the earlier findings of Blandy and Singh.

Q. The patient opts for percutaneous nephrolithotomy (PCNL). What are the indications and contraindications for this procedure?

A. *Indications*

1. Stone size
    a. Stones >3 cm diameter.
    b. Renal pelvis stones >2 cm.
    c. Lower pole stones >1 cm.
    d. Staghorn stones.
2. Obstruction
    a. An anatomic abnormality is present that will prevent stone fragments from passing spontaneously, especially where extracorporeal shock wave lithotripsy (ESWL) is usually contraindicated.
3. Anatomical considerations
    a. Abnormal renal anatomy such as horseshoe kidney or calyceal diverticular stones.
    b. Abnormal patient anatomy such as kyphoscoliosis or obesity preventing ESWL.
4. Failed ESWL/ureteroscopy (URS)
5. Stones associated with a foreign body
6. Patient choice/desire for one treatment only

Contraindications

1. Absolute
    a. Uncorrected bleeding disorder
    b. Pregnancy
    c. Sepsis
    d. Poor kidney function (e.g. <15%), where nephrectomy would be indicated
    e. Need for coincidental open procedure
2. Relative
    a. Medical problems – Patient high risk for anaesthesia
    b. Anterior calyceal diverticulum

Q. Describe how you would take informed consent for this procedure.

A. Informed consent must include a discussion of available alternative treatment options, as described above, the intended benefit of the proposed procedure, and the potential complications, which are listed as follows with approximate percentages in parentheses:

- *Complications related to access*
  - Bleeding
    - Requiring transfusion (2%–3%)
    - Requiring embolisation (1%)
    - Requiring nephrectomy (rare)
  - Perforation of adjacent organs (bowel <1%, pneumothorax 0%–5%)
  - Access failure (up to 5%)
- *Complications related to stone removal*
  - Infection (bacteriuria 77%; sepsis 0.25%–1.5%)
  - Transurethral resection (TUR) syndrome
  - Irrigant extravasation (30%)
  - Renal pelvis injury
  - Residual stones (>10%), dependent upon stone complexity
- *Others*
  - Pleural effusion (10%)
  - Hypertension and fibrosis (late)
  - Mortality (0.3%)

Q. Are there any advantages of supine versus prone PCNL?

A. Patient positioning during supine PCNL is less time consuming and the potential risks of musculoskeletal injuries (e.g. cervical spine, brachial plexus), cardiovascular (increased cardiac output, venous stasis and thromboembolic events) and visual complications are decreased. The supine position also allows easy access to the urethral meatus for simultaneous retrograde procedures during PCNL, is more ergonomic for the surgeon during the procedure, may reduce radiation exposure, promotes spontaneous drainage of stone fragments due to the relatively downward direction of the tract and provides lower irrigating pressures. Prone PCNL provides more options and a wider surface area for puncture (upper pole/multiple punctures), may reduce the risk of damage to visceral organs (retro-renal colon and lateral rotation of spleen/liver away from puncture site), allows greater manipulation with the nephroscope and may reduce perirenal injury (excessive anterio-medial movement with supine increases risk of injury during dilation) [3].

Three meta-analyses have been carried out to date comparing outcomes of prone versus supine PCNL and have reported conflicting results [4–6]. Two of these reported similar stone-free rates (SFRs) (prone 81.6%–83.4% versus supine 83.5%–84.5%), length of stay and complication rates but shorter operative times with supine [4,5]. In contrast, Zhang et al. [6] found better SFRs with the prone position compared to supine (77.3% versus 72.9%).

Q. In this case what is this stone likely to consist of?

A. This is most likely to be a struvite stone, named after the nineteenth-century Russian diplomat Baron von Struve. They are also referred to as triple-phosphate stones (calcium, ammonium and magnesium, phosphate), infection stones or urease stones. The following conditions must coexist for crystallisation of struvite:

- Alkaline urine pH > 7.2
- Ammonia in urine
- The driving force is UTI with urease-producing bacteria. Urease-producing bacteria hydrolyse urea to ammonia molecules and carbon dioxide (Figure 10.2).

High urine pH with high ammonia concentration, abundant phosphate and magnesium lead to crystallisation of magnesium ammonium phosphate and the subsequent formation of large branched staghorn stones.

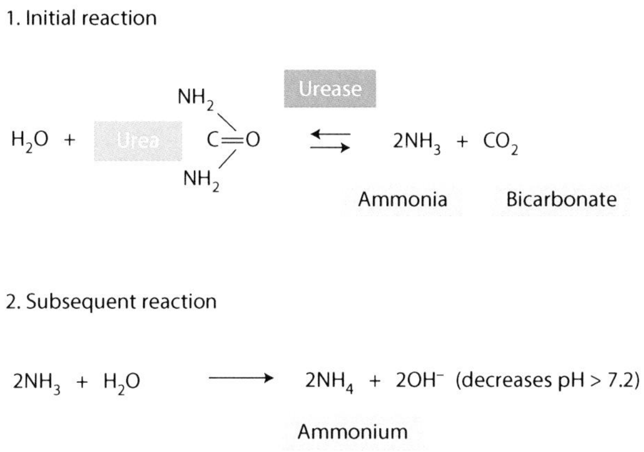

1. Initial reaction

$$H_2O + Urea \quad \begin{matrix} NH_2 \\ | \\ C=O \\ | \\ NH_2 \end{matrix} \quad \underset{Urease}{\rightleftarrows} \quad 2NH_3 + CO_2$$

Ammonia   Bicarbonate

2. Subsequent reaction

$$2NH_3 + H_2O \longrightarrow 2NH_4 + 2OH^- \text{ (decreases pH > 7.2)}$$

Ammonium

Figure 10.2 Urease-producing bacteria hydrolyse urea to ammonia molecules and carbon dioxide.

Q. Which bacteria produce urease?

A. Gram −ve
> *Proteus (mirabilis)*
> *Providencia*
> *Klebsiella*
> *Pseudomonas*

Gram +ve
> *Staphylococcus*

Mycoplasma
> *Ureaplasma urealyticum*

LOWER POLE STONES

Q. A 51-year-old man is referred to the one-stop haematuria clinic with occasional left loin ache and microscopic haematuria. He is otherwise well and takes no regular medication. Examination is unremarkable. His GP has requested a plain abdominal film. What does the KUB x-ray in Figure 10.3 show?

A. The x-ray in Figure 10.3 shows a 1.2 cm left lower pole calculus.

Q. He asks you what treatment options there are for the stone in the left kidney. What is the success rate of ESWL?

A. Available treatment options for this patient include ESWL, PCNL or flexible URS.

Lingeman et al. [7] reported the results of a meta-analysis that showed that the overall stone-free rate for ESWL when applied to lower pole stones (LPSs) was 59%, whereas ESWL for upper and middle pole calyces had a stone-free rate of up to 90%.

Stratified by stone size, LPSs fair worse than other sites. The meta-analysis showed stone-free rates for LPS (using ESWL), as follows:

Up to 10 mm	74%
11–20 mm	56%
Over 20 mm	33%

The European Association of Urology (EAU) 2017 treatment algorithm for renal stones [8] is summarised in Figure 10.4. LP stones >20 mm should be treated primarily by PCNL because ESWL will often require multiple treatments and it is associated with an increased

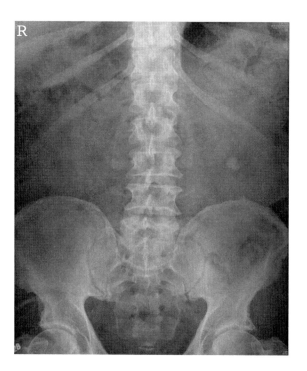

Figure 10.3

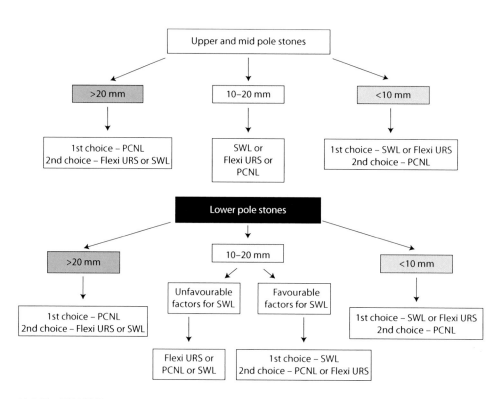

Figure 10.4 The EAU 2017 treatment algorithm for renal stones.

risk of ureteric obstruction (steinstrasse) with the need for additional procedures. URS should only be offered as first line for these stones if the patient is not suitable for PCNL, with the down side of reduced SFRs and the need for staged procedures. LP stones between 10 and 20 mm with unfavourable factors for ESWL should be offered either URS or PCNL. LP stones under <10 mm can be offered ESWL or URS as primary treatment options.

Q. **Are there any factors that predict outcome with ESWL?**

A. Clearance after ESWL may be influenced by lower pole collecting system anatomy. Sampaio and colleagues first described the spatial anatomy of the lower pole as a possible factor in stone passage [9].

The following factors negatively impact the stone-free rates for LP stones:

- Steep infundibular-pelvic angle
- Long calyx (>10 mm)
- Narrow infundibulum (<5 mm)
- Shockwave-resistant stones (calcium oxalate monohydrate, brushite or cystine)

Different studies address calculation of predictive angles in different ways, however, making direct comparison of results problematic.

Keeley et al. [10] measured the LIP (lower pole infundibulopelvic) angle as the angle created by the lower border of the pelvis with the medial border of the lower pole infundibulum. One hundred and sixteen patients underwent ESWL for LPS. The LIP angle was the only factor to attain significance in predicting stone-free status.

Elbahnasy et al. [11] published a retrospective study of 159 patients undergoing ESWL, PCNL and URS for LPS. These authors used an alternative method for measuring the angle between two lines: the central point of the renal pelvis to the central point of the proximal ureter – to determine the ureteropelvic axis and the central axis of the lower pole infundibulum. In this study, all patients with three favourable factors (LIP greater than 70°, infundibular length less than 3 cm, and width greater than 5 mm) became stone free. Conversely, in patients with a combination of three unfavorable factors only 16% became stone free. These data must be interpreted with caution, however, as results from other studies have provided conflicting evidence.

It is intuitive that an obtuse versus an acute angle in LPS is important in fragment clearance after ESWL, but further prospective randomised studies are required to clearly determine the role of intrarenal anatomy.

Q. **Is there anything else which can be done to improve the efficiency of stone clearance after ESWL for LPS?**

A. Pace et al. [12] described percussion, diuresis and inversion (PDI) to enhance stone-free rates. Three months after ESWL 69 patients with residual lower calyceal fragments <4 mm were randomised to either mechanical percussion and inversion or observation for 1 month. They were treated with a mechanical chest percussor applied to the flank while inverted to greater than 60° after receiving 20 mg furosemide. Thirty-five patients had PDI and 34 observation. In the observation group 28 subsequently received mechanical percussion and inversion after completing the observation period. Stone-free rates were PDI 40% versus 3% observation.

Q. **Are there any studies which compare ESWL, URS and PCNL for LPS?**

A. ESWL was compared with PCNL in the 'Lower Pole I' study, published in 2001 [13]. This was a prospective, randomised, multicentre trial comparing PCNL and ESWL for LPS smaller than 30 mm. One hundred and twenty-eight patients were randomised to undergo PCNL (60) and ESWL (68). Three-month stone-free rates overall were 95% for PCNL and 37% for ESWL. The direct comparison of stone-free rates, stratified by stone size is shown in Table 10.1.

Table 10.1 The direct comparison of stone-free rates, stratified by stone size

	Overall	<10 mm	11–20 mm	21–30 mm
ESWL	37%	63%	23%	14%
PCNL	95%	100%	93%	86%

Retreatment and ancillary rates in the ESWL and PCNL groups were 31% and 11%, respectively. The overall morbidity of both procedures was thought to be low.

Reported complication rates were 12% and 23% for ESWL and PCNL, respectively. Cost analysis has revealed PCNL and ESWL were equally effective for stones less than 10 mm, PCNL was more cost-effective for larger stones. The authors suggested that PCNL should be considered the primary approach for LPS larger than 10 mm. The drawback of this study is that URS was not considered.

This issue was addressed in the subsequent 'Lower Pole II' study [14]. Seventy-eight patients with 1 cm or less isolated lower pole stones were randomised to ESWL or URS. The operative time was significantly shorter for ESWL than URS. Intraoperative complications occurred in one ESWL case (unable to target stone) and in seven URS cases (failed access in five and perforation in two patients). This study did not show a statistically significant difference in stone-free rates between ESWL and URS for LPS, even though URS was 15% better. However, with continuing improvements in ureteroscopic technology and a study with a larger number of participants, a different outcome may be achieved if such a study were to be repeated. The Percutaneous nephrolithotomy, flexible Ureterorenoscopy and Extracorporeal shockwave lithotripsy (PUrE) study was therefore set up in the United Kingdom in 2015 to determine the clinical effectiveness and cost-effectiveness of the treatments for lower pole stones (URS versus ESWL for stones ≤10 mm and URS versus PCNL for stones >10 mm ≤25 mm) and will report their findings in 2020 [15].

URS could be proposed as the primary approach or as a less morbid treatment modality for patients with LPS who failed ESWL rather than proceeding to PCNL. The success rate (including 'insignificant' residual fragments) of URS for LPS is relatively high, with an average of 86% SFR for LPSs larger than 20 mm.

Anatomy of the lower pole may affect the results of URS for LPS, in a similar manner to ESWL as an acute angle may prevent passage of the laser fibre to the stone by limiting flexion.

ESWL is the preferred initial approach for most patients with LPS smaller than 1 cm, as it is a less invasive approach, not requiring general anaesthesia. Patients who failed ESWL, and patients known to have stones resistant to ESWL should be treated with PCNL or URS having considered the risks and benefits after an informed discussion with their urologist.

In contrast to URS and ESWL results, PCNL outcomes are independent of stone size and renal anatomy.

Q. Should a JJ stent be placed before considering ESWL in this patient?

A. Routine stenting is contraindicated prior to ESWL, and should be avoided.

ASYMPTOMATIC SMALL RENAL STONES

Q. A fit and well 60-year-old male is referred by his GP for an opinion on an asymptomatic 5 mm lower pole renal stone found incidentally on a CT scan. How common are asymptomatic renal stones and are they safe to monitor?

A. Historically the prevalence of asymptomatic renal stones was estimated to be between 3% and 5% within the United Kingdom [16]. There is now clear evidence that stone disease is increasing across all Western societies. Stamatelou et al. showed an increase in prevalence

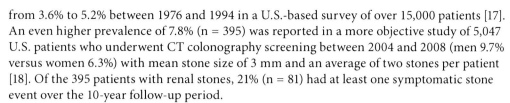

from 3.6% to 5.2% between 1976 and 1994 in a U.S.-based survey of over 15,000 patients [17]. An even higher prevalence of 7.8% (n = 395) was reported in a more objective study of 5,047 U.S. patients who underwent CT colonography screening between 2004 and 2008 (men 9.7% versus women 6.3%) with mean stone size of 3 mm and an average of two stones per patient [18]. Of the 395 patients with renal stones, 21% (n = 81) had at least one symptomatic stone event over the 10-year follow-up period.

The natural history of small asymptomatic renal stones has been described in a few key papers from mainly single institution case series which have reported conflicting results.

Glowacki et al. [19] prospectively followed up 107 patients for a mean of 31 months and reported a symptomatic event in only 32%, whereas 68% remained symptom free with the number of stones and a past history of stones being predictors of observation failure. Of the patients with symptoms, 47% passed their stone spontaneously, 26.5% required surgical intervention and 26.5% had ESWL.

Burgher et al. [20] retrospectively assessed 300 patients with a mean follow-up of 38 months and showed 77% of patients progressed with regards to stone size, number and symptoms, of which 26% required an intervention. Patients with stones larger than 4 mm or those with lower pole stones were more likely to increase in size, develop symptoms or require intervention.

A further retrospective study by Kang et al. [21] of 347 patients reported 53% having a symptomatic stone event within 31 months follow-up of which 24.5% required an intervention with only 5% needing surgery. A stone event was more likely in those who were young, male and had a stone history.

In a more contemporary series Dropkin et al. [22] followed up 110 patients for over 3 years (mean stone size 7 mm) with only 24% becoming symptomatic and 19% requiring surgical intervention. However, 19% increased in size and only 2.9% passed the stone spontaneously.

Finally, a prospective randomised controlled trial (RCT) comparing observation to prophylactic ESWL in asymptomatic renal stones less than 15 mm reported no significant difference in terms of symptoms, requirement for additional treatment, quality of life or hospital admission during a 2-year follow-up period, with only 9% requiring surgery [23].

In summary, the natural history of small asymptomatic renal stones remains unclear; however, a period of observation appears to be a safe initial treatment option. Long-term follow-up is necessary especially in patients with increased risk of stone progression where the need for future active treatment is higher.

Q. **The patient chooses a period of observation as his initial management. What is your follow-up regime and what are your indications for treatment?**

A. I would follow-up this patient initially on a 6-monthly basis in a dedicated stone clinic to assess for symptoms and stone growth. If the stone was visible on the initial CT scout film I would use an x-ray KUB to assess for stone progression. If there was no growth and the patient remained asymptomatic I would consider increasing the follow-up to 12 monthly and discharging after 5 years. If the patient became symptomatic I would arrange a repeat CT-KUB to accurately assess his stone burden and help guide further management.

The majority of articles previously discussed have shown that progression is linked to stone size. The spontaneous passage of stones appears higher for <5 mm compared to 5–10 mm with some authors recommending the treatment of all renal stones >5 mm [24,25]. The EAU 2017 guidelines recommend the treatment of renal stones in patients with stone growth (>5 mm), *de novo* obstruction, associated sepsis, patient preference, social situation (professional or travelling), stones in patients at high risk of recurrence, solitary kidneys, women planning on getting pregnant and in patients with chronic pain. The recommended treatment options are discussed previously [8].

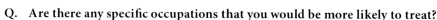

Q. Are there any specific occupations that you would be more likely to treat?

A. The Civil Aviation Authority (CAA) has a formalised guideline for the management of pilots diagnosed with one or more asymptomatic renal stones. They are deemed unfit to fly until they have been fully investigated and have been proven radiologically to be stone free after treatment. The UK Royal Air Force also requires the pilot's metabolic stone profile to be normal before the pilot can return to work. In addition, patients whose jobs have the potential to risk the safety of others during an episode of renal colic (driving heavy good vehicles, trains, buses, etc.) should be advised that they are not fit to carry out their work until they are stone free and they should inform their employer and the Driver and Vehicle Licensing Agency as soon as possible [26].

CALYCEAL DIVERTICULAR STONES

Q. Figure 10.5 is the KUB x-ray of a 36-year-old man. He complains of intermittent left loin pain and has microscopic haematuria. How would you treat this stone initially?

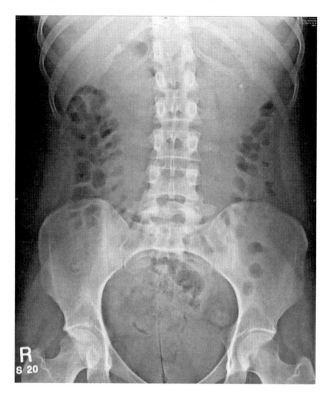

Figure 10.5

A. Figure 10.5 shows a 4–5 mm radiopacity in the left kidney, likely to be a stone.

The initial management of a stone of this size would be ESWL. There is a 70% chance that stone clearance would be achieved, if it is in anatomically normal calyx.

Q. This stone has been treated with two sessions of ESWL. While it appeared to have partially fragmented, the fragments did not clear. What are the possible reasons for this?

A. One possible reason is that this stone lies within a calyceal diverticulum. Other possibilities include that the stone is too hard to be fragmented with ESWL, and this might indicate that the stone is a calcium oxalate monohydrate stone.

Q. What is a calyceal diverticulum, and how would you manage this stone?

A. Calyceal diverticula are nonsecretory urothelial-lined compartments in communication with the renal collecting system, although the point of communication is often only very narrow. While it is reasonable to manage asymptomatic diverticular stones conservatively, those causing pain, infection or bleeding should be treated.

ESWL can been used to treat calyceal diverticular stones, but due to poor drainage of the fragments, the stone-free rates are low (often 20%–30% only), and are not comparable to that of PCNL, where stone-free rates are around 90%. Ureteroscopy can also be used, often with laser incision of the diverticular neck initially, allowing stone-free rates of up to 70%.

However, as well as clearance of the stone, obliteration of the diverticulum should be attempted. This is not possible with ESWL, and success at ureteroscopy is low. However, PCNL provides excellent access for this and obliteration rates of up to 80% are seen. Finally, laparoscopic and robotic-assisted laparoscopic approaches to calyceal diverticular stones have been reported with good success.

HORSESHOE KIDNEY STONES

Q. This 46-year-old man presented with left loin pain. What do you see in this CT slice in Figure 10.6?

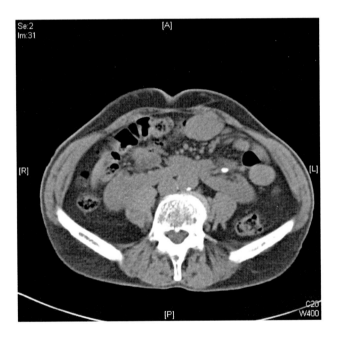

Figure 10.6

A. Figure 10.6 shows a CT slice in which there is a 7 mm stone in the left renal pelvis of a horseshoe kidney.

Q. What is the prevalence of a horseshoe kidney, and how do they arise embryologically?

A. The prevalence is approximately 1 in 400. This congenital anomaly results from abnormal medial fusion of the metanephric blastema causing failure of ascent and rotation of the kidneys. Ascent is arrested by the inferior mesenteric artery.

Q. **What do you know of the anatomic differences between a horseshoe kidney and a normal kidney?**

A. The fused horseshoe kidney lies more caudal in position compared with normal kidneys and, because of incomplete rotation, the renal pelvis is anterior to all of the calyces. The ureter is usually inserted high and lateral onto the renal pelvis. In a horseshoe kidney the calyces point posteriorly with the lower pole calyces pointing caudally and medially. In a normal kidney all calyces are located lateral to the renal pelvis and point laterally.

Q. **How would you manage this patient, and what problems might arise with the various management options?**

A. *ESWL* would be a reasonable first-line treatment option in this patient. Problems which might arise include difficulties with stone localisation with ultrasound scan (USS) due to the medial location of the kidney and the fact that intervening bowel gas may further impair visualisation. Fluoroscopy may be difficult because of overlying bony landmarks. Even if there is good visualisation and fragmentation, dilatation of the collecting system, relative urinary stasis and the relatively high insertion of the ureter on the renal pelvis all impair the drainage of fragments. However, with good patient positioning for a stone of this size there is a significant chance that ESWL would leave the patient stone free.

Ureteroscopy is a viable treatment option for small symptomatic stones which have not responded to ESWL. Because of the tortuous path of the ureter and the complicated intrarenal anatomy a flexible instrument will be needed, but if used with an access sheath to allow for continuous irrigation and the ability to remove small fragments, high stone-free rates are achievable, though not as high as in patients with normal kidneys.

PCNL should be used for large stones (>2 cm) and for stones where ureteroscopy or ESWL has failed. Because of the anterior location of the kidney, the track may be long, and the usual point of access is the upper pole posterior calyx. This means that to reach the lower pole calyces or PUJ, a flexible instrument will likely be required. The track is usually more medial than in normal kidneys, with a higher risk of retrorenal colon, but lower chance of pulmonary injury. High stone-free rates of over 70% are achievable.

URETERIC STONES

Q. **A 29-year-old man presents to the emergency department with a 72-hour history of right loin pain, radiating to the groin. He is otherwise well. Examination shows he is writhing in pain and is difficult to assess, but observations are stable and he is not pyrexial. Full blood count and creatinine and electrolytes are both normal and urine dipstick is positive for blood. What is your next step and why?**

A. This man should be given parental NSAIDs to relieve his pain unless contraindicated (history of gastric ulcer, severe asthma or renal impairment).

A Cochrane review of the management of pain in acute renal colic was published in 2005 [27]. RCTs comparing any opioid with any NSAID, regardless of dose or route of administration were included. Twenty trials from nine countries with a total of 1613 participants were identified. Both NSAIDs and opioids lead to clinically significant falls in patient-reported pain scores. Due to unexplained heterogeneity these results could not be pooled although 10/13 studies reported lower pain scores in patients receiving NSAIDs. Patients treated with NSAIDs were significantly less likely to require rescue medication. The majority of trials showed a higher incidence of adverse events, particularly vomiting, in patients treated with opioids (especially pethidine) [27]. NSAIDs are thought to work by prostaglandin-induced afferent arteriole vasoconstriction of the glomerulus therefore reducing diuresis, oedema and ureteric smooth muscle stimulation [28]. A further Cochrane review in 2015 was unable to determine which NSAID was the most effective [29].

Q. What is the imaging test of choice and why?

A. CT-KUB (non-contrast CT of kidneys, ureters and bladder) has now replaced IVU as the gold standard for investigating acute flank pain. CT-KUB (sensitivity 94%–100% and specificity 92%–100%) is significantly more accurate at detecting stones compared to IVU (sensitivity 51%–87% and specificity 92%–100%) with the added benefit of being able to measure their diameter, skin to stone distance and Hounsfield unit (HU) density [30]. CT-KUB is also much quicker to perform, does not require the delivery of intravenous contrast and if a stone is not detected it has the added benefit of being able to diagnose other causes of abdominal pain. Radiation risk can be reduced to similar levels as IVU by low-dose CT (3 mSv) with a recent meta-analysis of prospective studies a pooled sensitivity of 96.6% and specificity of 94.9% [31].

Q. What other imaging modalities are useful in the management of renal colic?

A. Ultrasound is a safe (no risk of radiation) and inexpensive imaging tool which is able to detect stones located in the kidney and at the vesicoureteric junction (with a filled bladder) as well as dilation of the upper tracts. It is the imaging modality of choice for suspected renal colic in children and pregnant patients. It has a sensitivity and specificity of 45% and 94% for the detection of ureteric stones and 45% and 88% for renal stones, respectively [32]. X-ray KUB has a sensitivity of 44%–77% and specificity of 80%–87% and is helpful in the follow-up of radiopaque stones [33].

Q. Which stones are not visible on CT-KUB and what is the benefit of performing the scan with the patient in the prone position?

A. Ninety-nine per cent of stones in the urinary tract are visible on CT-KUB. Indinavir stones (HIV drug with poor solubility and excessive excretion in urine leading to crystallisation) and pure matrix stones (consist of protein and cellular debris) are the only two stones which are radiolucent on CT-KUB.

One of the most common sites for stones to become obstructed is at the vesicoureteric junction (VUJ). Scanning the patients prone allows for clinicians to establish if the stone is still contained within the VUJ or if it has already passed into the bladder. If it has passed into the bladder, then the stone will fall away from the VUJ on the prone CT.

Q. How does a CT scan work?

A. A fixed x-ray tube is positioned opposite a banana-shaped x-ray detector inside a rotating frame which rotates around the patient. The x-ray tube is configured to produce a thin fan-shaped beam of x-rays towards the detectors. Each time the x-ray tube and detector rotates 360° around the patient an image or slice is acquired. Each slice is collimated (focused) to a thickness between 1 and 10 mm using lead shutters which are situated just in front of the x-ray tube. The patient moves through the rotating frame in the horizontal plane on a bed allowing a slice to be obtained at each level. Typically, during one 360° rotation approximately 1000 profiles of x-ray beam are sampled by each detector. Each profile is subsequently reconstructed by sophisticated software into a two-dimensional image of the slice. Individual attenuation values (Hounsfield units) can be generated for a particular area of tissue.

Q. What is the radiation risk associated with CT and other imaging modalities?

A. Table 10.2 shows the relative radiation exposure of various radiological investigations.

Table 10.2 Relative radiation exposure of common radiological investigations

Diagnostic procedure	Typical effective dose (mSv)	CXR equivalent for effective dose	Time for equivalent dose from natural background radiation
CXR (PA)	0.02	1	2.4 days
Skull XR	0.07	4	8.5 days
Lumbar spine	1.3	65	158 days
IVU	2.5	125	304 days
Ba swallow	3.0	150	1 year
CT-KUB (non-contrast)	4.7	250	1.6 years
Low-dose CT-KUB	3	150	1 year
CT abdomen with contrast	10.0	500	3.3 years

With regard to the associated increased risk of cancer related to such exposure, the U.S. Food and Drug Administration has stated that the natural incidence of fatal cancer is one in five. A 10 mSv dose increases this by 1 in 2000.

Hence an IVU of 1.5–3 mSv increases the risk by 1 in 10,000, whereas a CT-KUB of 4.5–5 mSv increases risk by 1 in 4000.

Q. What are the signs of obstruction on CT-KUB?

A. Hydronephrosis, increased renal size (nephromegaly), unilateral perinephric stranding, periureteric stranding and ureteric wall oedema/soft tissue cuff/ring around stone (Rim sign).

Q. What is a Hounsfield unit? How can this property be utilised in the management of stone disease?

A. A Hounsfield unit is a quantitative scale for measuring radiodensity. Zero HU is the radiodensity of distilled water at standard pressure and temperature. The radiodensities of common substances in the body are summarised in Table 10.3.

Table 10.3 Radiodensities (HU) of common substances in the body

Substances	Hounsfield unit (HU)
Air	−1000
Lung	−500
Fat	−100 to −50
Water	0
CSF	+15
Kidney	+30
Blood	+30 to +45
Muscle	+10 to +40
Liver	+40 to +60
Soft tissue with contrast	+100 to +300
Bone	+700 (cancellous) +3000 (cortical)

CT attenuation values (HU) have shown some promise in predicting stone composition which plays an important role in helping clinicians determine the most effective treatment for an individual patient. Uric acid stones have a low density (200–450 HUs) and can sometimes be successfully treated non-surgically with urine alkalinisation. Calcium base stones, however, have a higher density (1000 + HUs) making them more resistant to ESWL and therefore more likely to require surgical management. CT attenuation values prior to ESWL have been shown to help predict treatment success (threshold of ≤815 HUs has significantly better stone clearance than ≥815 HUs) [34].

The HUs of common pure stones can be predicted by CT HUs during *in vitro* studies to an accuracy between 64% and 81% and usually fall within certain ranges (Table 10.4) [35]. The accuracy of HUs in clinical practice is much more complicated and less reliable as factors such as stone size, accurate placement of area of interest (average HU) and mixed stones (35%–65% of all stones) reduce its effectiveness. Dual-energy CT is a new technique which measures stone attenuation much more accurately and has been shown in a recent meta-analysis to have a pooled sensitivity of 96% and specificity of 99% at predicting uric acid stones [36].

Table 10.4 The attenuation values of common stones during *in vitro* studies

Stone composition	Hounsfield units
Uric acid	200–450
Struvite	600–900
Cystine	600–1100
Calcium phosphate	1200–1600
Calcium monohydrate and brushite	1700–2800

Source: Adapted from Bellin MF et al. *Eur Radiol* 2004; 14(11): 2134–2140.

Q. A 22-year-old man would like to try conservative management in the first instance for a 5 mm distal ureteric stone. He is also aware that certain medications may help the stone to pass. However, his friends have also had stones treated with ESWL and URS. What evidence is there for the optimum management of ureteric calculi?

A. The evidence regarding spontaneous stone passage (SSP) of ureteric stones according to stone size is based historically on the 2007 joint EAU/American Urological Association (AUA) Guideline for the Management of Ureteral Calculi [37,38].

This meta-analysis concluded that the median probability of spontaneous passage of ureteric stones <5 mm is 68% versus 47% for those stones of 5–10 mm and estimated that a stone of up to 4 mm has a 95% chance of passing spontaneously within 40 days. A more recent systematic review of 37 studies by Skolarikos et al. [39] concluded that symptomatic ureteric calculi <4 mm has a 38%–71% chance of passing spontaneously while only 4.8% of stones <2 mm will need intervention. Data from the placebo arms of recent RCTs assessing the effect of medical expulsion therapy (MET) have provided further insights with overall SSP rates for ureteric stones being as high as 86%–90% for stones <5 mm and 61% for stones >5 mm [40,41]. A period of observation is therefore recommended by the 2017 EAU guidelines panel in patients with small stones (<6 mm) who are fully informed and have no evidence of complications such as infection, deteriorating renal failure or uncontrolled pain [8].

The role of medical expulsive therapy (MET) in the spontaneous passage of ureteric calculi has recently been called into question by new high-quality data from three well-designed, multicentre, placebo-controlled, double-blinded RCTs which have shown limited or no benefit using alpha-blockers.

Pickard et al. [41] recruited 1167 patients with CT confirmed ureteric stones (<5 mm or >5 mm) and randomised them to either placebo, tamsulosin or nifedipine with the primary outcome measure being the requirement for treatment within 4 weeks of randomisation. They showed no difference in the number of patients requiring intervention at 4 weeks in each group (placebo 20%; tamsulosin 19%; and nifedipine 20%) but did show a trend towards a benefit in larger stones (>5 mm, P = 0.3) in the distal ureter (P = 0.09) which did not reach significance. The authors concluded that MET should no longer be offered, giving healthcare providers an opportunity to reallocate funds elsewhere. Critiques of this study have raised a number of concerns including the choice of the primary endpoint being the need for treatment rather than CT confirmation of stone passage; the high rate of stone passage in the placebo arm potentially reducing the statistical power to show a difference; and that the majority of the stones were <5 mm which were likely to pass spontaneously anyway [42].

The second RCT by Furyk et al. [40] randomised 403 patients with distal ureteric stones <1 cm detected on CT to MET or placebo, with the primary outcome measure assessing stone expulsion on CT at 28 days. They also showed no difference in overall passage rates (tamsulosin 87% versus placebo 82%) but did find a 22.4% increased chance of passage for larger (>5 mm) and more distal stones. The third RCT was published by Sur et al. [43] who randomised 239 patients with CT confirmed stones (4–10 mm) to received silodosin or placebo with the primary outcome measure being stone passage at 4 weeks confirmed by imaging or reported by the patient. Once again, no overall difference in stone passage rates was observed between treatment groups (52% versus 44%, P = 0.2), however, silodosin achieved a significantly greater rate of distal stone passage than placebo (P = 0.01).

Hollingsworth et al. [44] subsequently published a meta-analysis of 55 trials which including the new studies previously discussed and concluded that MET promotes stone passage of large stones located in any part of the ureter. Opponents of this analysis contest their findings as the majority of studies included were small and from single centres with poor methodological quality which therefore limits the strength of their conclusions. Although the majority of UK urologists have now moved away from using MET in their practice, the EAU 2017 guideline panel have concluded that MET seems to be efficacious in patients with ureteric stones with the greatest benefit in larger and more distal stones [8]. If considering to offer MET, patients should be informed that the evidence is controversial, its use is 'off label' and be made aware of the potential side effects (low blood pressure, retrograde ejaculation and stuffy nose).

Finally, with regards to intervention, the stone-free (clearance) rates of ureteric stones when treated with ESWL or with URS, the guidelines addressed proximal, mid and distal stones separately. The overall stone-free figures, according to location and size, are presented in Table 10.5.

Briefly, for proximal ureteric stones, it appears that ESWL may be superior for stones <10 mm, but that URS is better for stones >10 mm. In patients with distal ureteric stones, URS is considered superior irrespective of size. Finally, for mid-ureteric stones the treatments are generally considered equivalent. Importantly, it should be understood that the data from the guidelines have been based on the 'index patient', designed to reflect the typical individual with a ureteric stone. The definition of an index patient is a non-pregnant adult with a unilateral non-cystine/non-uric acid radiopaque ureteral stone without renal calculi requiring therapy whose contralateral kidney functions normally and whose medical condition, body habitus, and anatomy allow any one of the treatment options to be undertaken.

Table 10.5 The overall stone-free figures, and the breakdown for stones <10 and >10 mm in size, according to joint EAU and AUA guidelines

		ESWL (%)	URS (%)
Proximal	Overall	82	81
	<10 mm	90	80
	>10 mm	68	79
Middle	Overall	73	86
	<10 mm	84	91
	>10 mm	76	78
Distal	Overall	74	94
	<10 mm	86	97
	>10 mm	74	93

Q. **While under observation, this patient develops a temperature of 39° Celsius. What is your further management?**

A. An infected obstructed system is a urological emergency and must be drained expeditiously after initial resuscitation of the patient and administration of intravenous antibiotics according to local microbiology department guidelines.

The question of whether to use nephrostomy tube drainage or pass a retrograde JJ stent under anaesthesia cystoscopically has been addressed in two studies. Pearle et al. [45] compared the efficacy of percutaneous nephrostomy with retrograde ureteral catheterisation for renal drainage in cases of obstruction and infection associated with ureteral calculi. Forty-two patients presenting with obstructing ureteral calculi and clinical signs of infection were randomised to nephrostomy or stenting. There was no significant difference in the time to treatment between the two groups. Procedural and fluoroscopy times were significantly shorter in the retrograde ureteral catheterisation group. One treatment failure occurred in the percutaneous nephrostomy group, which was successfully salvaged with retrograde ureteral catheterisation. Time to normal temperature was 2.3 days in the percutaneous nephrostomy and 2.6 in the retrograde ureteral catheterisation group. The authors concluded that stenting and percutaneous nephrostomy both effectively relieved obstruction and infection due to ureteral calculi. Neither modality demonstrated superiority in promoting a more rapid recovery after drainage. The decision of which mode of drainage to use may be based on logistical factors, surgeon preference and stone characteristics.

In a similar study, Mokhmalji and co-workers [46] observed that those randomised to nephrostomy tube drainage required antibiotics for a shorter time after drainage, and that this mode of drainage appeared to be superior to stent insertion, especially in those with a high temperature, males and juveniles. In addition, stent insertion was unsuccessful in 20% of cases, compared to 100% success with percutaneous nephrostomy.

Q. **What are the advantages and disadvantages of JJ stents and nephrostomy tube?**

A. These are listed in Table 10.6.

Table 10.6 Advantages and disadvantages of stents and nephrostomies

Stent advantages	Stent disadvantages	Nephrostomy advantages	Nephrostomy disadvantages
Resources and availability – There is no need for radiologist, as urologist can do procedure	Renal pelvis pressure remains elevated	Rapid and maintained decrease in renal pelvis pressure	Resources and availability – There is a need for a radiologist
No risk of injury to adjacent organs	Usually has to be performed under general anaesthesia, which may be risky, particularly in a sick/unwell patient	Can be performed under local anaesthesia/sedation, hence not requiring general anaesthesia	Risk of injury to adjacent organs
No need for nephrostomy bag	Risk of ureteric manipulation and resulting bacteraemia/ureteric injury	Avoids ureteric manipulation and risk of bacteraemia/ureteric injury	Need for nephrostomy bag
Better 'functional' information, especially in obstructed systems	Failure rate (impacted stone)	Low failure rate	Signs may be subtle especially in obstructed systems
	Cannot monitor urine output from kidney	Can monitor urine from kidney	
	No access available for subsequent tract, if required	Access available for subsequent tract, if required	

Q. Describe how you would take informed consent for ureteroscopy.

A. Informed consent must include a discussion of available alternative treatment options, as described previously, the intended benefit of the proposed procedure, and the potential complications, which are listed as follows with approximate percentages in brackets, based on complications of 3000 semi-rigid ureteroscopies performed by Geavlete et al. [47]:

Intraoperative complications (3.5%)	
Mucosal injury or abrasion	1.5%
False passage	1.0%
Ureteric perforation	0.6%
Extraureteric stone migration	0.2%
Ureteral avulsions	0.1%
Bleeding	0.1%
Early complications (10%)	
Fever or sepsis	1.0%
Persistent haematuria	2.0%
Renal colic	2.0%
Transient vesico-ureteric reflux (VUR)	4.5%
Late complications	
Ureteric stricture	0.5%
Persistent VUR	Rare
Intraoperative incidents	
Stone migration	4.2%
Unable to access calculi	3.7%
Trapped stone extractors	0.7%
Equipment damage	0.7%
JJ stent malpositioning	0.7%
Migrated JJ stent	0.66%

Q. What laser do you use in your practice and what settings do you use for dusting and fragmenting stones?

A. I use a Holmium:YAG laser to treat stones. This is a solid-state pulsed laser, with a wavelength of 2.1 microns. The shallow penetration depth minimises the collateral damage to sensitive surrounding tissue. The combination of the controlled penetration depth and the water absorption characteristics reduce the energy that can reach the non-target tissue, contributing to the safety profile of the procedure.

There are three parameters which are important to consider when fragmenting stones. These are frequency (measured in Hz), the energy (measured in J) and the pulse duration. The frequency multiplied by the energy gives the power of the laser. For dusting stones, the optimal settings are low energy, such as 0.3 or 0.4 J, a high frequency, such as 30–50 Hz, and a long pulse duration (such as 800 microseconds).

Q. When would you insert a stent following ureteroscopy?

A. Routine stenting after complete stone removal during an uncomplicated URS is not necessary and may be associated with higher post-operative morbidity [8]. A meta-analysis by Nabi et al. [48] reviewed nine RCTs (831 patients) that reported outcomes after stenting post-ureteroscopy and showed higher morbidity in the form of storage lower urinary tract symptoms, with no influence on SFRs, requirement for analgesia, rate of urinary tract infection, or long-term ureteric stricture.

The EAU 2017 guidelines recommend JJ stent insertion in the following circumstances:

- Ureteric trauma during the procedure
- Residual stone fragments greater than 2 mm remaining in ureter
- Bleeding (potential for clot colic)
- Pregnancy
- If treating an impacted stone (usually ureter very oedematous at site of impaction)
- Prolonged manipulation within ureter, particularly upper third
- After flexible ureteroscopy and use of an access sheath
- All doubtful cases, to avoid stressful emergencies

Stone disease in pregnancy

Q. How common are stones in pregnancy?

A. Pregnant patients do not appear to be at increased risk of stone formation compared to non-pregnant females of childbearing age [49]. Urolithiasis affects 1 in 200–1500 pregnancies [50,51] with 80%–90% being diagnosed after the first trimester [52]. The top reason for non-obstetric admissions during pregnancy is acute urolithiasis with symptomatic stones being found in the ureter twice as often as in the renal pelvis [53].

Q. What changes occur in pregnancy that affect the risk of forming stones?

A. The anatomical and physiological changes that may affect stone formation in pregnancy are summarised in Table 10.7 [54,55]. The net effect of these changes is no increased risk of stone formation.

Table 10.7 The anatomical and physiological changes that may affect stone formation in pregnancy

Promoting stone formation	Inhibiting stone formation
Physiological hydronephrosis and urinary stasis due by progesterone (ureteric smooth muscle dilation) and mechanical obstruction	Increased filtration of magnesium, citrate, uromodulin, nephrocalcin and urinary glycosaminoglycans due to increased eGFR
Increased excretion of glucose, sodium, uric acid and urea due to increased eGFR	
Absorptive hypercalcuria caused by placental formation of 1,25 dihydroxycholecalciferol and suppressed parathyroid hormone	

Q. A 28-year-old female who is 20 weeks pregnant presents to the A+E department with acute right loin pain. What is the differential diagnosis and what is your initial management?

A. The common causes of acute abdominal pain in a pregnant patient include ureteric colic, placental abruption, pyelonephritis, colitis and appendicitis. I would provide immediate pain relief and arrange some investigations, including a urine dipstick (haematuria, pyuria and pH), urine culture and sensitivity, baseline bloods and imaging of the upper tracts. I would also request urgent review by the obstetric team.

Q. What imaging modality would you use for suspected ureteric colic and why?

A. The 2017 EAU guidelines recommend transvaginal/transabdominal ultrasound with a full bladder as the primary diagnostic tool in evaluating pregnant patients with suspected renal colic [8]. Ultrasound has a poor sensitivity at identifying ureteric stones and is unable to differentiate between physiological hydronephrosis of pregnancy and acute obstruction. Transvaginal ultrasound can be helpful to assess the distal ureter. Magnetic resonance imaging (MRI) is advised as a second-line investigation when results are equivocal and is able to define the level of urinary obstruction, visualise stones as a filling defect and can assess non-urological organ systems. Low-dose non-contrast CT-KUB (fetal exposure 0.05 versus 2.5 Gy) is increasing in popularity with a high sensitivity and specificity but still is last-line as exposure to ionising radiation can be associated with teratogenic risks and development of childhood malignancies. The importance and need for more accurate diagnosis was illustrated by White et al. who assessed the outcomes of 51 pregnant patients who underwent ureteroscopy for suspected ureteric stones on pre-op imaging. They reported an overall 14% (n = 7) negative ureteroscopy rate with the lowest rate in those who underwent pre-op low-dose CT (4%) and the highest rate in those who had ultrasound (23%) and MRI (20%) [56].

Q. **Which side does physiological hydronephrosis occur on more commonly and why?**

A. Physiological hydronephrosis is more prominent on the right side (right 90%: left 10%) because of compression by the dilated right ovarian vein and uterine dextro-rotation and protection of the left ureter by the gas-filled sigmoid colon [57]. Mechanical compression is probably more significant than progesterone-mediated dilatation as studies have shown that dilation is not seen when the ureter does not cross the pelvic brim, as in patients with a pelvic kidney or urinary diversion [58,59]. Hydronephrosis can be seen as early as 6 weeks' gestation and has usually resolved by 6 weeks' post-partum [60].

Q. **The USS suspects a 7 mm upper ureteric stone. Her pain is controlled with analgesia, she is eating and drinking normally and has normal observations. Her bloods revealed a raised WCC of 13, CRP 7 and an estimated glomerular filtration rate (eGFR) of >90. How would you manage this patient?**

A. The management of this patient is complex and should involve close collaboration between the patient, obstetrician, radiologist and urologist given the potential complications that can occur. Expectant therapy is appropriate in this situation as her pain is controlled, there is no sign of infection and she is tolerating food and liquid orally. In addition, previous studies have shown 60%–80% will pass spontaneously due to the physiologically dilated upper tracts [50,61]. Conservative management consists of rest, adequate hydration, analgesia and anti-emetics. Prophylactic antibiotics may also be required as up to half of pregnant patients with stones have concomitant infection [62]. The patient should be closely followed-up by the urology and obstetric team with regular examination, bloods and repeat ultrasound.

Q. **What pain killers and antibiotics would you recommend?**

A. Paracetamol and opioids are first line because of the potential harmful effects of other medications. Oral opioid agents such as codeine, oxycodone and morphine are all considered safe to use in pregnancy. NSAIDs should be avoided because of the potential risk of closure of the ductus arteriosus due to blocking prostaglandin release as well as the increased risk of hypertension and early spontaneous abortion. Severe pain can be managed with patient-controlled analgesia, an epidural or segmental blocks (T11 and L2) [57].

Antibiotics treatment should be guided based on culture and sensitivity with specialist microbiology advice requested in more severe infections. Penicillin, cephalosporin and macrolide antibiotics are considered safe to use in pregnancy. Nitrofurantoin is also safe for most of pregnancy but should be avoided towards term due to an increased risk of neonatal haemolysis. Trimethoprim is a folate antagonist and should be avoided especially in the first trimester during organogenesis. There is a risk of auditory or vestibular nerve damage with gentamicin. There is limited information on Tazocin or carbapenems with manufactures advising to use only if the potential benefit outweighs the risk in more severe infections [63].

Q. **What are the risks associated with renal colic in the pregnant patient?**

A. There are multiple potential risks to the mother and fetus, including recurrent miscarriages, preterm labour, premature rupture of membranes and pre-eclampsia [54].

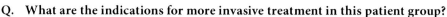

Q. **What are the indications for more invasive treatment in this patient group?**

A. Approximately 15%–30% of pregnant patients' stones will need some form of active intervention [52]. Indications for treatment include uncontrolled pain, sepsis, obstructed single kidney or bilateral obstruction, social and psychological reasons and obstetric complications (pre-eclampsia or premature onset of labor) [57].

Q. **What are the potential active treatment options and associated risks?**

A. Prior to any active therapy the patient must be made aware of the nature of the proposed treatment, alternative options, the potential risks to mother and fetus and local available expertise. An infected and obstructed kidney must be drained with either a retrograde stent or antegrade nephrostomy. Ureteric stent insertion usually requires a general anaesthetic and use of fluoroscopy. They are also associated with storage lower urinary tract symptoms and an increased risk of stent encrustation due to hypercalcuria and hyperuricosia of pregnancy. They should therefore be changed every 4 weeks initially with increasing time between procedures if no encrustation is observed [57].

Percutaneous nephrostomy (PNL) is especially useful in pregnancy as it is minimally invasive (ultrasound guidance under local anaesthetic), provides immediate and effective drainage of an obstructed system (success rate >90%), allows urine collection for culture and sensitivity, avoids ureteral manipulation and provides access for future percutaneous nephrolithotomy or stone dissolution [57]. PNL is also more cost effective than ureteric stents and is easily exchanged over a guidewire without the need for local anaesthetic [52]. Its disadvantages include pain or bleeding during placement, dislodgement, recurrent blockages, bacterial colonisation and the social and psychological issues associated with an external drainage tube. PNL should be exchanged every 4 weeks [57] initially, due to increased risk of encrustation.

Ureteroscopy and stone removal is the procedure of choice if conservative measures fail and should be performed in experienced centres [8]. It has been shown to be safe, effective (stone-free rates 70%–100%) and is associated with significantly shorter lengths of hospital stay when compared with ureteral stenting [64–66]. The procedure is performed under a general or spinal anaesthetic with the patient placed in the modified dorsal lithotomy. A stent should be placed post-procedure and left on a string to be removed a few days later if there were no complications. The potential complications associated with ureteroscopy were previously discussed. Although PCNL is feasible in early pregnancy [67–69] this procedure is usually not recommended due to the increased maternal and fetal risk secondary to prolonged general anaesthesia, use of fluoroscopy and patient positioning. The ESWL is an absolute contraindication in pregnancy because of the risk of foetal death during shockwave delivery [8].

METABOLIC STONES

Q. **A 26-year-old man comes to see you having had his second episode of renal colic. He has passed his stone and presents it to you. He is presently symptom free. There is no family history of renal stones. What might the stone be made of?**

A. The majority of stones have more than one constituent, but the major constituents of stones with their relative percentages are as follows:

Calcium oxalate	70%–80%
Struvite (magnesium ammonium phosphate)	10%
Uric acid	8%–10%
Cystine	1%–2%
Calcium phosphate	1%

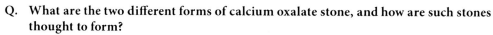

Q. **What are the two different forms of calcium oxalate stone, and how are such stones thought to form?**

A. Calcium oxalate stones occur in two different forms: calcium oxalate monohydrate (whewellite) and calcium oxalate dihydrate (weddellite). The former are much harder to break than the latter.

Calcium oxalate stones are thought to develop as a result of a number of factors. There is an imbalance between promoters of stone formation, which are increased, and inhibitors of stone formation, which are decreased. Thus a decreased urinary volume, decreased urinary pH, and decreased urinary citrate, magnesium and glycosaminoglycans, with increased urinary uric acid, oxalate and calcium are all risk factors for urinary supersaturation with calcium oxalate. The more supersaturated the urine is, the higher the risk of stone formation. If the saturation is below the *solubility product*, then a stone will not form. Once it goes above this, however, crystal growth will occur, and crystals will aggregate, but *de novo* nucleation is very slow. An increase in inhibitors in the urine at this level may prevent stone formation. However, as the saturation of calcium oxalate in the urine increases above the *formation product*, nucleation can occur and inhibitors are not effective.

Q. **What investigations does this man need?**

A. There is debate as to how stone formers should be evaluated metabolically. One way to approach this is to determine the patient's risk of developing a further stone, so that resources are directed to where they are likely to have the most benefit.

Thus, first-time stone formers who are at lower risk of developing a further stone can undergo an abbreviated workup, whereas higher-risk patients should have a more thorough workup.

The following are risk factors for recurrent stone formation, which necessitate a thorough metabolic workup:

- Children
- White patients with a positive family history
- Black patients
- Patients with chronic diarrhoea or malabsorptive states
- History of gout
- Osteoporosis
- Nephrocalcinosis
- Recurrent UTIs
- Pathologic skeletal fractures
- Patients with stones composed of uric acid, cystine or struvite

An abbreviated workup consists of

- *Bloods* – U and Es (renal function, hypokalaemia in distal renal tubular acidosis), urate (hyperuricaemia in patients with uric acid stones), serum calcium and serum phosphate (hypercalcaemia and hypophosphataemia in patients with hyperparathyroidism)
- *Urine* – MSU (C and S and microscopy of the sediment to look for crystals), spot cystine, urine pH (high in infection stones, <5.5 in patients with uric acid stones)
- *Stone* – Analysis of the stone

An extensive workup consists of the previous list plus the following:

- *24-hour urine collections* – The standard in the United Kingdom is for patients to provide two 24-hour urine collections, one in a bottle with hydrochloric acid (looking for 24-hour calcium, oxalate, phosphate, citrate and magnesium) and one plain bottle (looking for 24-hour uric acid and electrolytes and pH). Also measured is 24-hour urine volume.
- A dietary diary is useful to help address with patients changes which need to be made. Furthermore, some urologists would advocate the collection of a 24-hour urine after

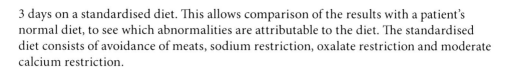

3 days on a standardised diet. This allows comparison of the results with a patient's normal diet, to see which abnormalities are attributable to the diet. The standardised diet consists of avoidance of meats, sodium restriction, oxalate restriction and moderate calcium restriction.

Q. How do you tell your patients to perform a 24-hour urine collection?

A. It is important to get a complete 24-hour collection of urine, and to ensure that patients understand how to perform a 24-hour collection. Many will not really understand what you tell them in the clinic, and thus it is imperative to give them some written information to take home with them to read.

On the day that patients decide they are going to do their collection, they should wake up in the morning as usual. They should then void into the toilet and note the time (i.e. discard first void on the day of starting the collection). Every time they pass urine for the next 24 hours, including the first void of the following day (which should be at the same time as the void into the toilet at the start of the collection) should be collected in the bucket/collection bottle. The urine should then be kept in a cool place until it is analysed, ideally as soon as possible after the collection is complete.

Q. What is different about the metabolic management of patients with uric acid stones?

A. Uric acid stones are only formed in acid urine. Diet may be especially important in patients with uric acid stones, as a diet rich in purines and proteins with a high consumption of alcohol increases uric acid excretion and lowers urinary pH. Over 20% of patients who have gout will get uric acid stones, due to hyperuricosuria.

Uric acid stones are the only stones that can be dissolved by medical agents. This can be successful in the majority of patients. Oral chemolysis is carried out by alkalinising the urine, preferably using potassium citrate. The dosage of agent should be determined by the pH response in the urine. In patients who have high uric acid excretion, hyperuricosuria, prescription of allopurinol should be considered. Finally, as with all stone formers, diuresis should be promoted by increasing fluid intake.

Q. Tell me what you know about cystinuria.

A. Cystine stones are caused by an autosomally recessive inherited inborn error of metabolism, such that the proximal tubular reabsorption of the dibasic amino acids Cystine, Ornithine, Lysine and Arginine (COLA) is decreased. However, cystine is the only poorly soluble amino acid out of these, and thus these patients form only cystine stones.

Cystine stones account for about 1% of adult renal tract stones. The peak incidence of stone formation is in the second to third decades of life, but these patients get recurrent stones, which typically have a ground glass appearance. The crystals are hexagonal.

Diagnosis is made based on stone examination, microscopy of urinary sediment or measurement of urinary cystine levels. The cyanide-nitroprusside test (Brand's test) is a spot test to detect cystinuria, but in patients with a suspected diagnosis a 24-hour collection is performed, which will determine if the patient is homozygous or heterozygous.

Medical care of these patients consists of advice to drink copious amount of fluid, aiming for 4 or more litres of fluid intake a day. Alkalinisation of the urine to a high pH increases solubility of cystine, and further medical treatment includes the use of complexing agents to bind with cystine forming soluble compounds. Such agents include D-penicillamine and α-mercaptopropionylglycine (Thiola). Finally captopril can be used. Captopril is a first-generation angiotensin-converting enzyme (ACE) inhibitor and has been shown to form a complex with cystine that is 200 times more soluble.

Surgical care of these patients is similar to that of patients with other types of stone, except that it should be noted that cystine stones are more resistant to ESWL than many other stone types.

Q. How does Brand's test work? What levels of cystine in the urine would indicate that the patient was a homozygote?

A. Cyanide-nitroprusside test: This is a rapid, simple and qualitative determination of cystine concentration. Cyanide converts cystine to cysteine. Nitroprusside then binds, causing a purple hue in 2–10 minutes. The test detects cystine levels of higher than 75 mg/L. False-positive test results occur in some individuals with homocystinuria or acetonuria and in people taking sulfa drugs, ampicillin, or N-acetylcysteine. The normal excretion rate is 40–80 mg/day. Heterozygotes excrete 200–400 mg/day. Homozygotes usually excrete >600 mg/day.

Q. What are the principles of treatment of patients with cystine stones?

A. The main considerations are that these patients are young, will tend to have recurrent stone episodes and hence may require multiple interventions. As such prevention is vitally important, bearing in mind the significant risk of poor compliance.

- Diet
  - As cystine is produced from the essential amino acid methionine, attempts are made to reduce foods high in methionine, such as red meat, fish and poultry.
- High fluid input
  - Ideally >3–4 L/day, as it is known that 250 mg cystine will dissolve in 1 L of fluid.
- Alkalinisation
  - Using potassium citrate, sodium bicarbonate ($NaHCO_3$) or in some cases acetazolamide, which is a carbonic anhydrase inhibitor and thus increases HCO_3 excretion.
- Oral chelators
  - These drugs combine with cystine to form a soluble complex thus preventing stone formation and possibly even dissolving existing cystine stones, and include D-penicillamine, α-mercaptopropionylglycine and captopril.

Q. How would you make a clinical diagnosis of renal tubular acidosis (RTA)?

A. Patients with RTA are unable to acidify their urine, and thus the pH of the urine never goes below 5.8. Confirmation of the diagnosis requires ammonium chloride loading test. In addition there is a decrease in blood pH, lowered plasma bicarbonate and raised serum chloride. Urinary calcium and phosphate levels are raised.

Q. Why do you get these findings with RTA?

A. RTA results from a disturbed secretion of H^+ ions in the renal tubules, with too few H^+ ions available for adequate bicarbonate reabsorption in exchange for acid ions. Instead, chloride ions are reabsorbed and a hyperchloremic metabolic acidosis develops which in turn leads to resorption of apatite from bone and thus increased serum calcium. Hypercalcuria follows, with recurrent stone formation and often nephrocalcinosis. Only distal RTA is of importance in stone formers.

REFERENCES

1. Blandy JP, Singh M. The case for a more aggressive approach to staghorn stones. *J Urol* 1976; 115(5): 505–506.
2. Teichman JM, Long RD, Hulbert JC. Long-term renal fate and prognosis after staghorn calculus management. *J Urol* 1995; 153(5): 1403–1407.
3. Ghani KR et al. Percutaneous nephrolithotomy: Update, trends, and future directions. *Eur Urol* 2016; 70(2): 382–396.

4. Liu L, Zheng S, Xu Y, Wei Q. Systematic review and meta-analysis of percutaneous nephrolithotomy for patients in the supine versus prone position. *J Endourol* 2010; 24(12): 1941–1946.

5. Wu P, Wang L, Wang K. Supine versus prone position in percutaneous nephrolithotomy for kidney calculi: A meta-analysis. *Int Urol Nephrol* 2011; 43(1): 67–77.

6. Zhang X, Xia L, Xu T, Wang X, Zhong S, Shen Z. Is the supine position superior to the prone position for percutaneous nephrolithotomy (PCNL)? *Urolithiasis* 2014; 42(1): 87–93.

7. Lingeman JE, Siegel YI, Steele B, Nyhuis AW, Woods JR. Management of lower pole nephrolithiasis: A critical analysis. *J Urol* 1994; 151(3): 663–667.

8. European Association of Urology Guidelines on urolithiasis. 2017. http://uroweb.org/guideline/urolithiasis/

9. Sampaio FJ, Aragao AH. Inferior pole collecting system anatomy: Its probable role in extracorporeal shock wave lithotripsy. *J Urol* 1992; 147(2): 322–324.

10. Keeley FX, Jr., Moussa SA, Smith G, Tolley DA. Clearance of lower-pole stones following shock wave lithotripsy: Effect of the infundibulopelvic angle. *Eur Urol* 1999; 36(5): 371–375.

11. Elbahnasy AM et al. Lower caliceal stone clearance after shock wave lithotripsy or ureteroscopy: The impact of lower pole radiographic anatomy. *J Urol* 1998; 159(3): 676–682.

12. Pace KT, Tariq N, Dyer SJ, Weir MJ, Dah RJ. Mechanical percussion, inversion and diuresis for residual lower pole fragments after shock wave lithotripsy: A prospective, single blind, randomized controlled trial. *J Urol* 2001; 166(6): 2065–2071.

13. Albala DM et al. Lower pole I: A prospective randomized trial of extracorporeal shock wave lithotripsy and percutaneous nephrostolithotomy for lower pole nephrolithiasis-initial results. *J Urol* 2001; 166(6): 2072–2080.

14. Pearle MS et al. Prospective, randomized trial comparing shock wave lithotripsy and ureteroscopy for lower pole caliceal calculi 1 cm or less. *J Urol* 2005; 173(6): 2005–2009.

15. McClinton S. PUrE: percutaneous nephrolithotomy, flexible ureterorenoscopy and extracorporeal shockwave lithotripsy for lower pole kidney stones. https://ukctg.nihr.ac.uk/trials/trial-details/trial-details?trialNumber=ISRCTN98970319. 2015. Accessed 15/04/2017, 2017.

16. Pak CY. Kidney stones. *Lancet (London, England)* 1998; 351(9118): 1797–1801.

17. Stamatelou KK, Francis ME, Jones CA, Nyberg LM, Jr., Curhan GC. Time trends in reported prevalence of kidney stones in the United States: 1976–2013; 1994[1]. *Kidney Int* 2003; 63(5): 1817–1823.

18. Boyce CJ, Pickhardt PJ, Lawrence EM, Kim DH, Bruce RJ. Prevalence of urolithiasis in asymptomatic adults: Objective determination using low dose noncontrast computerized tomography. *J Urol* 2010; 183(3): 1017–1021.

19. Glowacki LS, Beecroft ML, Cook RJ, Pahl D, Churchill DN. The natural history of asymptomatic urolithiasis. *J Urol* 1992; 147(2): 319–321.

20. Burgher A, Beman M, Holtzman JL, Monga M. Progression of nephrolithiasis: Long-term outcomes with observation of asymptomatic calculi. *J Endourol* 2004; 18(6): 534–539.

21. Kang HW et al. Natural history of asymptomatic renal stones and prediction of stone related events. *J Urol* 2013; 189(5): 1740–1746.

22. Dropkin BM, Moses RA, Sharma D, Pais VM, Jr. The natural history of nonobstructing asymptomatic renal stones managed with active surveillance. *J Urol* 2015; 193(4): 1265–1269.

23. Keeley FX, Jr. et al. Preliminary results of a randomized controlled trial of prophylactic shock wave lithotripsy for small asymptomatic renal calyceal stones. *BJU Int* 2001; 87(1): 1–8.

24. Inci K, Sahin A, Islamoglu E, Eren MT, Bakkaloglu M, Ozen H. Prospective long-term followup of patients with asymptomatic lower pole caliceal stones. *J Urol* 2007; 177(6): 2189–2192.

25. Monga M. Does treatment of asymptomatic, small renal calculi depend on the patient population? *J Urol* 2015; 193(4): 1086.

26. Borley NC, Rainford D, Anson KM, Watkin N. What activities are safe with kidney stones? A review of occupational and travel advice in the UK. *BJU Int* 2007; 99(3): 494–496.

27. Holdgate A, Pollock T. Nonsteroidal anti-inflammatory drugs (NSAIDs) versus opioids for acute renal colic. *Cochrane Database Syst Rev* 2005; Apr 18(2): CD004137.

28. Teichman JMH. Acute renal colic from ureteral calculus. *N Engl J Med* 2004; 350(7): 684–693.

29. Afshar K, Jafari S, Marks AJ, Eftekhari A, MacNeily AE. Nonsteroidal anti-inflammatory drugs (NSAIDs) and non-opioids for acute renal colic. *Cochrane Database Syst Rev* 2015; Jun 29(6): CD006027.

30. Worster A, Preyra I, Weaver B, Haines T. The accuracy of noncontrast helical computed tomography versus intravenous pyelography in the diagnosis of suspected acute urolithiasis: A meta-analysis. *Ann Emerg Med* 2002; 40(3): 280–286.

31. Niemann T, Kollmann T, Bongartz G. Diagnostic performance of low-dose CT for the detection of urolithiasis: A meta-analysis. *AJR Am J Roentgenol* 2008; 191(2): 396–401.

32. Smith-Bindman R et al. Ultrasonography versus computed tomography for suspected nephrolithiasis. *N Engl J Med* 2014; 371(12): 1100–1110.

33. Heidenreich A, Desgrandschamps F, Terrier F. Modern approach of diagnosis and management of acute flank pain: Review of all imaging modalities. *Eur Urol* 2002; 41(4): 351–362.

34. Nakasato T, Morita J, Ogawa Y. Evaluation of Hounsfield units as a predictive factor for the outcome of extracorporeal shock wave lithotripsy and stone composition. *Urolithiasis* 2015; 43(1): 69–75.

35. Bellin MF et al. Helical CT evaluation of the chemical composition of urinary tract calculi with a discriminant analysis of CT-attenuation values and density. *Eur Radiol* 2004; 14(11): 2134–2140.

36. Zheng X, Liu Y, Li M, Wang Q, Song B. Dual-energy computed tomography for characterizing urinary calcified calculi and uric acid calculi: A meta-analysis. *Eur J Radiol* 2016; 85(10): 1843–1848.

37. Preminger GM et al. 2007 Guideline for the management of ureteral calculi. *Eur Urol* 2007; 52(6): 1610–1631.

38. Preminger GM et al. 2007 Guideline for the management of ureteral calculi. *J Urol* 2007; 178(6): 2418–2434.

39. Skolarikos A, Laguna MP, Alivizatos G, Kural AR, de la Rosette JJ. The role for active monitoring in urinary stones: A systematic review. *J Endourol* 2010; 24(6): 923–930.

40. Furyk JS et al. Distal ureteric stones and tamsulosin: A double-blind, placebo-controlled, randomized, multicenter trial. *Ann Emerg Med* 2016; 67(1): 86–95.e82.

41. Pickard R et al. Medical expulsive therapy in adults with ureteric colic: A multicentre, randomised, placebo-controlled trial. *Lancet (London, England)* 2015; 386(9991): 341–349.

42. Dauw CA, Hollingsworth JM. Medical expulsive therapy: PRO position. *Int J Surg* 2016; 36: 655–656.

43. Sur RL et al. Silodosin to facilitate passage of ureteral stones: A multi-institutional, randomized, double-blinded, placebo-controlled trial. *Eur Urol* 2015; 67(5): 959–964.

44. Hollingsworth JM et al. Alpha blockers for treatment of ureteric stones: Systematic review and meta-analysis. *The BMJ* 2016; 355: i6112.

45. Pearle MS et al. Optimal method of urgent decompression of the collecting system for obstruction and infection due to ureteral calculi. *J Urol* 1998; 160(4): 1260–1264.

46. Mokhmalji H, Braun PM, Martinez Portillo FJ, Siegsmund M, Alken P, Kohrmann KU. Percutaneous nephrostomy versus ureteral stents for diversion of hydronephrosis caused by stones: A prospective, randomized clinical trial. *J Urol* 2001; 165(4): 1088–1092.

47. Geavlete P, Georgescu D, Nita G, Mirciulescu V, Cauni V. Complications of 2735 retrograde semirigid ureteroscopy procedures: A single-center experience. *J Endourol* 2006; 20(3): 179–185.

48. Nabi G, Cook J, N'Dow J, McClinton S. Outcomes of stenting after uncomplicated ureteroscopy: Systematic review and meta-analysis. *BMJ* 2007; 334(7593): 572.

49. Coe FL, Parks JH, Lindheimer MD. Nephrolithiasis during pregnancy. *N Engl J Med* 1978; 298(6): 324–326.

50. Drago JR, Rohner TJ, Jr., Chez RA. Management of urinary calculi in pregnancy. *Urology* 1982; 20(6): 578–581.

51. Hendricks SK, Ross SO, Krieger JN. An algorithm for diagnosis and therapy of management and complications of urolithiasis during pregnancy. *Surg Gynecol Obstet* 1991; 172(1): 49–54.

52. Biyani CS, Joyce AD. Urolithiasis in pregnancy. II: Management. *BJU Int* 2002; 89(8): 819–823.

53. Strong DW, Murchison RJ, Lynch DF. The management of ureteral calculi during pregnancy. *Surg Gynecol Obstet* 1978; 146(4): 604–608.

54. Semins MJ, Matlaga BR. Management of urolithiasis in pregnancy. *Int J Womens Health* 2013; 5: 599–604.

55. Biyani CS, Joyce AD. Urolithiasis in pregnancy. I: Pathophysiology, fetal considerations and diagnosis. *BJU Int* 2002; 89(8): 811–818.

56. White WM et al. Predictive value of current imaging modalities for the detection of urolithiasis during pregnancy: A multicenter, longitudinal study. *J Urol* 2013; 189(3): 931–934.

57. Srirangam SJ, Hickerton B, Van Cleynenbreugel B. Management of urinary calculi in pregnancy: A review. *J Endourol* 2008; 22(5): 867–875.

58. Roberts JA. Hydronephrosis of pregnancy. *Urology* 1976; 8(1): 1–4.

59. Swanson SK, Heilman RL, Eversman WG. Urinary tract stones in pregnancy. *Surg Clin North Am* 1995; 75(1): 123–142.

60. Peake SL, Roxburgh HB, Langlois SL. Ultrasonic assessment of hydronephrosis of pregnancy. *Radiology* 1983; 146(1): 167–170.

61. Stothers L, Lee LM. Renal colic in pregnancy. *J Urol* 1992; 148(5): 1383–1387.

62. Lifshitz DA, Lingeman JE. Ureteroscopy as a first-line intervention for ureteral calculi in pregnancy. *J Endourol* 2002; 16(1): 19–22.

63. Hadjipavlou M, Tasleem A, Santos FD, Smith D, Sriprasad S. Urolithiasis in pregnancy. *J Clin Urol* 2017; 10(2): 93–104.

64. Ulvik NM, Bakke A, Hoisaeter PA. Ureteroscopy in pregnancy. *J Urol* 1995; 154(5): 1660–1663.

65. Watterson JD et al. Ureteroscopy and Holmium:YAG laser lithotripsy: An emerging definitive management strategy for symptomatic ureteral calculi in pregnancy. *Urology* 2002; 60(3): 383–387.

66. Shokeir AA, Mutabagani H. Rigid ureteroscopy in pregnant women. *Br J Urol* 1998; 81(5): 678–681.

67. Giusti G, Abate D, De Lisa A. Percutaneous approach to a complicated case of nephrolithiasis in a pregnant woman: A case study. *J Endourol Case Rep* 2016; 2(1): 84–86.

68. Shah A, Chandak P, Tiptaft R, Glass J, Dasgupta P. Percutaneous nephrolithotomy in early pregnancy. *Int J Clin Pract* 2004; 58(8): 809–810.

69. Tóth C, Tóth G, Varga A, Flaskó T, Salah MA. Percutaneous nephrolithotomy in early pregnancy. *Int Urol Nephrol* 2005; 37(1): 1–3.

CHAPTER 11
FEMALE UROLOGY
AND NEUROUROLOGY

Christian Nayar, Vinay Kalsi, Rizwan Hamid,
Julian Shah and Tina Rashid

Contents

OVERACTIVE BLADDER

Q. A 35-year-old woman is referred to your clinic with problems of urinary frequency, urgency, urgency incontinence and nocturia. How will you approach this patient's problems?

A. I will review her in my specialist clinic. I would like to elucidate the following points from her history:

- When did the symptoms first appear?
- Are there any exacerbating factors?
- Are there any associated obstructive symptoms or proven urinary tract infections (UTIs)?
- How many (if any) pads does she have to wear throughout the day, are they damp or soaked through?
- How is this problem impacting on her quality of life?
- Is there any history of neurological disease?
- Is there any history of previous pelvic surgery/pelvic cancer/pelvic radiotherapy?
- Is there any relevant smoking history?
- Ask for information about fluid intake including caffeinated beverages.
- What medications is she taking?
- What has she tried in the past to improve the problem, i.e. conservative methods/lifestyle changes/medications?

Q. What initial tests would you perform?

A. I would request the following:

- Urine dipstick analysis and urinary culture if appropriate.
- Uroflowmetry and post-void bladder scan.

- A bladder diary of at least 3 days' duration.
- If suprapubic pain or non-visible haematuria is present then I will organise urine cytology and a flexible cystoscopy.

Note: *If an elderly woman presents with these symptoms then I would perform urine cytology and a flexible cystoscopy initially, in order to exclude bladder pathology, e.g. bladder stone, carcinoma in situ or overt bladder cancer.*

Q. What is the difference between a bladder diary and a frequency-volume chart?

A. A bladder diary records the type and volume of fluid intake, incontinence episodes and number of pads used along with a recorded chart of urinary frequency and voided urine volume (i.e. functional bladder capacity). A frequency volume chart records only the volume of fluid intake, urinary frequency and incontinence episodes.

Q. How would you diagnose nocturnal polyuria from a bladder diary?

A. Nocturnal polyuria is present when an increased proportion of the 24-hour output occurs at night (normally during the 8 hours when the patient is in bed). The nighttime urine output excludes the last void before sleep but includes the first void of the morning. The International Continence Society (ICS) standardisation committee defines nocturnal polyuria as nocturnal urine production exceeding 20% of 24-hour urine output in younger adults and 33% in older adults [1].

Q. What do you understand by the term *overactive bladder* (OAB)?

A. The ICS/International Urogynecological Association (IUGA) defines OAB as a symptom syndrome of urgency with or without incontinence usually accompanied by urinary frequency and nocturia, in the absence of pathological (e.g. UTI, stones, bladder tumour) and metabolic factors (e.g. diabetes).

ICS definitions as related to urinary incontinence are given in Table 11.1.

Table 11.1 Definitions of terminology in overactive bladder and urinary incontinence

Overactive bladder syndrome	A symptom syndrome of urgency with or without incontinence usually accompanied by urinary frequency and nocturia, in the absence of pathological (e.g. UTI, stones, bladder tumour) and metabolic factors (e.g. diabetes).
Urgency	A sudden and compelling desire to pass urine that cannot be deferred.
Urge urinary incontinence	Involuntary leakage of urine accompanied by or immediately preceded by urgency. Usually represents a severe form of overactive bladder syndrome.
Stress urinary incontinence	Involuntary leakage of urine on effort or exertion, or on coughing or sneezing.
Mixed urinary incontinence	Involuntary leakage of urine associated with urgency and also with exertion, effort, sneezing and coughing.
Increased daytime frequency	This is the complaint by the patient who considers that he/she voids too often by the day.

Q. What is the difference between OAB and idiopathic detrusor overactivity (IDO)?

A. OAB is a symptomatic diagnosis while IDO is a urodynamic diagnosis, i.e. *urodynamic evidence* of detrusor contraction which may be spontaneous or provoked (in the absence of any other pathology OAB is presumed to be the result of IDO).

Q. What is the differential diagnosis for this patient's symptoms?

A. They can be divided into
- Urological
  - UTI
  - Detrusor overactivity
  - Urethral syndrome

- Urethral diverticulum
- Interstitial cystitis
- Bladder cancer
- Bladder dysfunction
- Gynaecological
  - Cystocele
  - Pelvic mass
- Genital
  - Vulvo-vaginitis
  - Urethritis
  - Urethral caruncle
  - Atrophy
- Medical
  - Upper motor neuron lesion
  - Diabetes mellitus
- General
  - Excessive fluid/caffeine intake
  - Anxiety
  - Pregnancy

Q. What are the treatment options for this patient if she has an OAB?

A. The management of OAB should be initiated in a stepwise manner starting with

- Lifestyle changes (eliminate caffeinated drinks, stop smoking, lose weight if obese).
- Bladder re-training and pelvic floor muscle exercises (both shown to be effective in OAB).
- Pharmacotherapy (efficacy 50%–75%).
- Intravesical injection of botulinum toxin A (efficacy 36%–89%, mean 70%, up to a mean time of 6 months).
- Neuromodulation (50% cure, 25% significant improvement of symptoms, 25% failure rate).
- Clam (augmentation) cystoplasty (50% cure, 25% significant improvement of symptoms, 25% failure rate).
- Urinary diversion is an option if all else fails in very severe cases.

Note: *The first three options in the previous list may be tried in the absence of urodynamic investigation. However, prior to any invasive procedure, urodynamic confirmation of the diagnosis of detrusor overactivity should be sought.*

Q. What do you understand by bladder re-training and pelvic floor muscle training (PFMT)?

A. Bladder re-training works on the idea that the central control can be re-learned as it was learnt in infancy. It is done by setting a target time for using the toilet before which the patient should not void. Once this is achieved the time is increased. The patient has to maintain a normal fluid intake.

PFMT was originally described by Kegel. The purpose is to strengthen and rehabilitate the pelvic floor. The aim is to increase the urethral resistance and improve the tone of the pelvic floor. It is performed by long slow contractions and short sharp pull-ups at regular intervals. Generally several sets consisting of 8–10 contractions of each are performed daily.

Q. What is the efficacy of anticholinergics?

A. It varies between 50% and 75%. They help to reduce urgency and incontinence episodes along with reducing frequency of micturition. The voided volume is also increased.

Q. How do anticholinergics work?

A. Anticholinergics are competitive muscarinic receptor antagonists, they have a high binding affinity for the cholinergic muscarinic receptors that mediate contraction of the urinary bladder (and enhance salivation). The majority of muscarinic receptors expressed in the detrusor muscle are M2, however, *M3 are the functionally important* ones in the detrusor muscle. Anticholinergics in general have a low affinity for other neurotransmitter receptors and other possible targets like calcium channels. Selective anticholinergics result in selective blockade of M2 or M3 muscarinic receptors, with the particular advantage of not affecting brain M1 receptors, and thus having a better side-effect profile than non-selective agents.

Anticholinergics exert a significant effect on the lower urinary tract by reducing spontaneous detrusor muscle activity during the filling phase, decreasing detrusor pressure (and increasing the residual urine).

Q. Which anticholinergics do you know?

A. See Table 11.2.

Table 11.2 Different anticholinergic drugs and their properties

Trade name/generic name	Dose (mg)	Frequency	Receptor subtype selectivity	Active metabolite	Elimination half-life of drug (hours)
Pro-Banthine/Propantheline	15	tds	Non-selective	No	<2
Detrusitol/Tolterodine tartrate	2	bd	Non-selective	Yes	2.4
Detrusitol XL/Tolterodine tartrate	4	od	Non-selective	Yes	8.4
Regurin/Trospium chloride	20	bd	Non-selective	No	20
Ditropan/Oxybutynin chloride	2.5–5	bd-qds	Non-selective	Yes	2.3
Lyrinel XL/Oxybutynin chloride XL	5–30	od	Non-selective	Yes	13.2
Detrunorm/Propiverine hydrochloride	15	od-qds	Non-selective	Yes	4.1
Emselex/Darifenacin	7.5–15	od	Selective muscarinic M3 receptor antagonist	Yes	3.1
Vesicare/Solifenacin	5–10	od	Selective muscarinic M2 and M3 receptor antagonist	Yes	40–68

Q. What are the side effects of anticholinergics?

A. Common side effects of muscarinic receptor blockade include a dry mouth, dyspepsia, constipation, blurred vision and drowsiness. Serious side effects include anaphylaxis, drowsiness/cognitive and memory impairment particularly in the elderly, dementia and cardiac arrhythmias through prolongation of the QT interval. Selective M3 agents are least likely to cause side effects.

Q. What are the contraindications of anticholinergics?

A. The following conditions are contraindications to the use of anticholinergics:

- Myasthenia gravis
- Narrow-angle glaucoma, uncontrolled
- Significant bladder outflow obstruction or urinary retention
- Severe/active ulcerative colitis
- Toxic megacolon
- Gastrointestinal obstruction or intestinal atony
- Hypersensitivity to the agent

Q. Are you aware of any studies linking use of anticholinergics and dementia?

A. The association between anticholinergic drugs and dementia/cognitive impairment has been established for some time, but was thought to be reversible on stopping the drugs. However

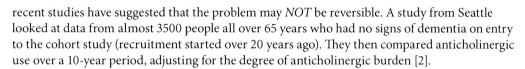

recent studies have suggested that the problem may *NOT* be reversible. A study from Seattle looked at data from almost 3500 people all over 65 years who had no signs of dementia on entry to the cohort study (recruitment started over 20 years ago). They then compared anticholinergic use over a 10-year period, adjusting for the degree of anticholinergic burden [2].

- For those using anticholinergics regularly there was increased risk of dementia and Alzheimer's compared with no use.
- The risk increase was small: A 1.5-fold increased risk of dementia in those using anticholinergics regularly for 3 years.
- The relationship was dose dependent – so the more anticholinergics you use the greater the risk of dementia/Alzheimer's.
- During the 10 years of study, when you took the medication was not important – so the effect is not related to recent use. Having ever taken these drugs is related to the same risk as being on them now.

Importantly though, this is an *ASSOCIATION* not a causation.

Q. Are there any other medications that could be tried?
A. If anticholinergics are not tolerated, ineffective or contraindicated then mirabegron (a ß-3 adrenergic agonist) may be an option.

Q. How does mirabegron work?
A. Mirabegron activates the ß-3 adrenergic receptor in the detrusor muscle in the bladder, which leads to muscle relaxation and an increase in bladder capacity helping the bladder to fill and store urine. The recommended dose is 50 mg once daily and 25 mg in renal or hepatic impairment.

Q. What are the side effects of mirabegron?
A. Tachycardia and UTI have been reported, less commonly reported are dyspepsia, palpitations, atrial fibrillation, hypertension, joint swelling, rash and pruritus.

Q. What are the contraindications to mirabegron?
A. The main contraindications are

- Hypersensitivity to the active ingredient
- Severe uncontrolled hypertension defined as systolic BP > 180 and or diastolic BP > 110 mm Hg

Q. What is the next step if medical therapy fails?
A. The next step will be to perform a urodynamic study (also known as cystometrogram [CMG]) as further treatment options involve invasive therapies.

Q. What are the aims of urodynamics studies?
A. Urodynamics has two basic aims:

- To reproduce the patient's symptomatic complaints
- To give a pathophysiological explanation by correlating the patients' symptoms to the urodynamics findings

Q. How will you perform urodynamics also known as cystometrogram (CMG)?
A. This is performed in a dedicated room with specialised urodynamic equipment or in the radiology department where fluoroscopy facilities are available (for videourodynamic studies). The test takes about 40–60 minutes and the aim is to duplicate the patient's symptoms. An initial urine dipstick is performed in order to exclude possible UTI. A flow test may then be performed and subsequently, following verbal consent a 6–8 F dual lumen catheter is inserted into the bladder having cleaned the external urethral meatus and anaesthetised the urethra – this records

the intravesical pressure. Using a dual lumen catheter avoids the need for two separate urethral catheters. The bladder is drained of urine and this initial volume recorded. A 6–8 F single lumen catheter is placed into the rectum – this records the intra-abdominal pressure (true detrusor pressure is calculated by measuring the intravesical pressure and subtracting the abdominal pressure). The lines are then connected to the urodynamic transducers and all lines are flushed through with saline thereby removing all air bubbles from both the tubing and the transducer chambers. All systems are zeroed at atmospheric pressure; the external transducers are placed at the level of the superior edge of the pubis symphysis. An initial cough ensures good subtraction. Contrast medium (or saline in a non-video study) at room temperature is then instilled via a peristaltic pump – medium and fast fill (50–100 mL/min) is often used, however, slower fill rates (10–30 mL/min) approaching the physiological range are mandatory when assessing a neuropathic bladder. During the study notes are made of the initial bladder residual volume, bladder volume at the time of patient's first sensation of filling, final tolerated bladder volume and final residual volume. During bladder filling the patient is asked to consciously suppress bladder contraction and filling is discontinued at maximum tolerated capacity. Quality control is obtained by asking the patient to cough at regular intervals (usually every minute during the study and at the end of the study). In units where a tipping table is not available the study can be carried out in the sitting or standing position. Patients are asked to stand at the end of the study to assess if there is postural detrusor instability.

Q. What does one look for in the filling phase of a CMG?

A. During the filling phase one notes:

- Subtraction of the lines as an indicator of study quality control
- Infused volume at which sensations are felt
- Evidence of detrusor overactivity (non-provoked or provoked)
- Evidence of stress urinary incontinence (e.g. on coughing)
- Bladder compliance (see case study on neurourology presented later in this chapter)
- Maximum bladder capacity

Q. What are the different-coloured traces seen in Figure 11.1?

A. Figure 11.1 demonstrates four traces. These show (from above down) the intra-abdominal (P_{abd}) and intravesical (P_{ves}) pressures, subtracted pressure, i.e. detrusor pressure ($P_{det} = P_{abd} - P_{ves}$), flow trace ($Q_{ura}$). A filling trace is also seen (V_{in}). For quality control purposes a cough is seen approximately every minute. Ideally there should be a cough every minute (ensures consistently good subtraction).

Q. What has happened in Figure 11.2?

A. Figure 11.2 is a CMG trace showing the filling phase only. The white arrow shows the point when the patient stood up.

Q. What has happened in Figure 11.3?

A. In Figure 11.3 there is a sharp decrease in P_{det} and P_{ves} (arrowed) due to the P_{ves} (bladder) catheter falling out (the adjacent short peak is the result of the catheter passing out through the external sphincter).

Q. Figure 11.4 is the filling phase of a CMG. What does it demonstrate?

A. Figure 11.4 shows idiopathic detrusor overactivity (white arrow) during the filling phase of a CMG (urgency symptoms in patient present).

Q. What type of botulinum toxin is normally used in urology?

A. Botulinum toxin is a neurotoxin derived from *Clostridium botulinum*. There are seven serotypes of botulinum toxin each with different antigenic profiles and biochemical actions;

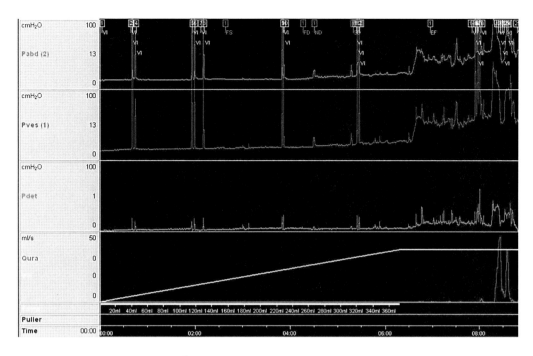

Figure 11.1 Urodynamics trace showing (from top down) intra-abdominal pressure trace, intravesical pressure trace, subtracted detrusor pressure trace and flow trace.

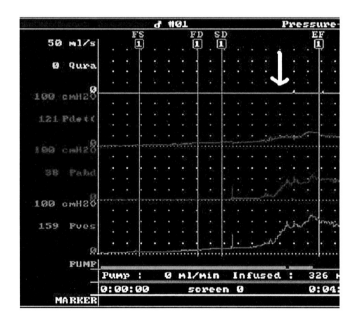

Figure 11.2 Urodynamics trace. The white arrow demonstrates a slight pressure rise (within normal limits) in subtracted detrusor pressure when the patient stands up.

however, they all have a similar pharmacological effect. Botulinum toxin types A (BoNT/A) and B (BoNT/B) have been developed for clinical use. The available formulations of BoNT/A are BOTOX (Allergan, United States), Dysport (Ipsen, United Kingdom), and Xeomin (Merz, Germany). Each formulation of BoNT/A has its own dosing regimen which is not interchangeable. BOTOX is most commonly used followed by Dysport (former is five times

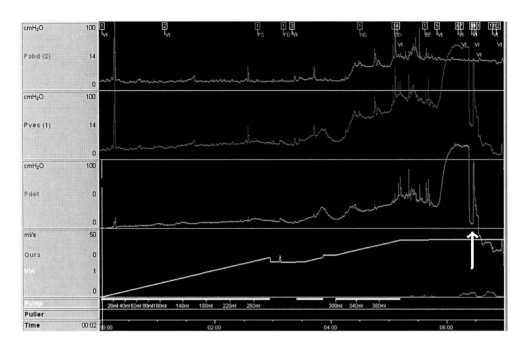

Figure 11.3 Urodynamics trace. The white arrow demonstrates a sudden decrease in detrusor and intravesical pressure as the vesical catheter is expelled from the bladder.

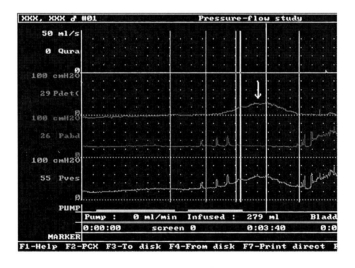

Figure 11.4 Urodynamics trace. The white arrow demonstrates a rise in detrusor and intravesical pressures which would be consistent with a detrusor contraction. Abdominal pressure remains constant at this point.

more potent than latter). The 2013 National Institute for Health and Care Excellence (NICE) guidelines for treatment of urinary incontinence in women suggest an initial dose of 200 units when offering botulinum toxin A, but consider 100 units in those women who would prefer a dose with a lower chance of catheterisation and accept a reduced chance of success.

Q. How does botulinum toxin work and how do you give the injections?

A. Botulinum neurotoxin type A (BoNT/A) temporarily blocks the presynaptic vesicular release of acetylcholine (ACh) at the neuromuscular junction of the parasympathetic nerves supplying the detrusor. This results in a temporary paralysis of the detrusor muscle. BoNT/A prevents the exocytosis of ACh by cleaving SNAP-25 off the SNARE proteins, a complex protein which when intact forms the core of the neuroexocytosis machinery. It is on this premise that intradetrusor injections of BoNT/A were introduced to treat intractable bladder symptoms of detrusor overactivity and is the basis of decrease in detrusor pressures and phasic contractions in both idiopathic and neuropathic bladders. However, patients also report a significant decrease in urgency and hence, it is hypothesised that botulinum toxin also modulates the sensory pathways. This is thought to work by its action on P2X receptors.

Administration of intradetrusor BoNT/A injections has been described under local, regional or general anaesthetic using a flexible or rigid cystoscope. For idiopathic detrusor overactivity typically 200 units of BOTOX (diluted in 20 mL of normal saline) or 750–1000 units of Dysport have been used. There is no standard injection technique. However, intradetrusor injections, as opposed to submucosal injections, with sparing of the trigone are favoured. Again, there is no consensus on the number of injection sites and the dilution of the toxin but generally 20 sites are injected and the volume per injection is usually 0.5–1 mL.

Q. What are the efficacy and potential side effects of intravesical injection of botulinum toxin?

A. The efficacy for idiopathic detrusor overactivity ranges from 36% to 89% (mean 70%). The effects last from 4 to 10 months (mean 6 months) (note BoNT/A is much more effective in neurogenic detrusor overactivity).

The local side effects include pain, UTI (<5%), bleeding (<5%), no benefit, need for further injections, need for temporary self-catheterisation (very variable, but approximately may be necessary in 10%–15%). The generalised side effects include flu-like symptoms, dry mouth and malaise.

Q. Are you aware of any long-term effects of repeated injections or that botulinum toxin loses its efficacy after repeated injections?

A. No significant bladder fibrosis has been reported on histological examination after repeated injections. Also seven repeat injections have not demonstrated any decrease in efficacy of BOTOX.

Q. What is the basis of sacral neuromodulation (SNM)?

A. The precise mechanism of action is not fully recognised. SNM can be used in the treatment of intractable detrusor overactivity and also women with urinary retention due to a primary disorder of sphincter relaxation (Fowler's syndrome). It is thought that the continuous use of mild electrical activity to stimulate the sacral afferents (mainly S3) to the bladder and pelvic floor modulates local neural reflexes and inhibits bladder contraction. There is also evidence to suggest that signals from higher brain centres involved in the control of micturition are also affected thus explaining its use in the mentioned conditions.

Q. How is the SNM delivered?

A. This is a minimally invasive procedure and can be performed under general or local anaesthesia. Generally a two-stage technique is used as it has been shown that the two-stage method improves the efficacy from 50% to 75% for refractory IDO. Initially a test implant (stimulation wire) is inserted into the S3 foramina. This is attached to a temporary pulse generator device that the patient wears externally. The patient goes home and keeps a bladder diary and records her symptoms for 2 weeks. This is compared with a pre-operative evaluation. A greater than 50% benefit in symptoms entitles the patient to have the second stage, i.e. permanent electrode fitted into the S3 foramen with the pulse generator being implanted in a pouch superficial to the posterior superior iliac crest.

Q. What are the efficacy/side effects and complications of SNM?

A. It is thought to be effective in 60%–75% of cases of IDO (efficacy rates are higher in women with Fowler's syndrome). Should the procedure prove to be efficacious then the beneficial effects should be long term; however, the battery life of the latest implants is about 7 years after which the unit will require revising. Previously the main complication was migration of the lead but this has reduced after introduction of the tined (barbed) lead. Occasionally the patient complains of pain at the site of implantation of the pulse generator or in the lower limb. The explantation rate is 10% and this is mainly due to infection or lack of sustained efficacy.

Q. What is a clam augmentation cystoplasty and how does it work?

A. The principle of an augmentation cystoplasty is to bivalve the bladder coronally (like a clam) and patch the defect with a piece of bowel, generally ileum is used (ileocystoplasty) however other bowel segments have been described (Figure 11.5). This impairs bladder contraction, lowers the detrusor pressures and increases the capacity of the bladder. It decreases the amplitude of contractions by preventing sustained detrusor contractions.

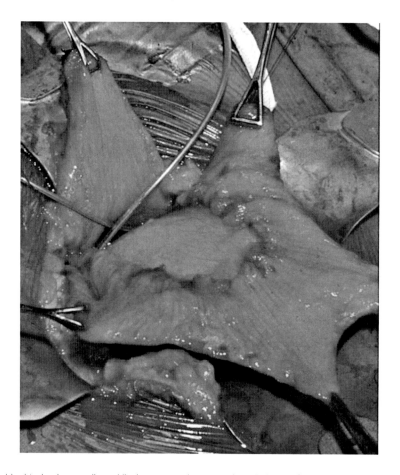

Figure 11.5 Bladder bivalved coronally and ileal augmentation cystoplasty being performed.

Q. What are contraindications for clam augmentation cystoplasty?

A. These include

- Severe inflammatory bowel disease, i.e. Crohn's disease
- Previous pelvic radiotherapy
- Critically short bowel
- A patient's unwillingness or inability (due to poor hand function) to perform self-catheterisation

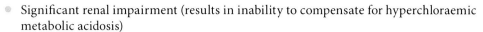

- Significant renal impairment (results in inability to compensate for hyperchloraemic metabolic acidosis)
- Significant hepatic impairment (results in inability to metabolise NH_3)

Q. What are the potential complications of clam augmentation cystoplasty (enterocystoplasty)?

A. These include

Major early complications:

1. *Mortality*: 0%–2.5% (especially in neurogenic patients due to bladder rupture)
2. *Myocardial infarction*: 0%–2.5%
3. *Thromboembolic events*: 1%–7%
4. *Re-operation for post-operative bleeding*: 0%–3%
5. *Wound infection* $\pm$ *dehiscence*: 5%–6.5%
6. *Small bowel obstruction due to adhesions*: 3%–5.5%
7. *Fistula*: 0.4%–30%

Long-term complications:

1. *The need for post-operative intermittent catheterisation* – The rate is approximately 50%–60% in idiopathic patients. This generally increases over time.
2. *Stones* – The reported rates are highly variable between 0% and 53%. It is generally thought to be approximately 15%. They are more common if there has been an associated Mitrofanoff procedure.
3. *Troublesome mucus production* – The average daily production from the incorporated bowel segment is 35–40 grams. This does not decrease over time and can lead to infections, stone formation and blockages. Bladder washouts might be required with acetylcysteine to dissolve excess mucus.
4. *Bacteriuria and UTI* – Almost 100% of patients will have asymptomatic bacteriuria. The incidence of clinically significant UTI is around 4%–43%.
5. *Biochemical abnormalities* – The presence of permeable bowel in the urinary tract leads to reabsorption of ammonium chloride and excretion of bicarbonate resulting in acid-base imbalance. Ammonium chloride (NH_4Cl) which is readily reabsorbed dissociates into ammonia (NH_3) and hydrochloric acid (HCl); the HCl in solution in turn dissociates into H^+ and Cl^- thereby resulting in hyperchloraemic acidosis. However, this is clinically important in few cases (15%) and in these the treatment is administration of bicarbonate. The biochemical changes explain the reason that augmentation cystoplasty is contraindicated in liver and significant renal failure – in these patients the NH_3 cannot be metabolized by the damaged liver and the acidosis cannot be corrected by the failing kidneys.

   Note: *The incidence of this biochemical abnormality happening in a patient with an ileal conduit is much less since the conduit is exactly that, a conduit for urine, and not a reservoir unlike the augmented bladder. Thus the urine in a conduit does not stay in it for sufficient time in order for the exchange to take place (i.e. absorption of NH_4Cl).*

6. *Renal function deterioration* – This can happen in 0%–15% of cases. It is more marked in patients who have a creatinine clearance of less than 15 mL/min (corrected for surface area) pre-operatively. However, it has been reported that the renal function has actually improved in 4% of cases.
7. *Perforation* – Spontaneous perforation is a rare complication (<1%) but carries a mortality of 25% mostly due to delay in diagnosis.
8. *Malignancy* – There is an increased incidence of cancer in augmented bladders. However, there is a long latent period (>10 years). This is associated with chronic inflammation, urinary stasis and recurrent UTIs. The tumours are generally

adenocarcinomas and in the region of the anastomosis. The mechanism seems to be related to bacteriuria. This leads to reduction of urinary nitrates to nitrites by colonic bacteria. This reacts with urinary amines to form N-nitrosamines, which are implicated in carcinogenesis.

9. *Bowel changes* – This usually results in diarrhoea. The symptom is troublesome in up to 30% of cases. Also there can be a decrease in absorption of vitamin B12 and folic acid leading to neurological complications (B12 deficiency may also be due to disruption of the absorptive terminal ileum).

10. *Reduced growth potential and increased incidence of fractures in growing children* – The hydrogen (from the acidosis) is buffered in exchange for calcium causing demineralisation of bone (this calcium is subsequently lost in the urine). The acidosis in growing children, if present, should be treated with sodium bicarbonate [3].

Q. How do you follow up a patient following an augmentation cystoplasty?

A. Once stable the patients are seen on a yearly basis with an ultrasound scan (USS) of kidneys and a kidneys, ureters and bladder (KUB) x-ray. The biochemical analysis includes evaluation of kidney and liver function and estimation of serum chloride, bicarbonate, vitamin B12 and folic acid levels. They are advised to contact the department urgently if they develop recurrent UTIs, haematuria, significant weight loss or severe lethargy. They will undergo yearly surveillance cystoscopies from 10 years after operation [4].

STRESS URINARY INCONTINENCE

Q. What is the ICS definition of stress urinary incontinence (SUI)?

A. SUI is the involuntary leakage of urine on cough or straining or exertion and effort. The prevalence ranges from 12% to 52%. Of all incontinence cases approximately 50% have SUI, 11% urge urinary incontinence and 36% have mixed urinary incontinence. SUI is bothersome in 20% of patients with this problem.

Q. What is urodynamic stress incontinence (USI)?

A. USI is noted during urodynamic testing (filling cystometry) and is defined as the involuntary leakage of urine during increases in abdominal pressure in the absence of a detrusor contraction.

Q. A 52-year-old fit woman presents with worsening complaints of urinary leakage, when coughing and lifting heavy items. How would you assess her?

A. I would see this patient in a specialist clinic, with my continence nurse specialist present, and with the following completed prior to being seen – a validated symptom questionnaire such as the International Consultation on Incontinence Modular Questionnaire Short Form (ICIQ-SF) (as recommended by the European Association of Urology [EAU]), a representative bladder diary (frequency-volume chart) over 3 days, urinalysis and a post-void residual volume.

Then, I would take a detailed history. In the history I would establish the type of incontinence (stress, urge or mixed), severity of incontinence (ICIQ-SF outcome and use of pads – how many, what type and how wet they were), effect on quality of life, treatments (surgical and non-surgical) already tried and the desire for further treatment and the patient's expectations. Furthermore, I would also enquire about associated voiding and bowel dysfunction (frequency, urgency, nocturia, dysuria, incomplete emptying, suprapubic pain, haematuria, UTIs, constipation and faecal leakage). A detailed gynaecological and obstetric history would be elicited including pregnancies (vaginal or caesarian section), menopausal status (including previous history of hysterectomy), use of Hormone Replacement Therapy

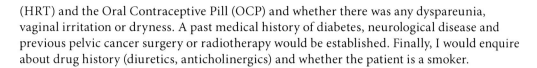

(HRT) and the Oral Contraceptive Pill (OCP) and whether there was any dyspareunia, vaginal irritation or dryness. A past medical history of diabetes, neurological disease and previous pelvic cancer surgery or radiotherapy would be established. Finally, I would enquire about drug history (diuretics, anticholinergics) and whether the patient is a smoker.

Q. **She has had three normal vaginal deliveries in the past and has not had a hysterectomy or any other abdominal or pelvic surgery. She does not complain of urinary infections or any other urinary symptoms. What will you look for on examination?**

A. I will obtain verbal consent and examine her in the presence of a chaperone. I would perform a general examination first, as this may have a bearing on subsequent management, looking specifically for obesity (BMI). Then, in the supine position, I would perform an abdominal examination looking for a palpable bladder. I would then perform a pelvic examination in the supine position initially inspecting the tissue state of the introitus (well oestrogenised or atrophic). I would then ask my patient to cough or perform a Valsalva manoeuver to elicit the sign of stress incontinence. I would assess for pelvic floor tone using the Oxford grading system. I will then ask the patient to turn to the left lateral position, I would ask my chaperone to help lift the upper leg. A warmed lubricated Sim's speculum would then be introduced and evaluation for cystocoele and rectocoele is performed. Finally, I check perineal sensation and assess anal tone to evaluate for any neurological abnormality. If present, lower limb neurological examination is also performed.

The Q-tip and Marshall tests which have been described to assess for urethral competence are not currently recommended by NICE.

Q. **Clinical examination revealed no significant abnormalities. What investigations would you like to perform?**

A. Initially, I would perform dipstick urinalysis to look for evidence of infection or non-visible haematuria. If a UTI is present, I would treat this and then re-assess the patient. I routinely perform a flow rate and estimation of post-void residual volume, as well as review a representative bladder diary, with the patient. Pad tests can be used to objectively confirm incontinence. Further investigations depend on causative factors in the history. Specifically, if neurological features are present, a renal USS and creatinine are requested.

Q. **How do you do a pad test?**

A. The objective of a pad test is to try to quantify the volume of urine lost by weighing a perineal pad before and after provocation testing. Pad tests can either be short term (over 1 hour) or longer term (over a 24-hour period). In a 1-hour test, the patient is required to drink 500 mL of fluid (non-saline based) and then perform a set series of exercises over the next 1 hour. The 24-hour test is a more physiological test where the patient is encouraged to perform the sort of normal daily activity which would cause her to leak urine. A weight gain of up to approximately 1.4 g for the 1-hour pad test and up to 8 g during the 24-hour pad test is considered normal (note that an increase in weight of the pad or pads of 1 g is considered equivalent to 1 mL of urine).

Pad testing is not recommended in the routine assessment of women with urinary incontinence (NICE).

Q. **Would you perform urodynamics in a woman with pure stress urinary incontinence?**

A. I do not perform urodynamics prior to starting conservative treatments for patients with urinary incontinence. I am aware that the NICE guidelines suggest that in the small group of women where pure SUI can be diagnosed on history and clinical examination alone that urodynamics are not necessary prior to considering invasive therapy. It is however my practice to perform urodynamics in all patients prior to surgery, for several reasons. First, there is evidence that 11%–16% of patients with history of stress incontinence also have detrusor overactivity on urodynamic testing and conversely, 22% of patients with a history of overactive bladder symptoms have demonstrable stress incontinence at urodynamics.

The NICE guidelines suggest that urodynamics should be undertaken if

- There are symptoms of OAB leading to a clinical suspicion of detrusor overactivity.
- Symptoms are suggestive of voiding dysfunction or anterior compartment prolapse.
- There has been previous surgery for SUI.

I would also consider urodynamics if the clinical diagnosis as unclear prior to surgery or there are neurological clinical features.

Q. What are the indications for video-urodynamics?

A. In my practice, it is used in those patients with previous failed surgery, those with neurological features and in children. Furthermore, I am aware that in specialist centres, video-urodynamics are used more widely than in my practice, because of the perceived advantages such as allowing better evaluation of bladder neck descent and urethra as well as quantifying anterior wall prolapse better.

Q. How do you describe a urodynamic trace?

A. I use a systematic method to describe the trace as follows:

- Establish which line is which on the trace (especially as the trace colours may be different to what you are used to normally)
  - P_{ves}
  - P_{abd}
  - P_{det}
  - Volume infused
  - Uroflowrate
- Quality control
- Are the baseline pressures correct?
  - Supine 5–20 cm H_2O
  - Sitting 15–40 cm H_2O
  - Standing 30–50 cm H_2O
  - Subtracted P_{det} 0–6 cm H_2O
  - Coughing – does it lead to good subtraction and a biphasic waveform in P_{det}?
- Are there any artefacts that need to be looked at?
- Filling phase
  - First desire
  - Normal desire
  - Strong desire
  - Cystometric capacity
  - Any detrusor overactivity?
  - Any stress incontinence?
  - Is quality control still OK? (see previous)
- Standing
  - Do the pressures increase on standing?
  - Is quality control still OK? (see previous)
- Provocative manoeuvres
  - Which have been used?
  - What are the effects of these?
  - Is quality control still OK? (see previous)
- Voiding phase
  - P_{det}
  - P_{det} at Q_{max}

- Q_{max}
- Volume voided
- Is quality control still OK? (see previous)

Q. Do you know of any theories for development of SUI?

A. The first theory was proposed by Kelly, Bonney and Enhorning known as the *urethral position theory*. It suggested that the urethra should remain above the pelvic floor so that the pressure from the abdomen could be equally transmitted to the urethra closing it.

The *intrinsic sphincter deficiency (ISD) theory* was proposed by McGuire in the 1970s. It proposed that the abnormality was the weakness of the sphincter itself. He introduced the concept of Valsalva leak point pressure (VLPP) and maximum urethral pressure (MUP). It was suggested that patients with VLPP <60 cm H_2O had ISD, while those with VLPP of >90 cm H_2O had an anatomical cause of SUI. The patients with pressures between 60 and 90 cm H_2O had a combination of two problems.

Hammock theory: This was suggested by Delancey in 1994. He described the urethra as resting on a supportive layer of endopelvic fascia and anterior vaginal wall. This was reinforced by the lateral attachments of this fascia with arcus tendineus.

Integral theory: This was proposed by Petros and Ulmsten. This proposed that laxity of the anterior vaginal wall and pubourethral ligaments causes hypermobility of the bladder neck and dissipation of urethral pressure resulting in urinary incontinence.

Lately, a *trampoline theory* has been offered which incorporates all of the above theories. This is applied to the female pelvis as acting as the outer ring, the fabric is the pelvic musculature and ligaments are the springs. This proposes that SUI is a multifactorial problem and all of the above are compromised to some extent in its aetiology.

Q. In this 52-year-old woman, a diagnosis of stress incontinence is made. What treatment options are available?

A. The following options are available:
- Non-surgical treatments
  - Lifestyle changes
    - Weight loss
    - Cessation of smoking
    - Modify high or low fluid intake
  - Supervised pelvic floor exercises
  - Bladder re-training
  - Oestrogen therapy if evidence of atrophy
  - Oral medical therapy in rare cases
- Surgical treatments
  - Occlusive
    - Bulking agents
    - Compressive (artificial urinary sphincter)
  - Supportive
    - Mid-urethral sling
    - Colposuspension

Q. She wants to know more about the medical therapy and especially how it works. What information will you give to her?

A. The only agent with published data is duloxetine (Yentreve), which is a combined norepinephrine and serotonin reuptake inhibitor at the spinal cord level (Onuf's nucleus). It increases the activity of the pudendal nerve and increases the urethral muscle tone. Its efficacy is about 20%–40%. However, it is limited by side effects and discontinuation rates are very high. The main adverse effects are nausea, dizziness, dry mouth, constipation, insomnia, somnolence and asthenia. Duloxetine is not recommended as a first-line treatment for women with predominant SUI, although it may be offered as second-line therapy if women prefer pharmacological therapy to surgery or who are not suitable for surgical treatment. In clinical practice, if duloxetine is prescribed, women should be counselled about its adverse effects, very carefully.

Q. Prior to offering this woman a surgical intervention or procedure is there anybody you would want to discuss your plans with?

A. Before offering invasive therapy for either OAB or SUI, each case should be discussed in a multidisciplinary team meeting (MDT) taking into account patient preference, past management, co-morbidities and treatment options.

Q. Who should be part of the MDT?

A. The MDT should comprise a urologist with a sub-specialist interest in female urology, a urogynaecologist, a specialist nurse, a specialist physiotherapist, a colorectal surgeon with a subspecialist interest in functional bowel problems for women with coexisting bowel problems and a member of the care of the elderly team for women with functional impairment [5].

Q. What are the indications for bulking agents?

A. The main indications will be symptomatic patients who are high risk for major surgery, elderly patients, previous multiple failed procedures and patient preference. I will offer this to patients with mild to moderate SUI with the understanding that although this is a minimally invasive technique, the success rate is between 50% and 70% but the effects are not long lasting. Women should be made aware that

- Repeat injections may be needed to achieve efficacy.
- Efficacy diminishes with time.
- Efficacy is inferior to that of synthetic tapes or autologous rectus fascial slings.

Q. What types of bulking agents are you aware of?

A. I am aware of macroplastique (silicone), durasphere (carbon-coated zirconium beads), Zuidex (cross-linked dextranomer) and coaptite (calcium hydroxylapatite). I use macroplastique as it is permanent and there is no significant risk of migration due to the size of the particles.

Q. What materials are mid-urethral slings made of?

A. Mid-urethral slings can be classified into

- Autologous
  - Rectus fascia
  - Fascia lata
- Synthetic
  - Prolene (polypropylene)
  - Dacron (Mersilene)
- Non-synthetic

Q. What is the efficacy of mid-urethral tension-free vaginal tape (TVT) slings?

A. Outcomes after TVT have shown that 90% of women were still objectively cured, from a study in which 11-year prospective follow-up data were available [6]. Similar data have been reported at 5- and 7-year follow-up [7].

Q. What are the complications of mid-urethral TVT slings?

A. These include

- Complications at insertion
  - Bladder perforation (0%–12%)
  - Significant haemorrhage (1.9%)

- Major vascular injury (<1%)
- Urethral laceration
- Bowel injury
- Nerve injury
- Material-related complication
  - Erosion (<1%)
  - UTI (4%–17%)
- Post-operative symptoms
  - Post-operative voiding dysfunction (30%)
  - *De novo* urgency (3%–9%)
  - Urinary retention (2.5%–5%)
  - Dyspareunia/pelvic pain

There have been serious concerns about the use of mesh in vaginal implants for prolapse and stress incontinence surgery, in Scotland this led to the use of mesh implants being banned. The MHRA (Medicines and Healthcare Products Regulatory Agency) has reviewed the currently available information on the safety of vaginal mesh implants and concluded that from a regulatory perspective the benefits of the use of these devices outweigh the risks.

Important issues which should be undertaken by those using vaginal mesh implants include

1. *Consent* – Consent guidance, consent forms and patient information are available from the specialist societies, e.g. British Association of Urological Surgeons (BAUS).
2. *Audit* – NICE recommends that all procedures using mesh insertion should be part of regular audit on a recognised database, e.g. BAUS surgical database.
3. *Adverse event reporting* – Mesh inserted for pelvic organ prolapse or SUI is considered a medical device and therefore any adverse events should be reported to the MHRA.
4. *Surgery for the removal of mesh* – Surgery for the removal of tapes or prolapsed mesh, or repeat surgery for prolapse or incontinence should be performed in centres which can demonstrate relevant specialist expertise.

Q. How is erosion treated?

A. The tape has to be removed if there is a urethral or vaginal erosion. The urethral defect can be buttressed with a Martius fat pad if there is a significant defect. A rectus facial sling can be inserted later on if the patient remains incontinent after tape removal. A bladder perforation is more difficult to treat. It is difficult to endoscopically remove the tape from inside the bladder. Laser can be used with some success, although it may require more than one sitting to remove the tape. If there is a considerable erosion a cystotomy is required. It has been suggested that mesh erosions and complications should be treated at specialist centres with greater experience in the management of these complications.

Q. How does TVT compare with other pubovaginal slings?

A. In a recent systematic review and meta-analysis of five randomised controlled trials (RCTs) comparing TVT and other pubovaginal slings, a comparable cure rate between the two procedures was found [8].

Q. How does TVT compare with transobturator tape (TOT)?

A. The effectiveness and complications of TOTs were assessed in a recent systematic review of five RCTs that compared TVTO with TVT and six RCTs that compared TOT with TVT [7]. Both techniques had similar efficacy, with regards to subjective cure. However, the risk of bladder perforation (odds ratio 0.12) and voiding difficulties (odds ratio 0.55) with TOT was lower, whereas groin/thigh pain (odds ratio 8.28), vaginal injuries or erosion of mesh (odds ratio 1.96) were significantly more common after tape insertion by the transobturator route.

Long-term follow-up on TOT is limited.

Q. **How does TVT compare with Burch colposuspension?**

A. A recent systematic review and meta-analysis of nine RCTs comparing TVT and Burch colposuspension, in which 1170 patients were followed up for 3–24 months, concluded that TVT had a significantly higher efficacy in terms of overall cure rate than Burch colposuspension [8].

   This was true for any definition of cure, namely, according to the presence of negative stress test (odds ratio 0.38) and according to the presence of negative pad test (odds ratio 0.59). Complication rates were similar after the two procedures, with the exclusion of bladder perforation, which was more common after TVT, and reoperation rate, which was significantly higher after Burch colposuspension.

   In summary, TVT appears to be significantly more effective with similar complication rates if compared to Burch colposuspension.

Q. **When will you offer colposuspension and what is its efficacy?**

A. I will recommend this to patients with *significant* urethral hypermobility (TVT/TOT in these cases is likely to fail with the patient representing with SUI in the future). This procedure has the longest follow-up and the cure rate at >10 years is 69%.

   I may consider offering a colposuspension to a young woman as an initial surgical treatment as there are currently concerns with the long-term complications of synthetic mesh and mesh erosions/complications.

Q. **What are the principles of a colposuspension?**

A. The surgical principle is the re-elevation of the bladder neck into the abdominal pressure zone so there is equal transmission of intra-abdominal pressure to the bladder neck, which closes off the urethra.

Q. **What are the main complications after Burch colposuspension?**

- Immediate complications
  - Retropubic space haemorrhage (transfusion risk is approximately 0.5%)
  - Bladder trauma (2%–3%)
- Long-term complications
  - Enterocele or rectocele (up to 20%)
  - Dyspareunia (4%)
  - Voiding dysfunction (up to 30% and need for CISC 0.5%)
  - *De novo* urgency (5%–15%)
  - Recurrent bacterial cystitis (1%–2%)

Q. **What are the causes of failure of anti-incontinence surgery?**

A. These include

- Anatomical failure due to technical reasons
- Functional failures due to poor tissue support
- Inappropriate patient selection
- Failure due to post-operative complications

FEMALE URETHRAL DIVERTICULUM

Q. **A 44-year-old woman is referred from her GP with a history of recurrent UTIs. Bimanual inspection reveals a tender mass on the anterior vaginal wall. What is your differential diagnosis?**

A. The differential diagnoses include

- Urethral diverticulum
- Skene's gland cyst or abscess

- Gartner's duct cyst
- Ectopic ureterocele
- Vaginal inclusion cyst
- Urethral or vaginal malignancy

Q. What is the pathogenesis of female urethral diverticula (UD)?

A. The causes of urethral diverticulum are not fully established; the most widely accepted theory is that they occur secondary to infection of the periurethral glands. The periurethral glands are tubular alveolar structures located posterolaterally to the periurethral fascia. They are found in the proximal two-thirds of the urethra and drain into the distal third. Infection leads to obstruction of the glands, local abscess formation and eventual rupture into the urethral lumen.

Q. How do female UD present?

A. Classically a urethral diverticulum was suspected if a woman presented with the triad of dysuria, post-void dribbling and dyspareunia. However, studies report a much broader spectrum of symptoms. According to a recent series up to 77% of cases would have been missed if the clinician relied upon this triad alone to make the diagnosis [9]. In reality patients present symptoms as shown in Table 11.3 [10].

Q. How would you investigate a potential urethral diverticulum?

A. *Clinical examination and cystoscopic evaluation* – A zero or 30° urethroscope is used, the anterior vaginal wall is compressed with a finger in the vagina and the urethral lumen is inspected for any expressed pus from the floor or the roof of the urethra. However often the os can be hidden between collapsed urethral folds and cystoscopy does not give any information about the size or shape or appearance of the diverticular wall.

VCUG – Voiding cystourethrogram is an invasive test which involves the use of ionizing radiation but has a sensitivity of 65% therefore further investigations are usually required.

Ultrasonography – Use of ultrasound has been described either transvaginally or trans-rectally but this investigation is operator dependent.

Magnetic resonance imaging (MRI) – MRI is the current gold standard in diagnostic imaging for UD. Endorectal or endovaginal coil MRI techniques differ from surface or body-coil techniques as the coil is placed within the body cavity adjacent to the tissue of interest; this leads to higher-resolution imaging of the urethra. Up to 100% sensitivity has been reported when MRI is used for the detection of UD. The signal intensity of fluid is high on the T2-weighted images. In addition MRI provides information on the size, location and complexity of the diverticulum allowing accurate surgical planning.

Retrograde positive-pressure urethrography – Reported to have a 90% diagnostic accuracy but is rarely used in current urological practice. It is an uncomfortable procedure and is technically difficult requiring a special catheter (Davis or Tratner catheter) which has a double balloon. One balloon is placed in the bladder. The distal balloon slides to occlude the external meatus during injection of contrast via ports located between the balloons.

Table 11.3 Presentations of urethral diverticulum

Frequency/urgency	40%–100%
Dysuria	30%–70%
Recurrent UTI	30%–50%
Post-micturition dribble	10%–30%
Dyspareunia	10%–25%
Haematuria	10%–25%

Q. What are the principles of repair of a female urethral diverticulum?

A. The key steps in the repair of the diverticulum are the following:

- Mobilisation of a well-vascularised anterior vaginal wall flap (or flaps)
- Preservation of periurethral fascia
- Identification and excision of the neck of the urethral diverticulum or ostia
- Remove of entire urethral diverticulum wall or sac (mucosa)
- Watertight urethral closure
- Multilayered, non-overlapping closure with absorbable sutures (Martius flap graft)
- Closure of dead space
- Preservation or creation of continence

Q. What are the principles of a Martius flap graft?

A. The Martius graft is a long band of adipose tissue taken from the labia majora, it has excellent strength and vascularity, its blood supply is threefold. Branches of the external pudendal supply the graft superiorly and anteriorly, obturator branches enter the graft at its lateral border. The inferior labial artery and vein supply the graft inferiorly; hence the graft may be mobilised superiorly or inferiorly depending upon the desired location of transfer.

Q. What are the possible complications of urethral diverticulum repair?

A. The complications are as follows:

- Urinary incontinence
- Urethrovaginal fistula
- Urethral stricture,
- Recurrent urethral diverticulum
- Recurrent UTI
- Bladder/ureteric injury
- Vaginal scarring/narrowing leading to dyspareunia

BLADDER PAIN SYNDROME/INTERSTITIAL CYSTITIS

Q. A 27-year-old woman presents with frequency and urgency associated with severe suprapubic pain. She also complains of cystitis-like symptoms and UTIs requiring repeated courses of antibiotics over the last 3 years. She has seen multiple specialists including pain consultants without much benefit. She appears to be very distressed by her symptoms and thinks she has got bladder pain syndrome/interstitial cystitis. How will you make this diagnosis?

A. By definition, bladder pain syndrome/interstitial cystitis is 'the complaint of suprapubic pain related to bladder filling, accompanied by other symptoms such as increased daytime and night-time frequency, in the absence of proven urinary infection or other obvious pathology'. It is distinctly possible that she has a diagnosis of bladder pain syndrome/interstitial cystitis (BPS/IC), but I am aware that this is a diagnosis by exclusion. Hence, I would perform a very detailed history, including ICSI score, careful clinical examination and then investigations such as 3-day frequency-volume diary, MSU, cystometrogram and cystodistention and biopsy. These patients require a very considerate approach and will have to be given a considerable time, especially during the first consultation.

Q. What is the National Institute of Diabetes and Digestive and Kidney Diseases (NIDDK) workshop research definition?

A. These criteria were devised in 1987–1988 and were for scientific studies. It appears that only one-third of the patients thought to have BPS/IC by experts fulfilled these strict criteria.

- *Automatic inclusions*
  - Hunner's ulcer
- *Positive factors*
  - Pain on bladder filling relieved by emptying
  - Pain (suprapubic, pelvic, urethral, vaginal or perineal)
  - Glomerulations on endoscopy
  - Decreased compliance on cystometrogram
- *Automatic exclusions*
  - <18 years old
  - Benign or malignant bladder tumours
  - Radiation cystitis
  - Tuberculous cystitis
  - Bacterial cystitis
  - Vaginitis
  - Cyclophosphamide cystitis
  - Symptomatic urethral diverticulum
  - Uterine, cervical, vaginal or urethral cancer
  - Active herpes
  - Bladder or lower ureteral calculi
  - Waking frequency < five times in 12 hours
  - Nocturia < two times
  - Symptoms relieved by antibiotics, urinary antiseptics, urinary analgesics
  - Duration < 12 months
  - Involuntary bladder contractions (urodynamics)
  - Capacity > 400 mL, absence of sensory urgency

Q. What are the types of BPS/IC according to the European Society for the Study of Interstitial Cystitis (ESSIC)?

A. They are classified on the basis of cystoscopic hydrodistention and biopsy. The hydrodistention is classified as normal, glomerulations or Hunner's ulcer denoted by 1, 2 or 3. The biopsy is classified as normal, inconclusive or positive represented by A, B or C. Hence BPS/IC can vary from both normal results as BPS/IC 1A or with Hunner's ulcer and positive biopsy denoted by 3C.

Q. What is Hunner's ulcer?

A. It is not a true ulcer but an inflammatory lesion which presents as deep rupture through mucosa and submucosa on hydrodistention. It appears as a reddened area with small vessels radiating to the centre and oozes blood like a waterfall after distention.

Q. What do you know about the pathogenesis of BPS/IC?

A. This is a multifactorial syndrome and none of the causes implicated in the aetiology have definitely been proved.

These include the following:

- *Urinary infections* – Initially recurrent UTI were thought to be the starting point but now this is doubtful.
- *Mast cells* – They are reported to be both a pathologic mechanism and a pathognomonic marker.
- *Epithelial permeability* – An abnormality in the glycosaminoglycan (GAG) layer leads to passage of urine causing inflammation.
- *Neurogenic mechanisms* – Neurogenic inflammation can lead to abnormal sensory nerve activity with release of neuropeptides.
- *Autoimmunity* – There is no clear evidence that this is the triggering factor of IC.

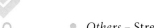

- *Others* – Stress.
- Female preponderance (10:1) hence role of hormones.

Q. How will you counsel this patient about her treatment?

A. I will explain to this patient that there is no cure for this condition but that the symptoms can be controlled with a variety of treatments. It is possible that we will have to try different treatment options before symptoms can be maintained on one. The patient should be made aware that there will be exacerbations and remissions in the long term. I will also tell her that 50% of patients achieve temporary remission without any treatment.

Q. What are the treatment options for her?

A. The treatment options are as follows:

- *Support* – Psychological support, e.g. IC support group.
- *Avoidance of triggers* – Drugs, chills, SMART diet, bubble bath, caffeine, etc.
- *Hydrodistention under anaesthesia* – This is done for 1–2 minutes at 80 cm H_2O.
- *Oral medical therapy* – Amitriptyline 75 mg daily (effects seen in 1–7 days)
  - Cimetidine 400 mg bd
  - Hydroxyzine 25 mg nocte
  - Dothiepin (also known as dosulepin) 75 mg daily
  - Diclofenac 75 mg bd
  - Pregabalin/Gabalin 100–300 mg daily increased to tds
  - Sodium pentosanpolysulphate (heparin analogue – 3%–6%) secreted in urine – 3- to 6-month trial is needed
- *Intravesical therapy*
  - *Dimethyl sulphoxide (DMSO)* – 50 mL 50% instilled for 15 minutes repeated at 2–4 weeks; response rate 50%–80%
  - *Pentosan polysulphate (Elmiron)* – Works as an exogenous GAG layer; response rate 16%–32%
  - *Hyaluronic acid* – Weekly instillations; response rate 70%
  - *Chondroitin sulphate* – Weekly for 6 weeks then monthly for 16 weeks; response rate 60%
- *Nerve stimulation*
  - *Transcutaneous nerve stimulation (TENS)* – Response rate 26%
  - Acupuncture
  - *Sacral nerve stimulation (SNS)* – An option but has not been widely tried
- *Surgery*
  - Transurethral resection of Hunner's ulcer
  - Transurethral resection by LASER of Hunner's ulcer
  - Denervation procedures
  - Supratrigonal cystectomy
  - Substitution cystoplasty with or without Mitrofanoff
  - Urinary diversion by conduit and cystourethrectomy

NEUROUROLOGY

Q. Please describe the motor innervation to the lower urinary tract.

A. The lower urinary tract (LUT) receives innervation from both the parasympathetic and the sympathetic branches of the autonomic nervous system. The parasympathetic preganglionic fibres are located in S2–4 spinal segments and these synapse with postganglionic cell bodies lying within the detrusor muscle. These parasympathetic nerves provide cholinergic excitatory input to bladder smooth muscle resulting in detrusor contraction. However, parasympathetic innervation of the outflow tract exerts an inhibitory effect resulting in relaxation of the bladder neck and urethra.

The sympathetic cell bodies are located in spinal segments T10–T12 and L1–L2. The preganglionic fibres synapse with postganglionic fibres in the hypogastric plexus. The predominant effect of the sympathetic innervation is inhibition of the parasympathetic pathways thus providing an inhibitory control on detrusor contraction. Additionally, sympathetic innervation results in contraction of the outflow tract (in males by stimulating contraction of the pre-prostatic sphincter and in females there is some, although relatively sparse, sympathetic innervation to the bladder neck).

The somatic nerve supply to the pelvic floor musculature and the external urethral rhabdosphincter originates from S2–S4 and is conveyed peripherally via the pudendal nerves. The cell bodies of the axons that innervate the external urethral rhabdosphincter lie in a distinct, medially placed motor nucleus at the same spinal level, called Onuf's nucleus.

Q. What is the sensory innervation of the bladder?

A. Sensory nerves have been identified in the suburothelial layer as well as in the detrusor muscle. This suburothelial plexus is particularly prominent at the bladder neck and relatively sparse at the dome of the bladder.

Sensations of bladder fullness are conveyed to the spinal cord in the pelvic and hypogastric nerves. The afferent components of these nerves contain myelinated (Aδ) and unmyelinated (C) axons. While the Aδ fibres respond to passive distension and active contraction and thus convey information about bladder filling, the C-fibres respond primarily to noxious stimuli such as chemical irritation of the urothelium or cooling. The cell bodies of both these classes of axons are located in the dorsal root ganglia (DRG) at the level of S2–S3 and T11–L2 spinal segments. Bladder afferent activity enters the spinal cord through the dorsal horn and ascends rostrally to higher brain centres involved in bladder control, i.e. the pontine micturition centre and then on to cerebral cortex.

Afferent fibres originating from the trigone and urethra run in the hypogastric and pudendal nerves, respectively.

Q. Please describe the micturition cycle.

A. The micturition cycle comprises filling and voiding phases:

- During the filling phase the intravesical pressure is kept low by the phenomenon of receptive relaxation. The extent to which a change in volume occurs as related to a change in pressure is known as bladder compliance (i.e. compliance = change in volume/change in pressure). Factors which contribute to bladder compliance are the vesicoelastic properties of the bladder and also the ability of detrusor smooth muscle cells to increase in length without significant increase in tension.

- During bladder filling, afferent activity from stretch receptors passes to the pons and cerebral cortex. If voiding is not to be initiated, activity within the external urethral rhabdosphincter is increased. Additionally, central inhibition decreases parasympathetic activity to the detrusor. Detrusor contraction is prevented by the 'gating mechanism'. This is inhibitory influence of interneurons via the sympathetics to prevent the transmission of afferent activity. This prevents the transmission of activity from preganglionic to postganglionic parasympathetic efferent neurons.

- When appropriate, voiding is initiated. The voiding phase begins first with relaxation of the external urethral sphincter followed by contraction of the detrusor muscle. Micturition is coordinated by Barrington's nucleus in the pons. The afferents from the bladder travel via parasympathetic nerves to the periaqueductal gray matter (PAG) in the pons. The PAG and cerebral cortical areas decide if it is appropriate to void. If so, the pontine micturition centre relays impulses resulting in external sphincter relaxation, and urine enters the posterior urethra. It also sends direct signals to the detrusor parasympathetics to initiate contraction. If this co-ordination is lost as in a suprasacral type of SCI, then the patient develops detrusor sphincter dyssynergia (i.e. uncoordinated contraction of the detrusor and external sphincter).

Q. What are the main urological characteristics of suprapontine, suprasacral and conus (S1–S5)/cauda equina/peripheral nerve (lower motor neurone) lesions?

A.

- *Suprapontine lesions (e.g. cerebrovascular accident [CVA], Parkinson's disease)* – In these the micturition reflexes are intact. Following a CVA, voiding at inappropriate times occurs (although voiding itself is normal) in addition to detrusor overactivity (latter also occurs in Parkinson's disease). These are 'safe' low-pressure bladders.
- *Suprasacral spinal cord injuries/lesions (i.e. lesions between the pons and spinal cord segment L5)* – These are characterised by neurogenic detrusor overactivity (NDO), detrusor sphincter dyssynergia (DSD; synchronous contraction of the detrusor and external urethral sphincter) and low-compliance bladders. In lesions above T6 autonomic dysreflexia may be a significant problem (see later discussion). Unlike suprapontine and conus/cauda equine/ peripheral nerve lower motor lesions, suprasacral injuries can result in 'unsafe' high-pressure bladders, as upper tract damage can result (due to DSD and low compliance).
- *Conus (S1–S5)/cauda equina/peripheral nerve lesions* – These tend to lead to a lower motor neurone type of injury and are characterised by an acontractile (areflexic) bladder with urethral sphincter weakness (leading to stress incontinence) (possible low compliance may also occur). The bladders tend to be 'safe' low-pressure bladders.

Q. What is detrusor sphincter dyssynergia (DSD)?

A. It is defined as involuntary contraction of the urethral and/or periurethral striated muscle simultaneously with a detrusor contraction. This usually is specific to a suprasacral neurological disorder.

Q. What do you know about detrusor leak point pressure (DLPP) and abdominal leak point pressure (ALPP)?

A.

- *The term DLPP must only be used in those with a neurological disorder/injury, i.e. those with a neuropathic bladder.* DLPP is the lowest detrusor pressure at which urine leakage occurs in the absence of either a detrusor contraction or increased abdominal pressure. McGuire observed, in spina bifida patients, that if the DLPP is greater than 40 cm H_2O then there is a significant risk of damage to the upper tracts [11].
- The ALPP (also called the Valsalva leak point pressure) is terminology used in *non-neuropathic females* as related to stress incontinence. It is the intravesical pressure at which urine leakage occurs due to increased abdominal pressure in the absence of a detrusor contraction. If the ALPP is <60 cm H_2O then stress incontinence is likely to be due to intrinsic sphincter deficiency. If the ALPP is >90 cm H_2O, stress incontinence is likely to be due to urethral hypermobility. An ALPP between 60 and 90 cm H_2O is an equivocal result. If the ALPP is >150 cm H_2O, then the urethra is unlikely to be the cause of urinary incontinence.

Q. A 28-year-old man sustained a T5 spinal cord injury (SCI) a year ago. He can walk and has been emptying his bladder by strain voiding and complains of recurrent UTIs and urinary leakages. What type of injury has he got?

A. He has sustained a suprasacral type of injury and is likely to have neurogenic detrusor overactivity, poorly sustained bladder contractions, DSD, low bladder compliance and reflex bladder voiding. As the lesion is above T6 he may also suffer from autonomic dysreflexia (see later discussion).

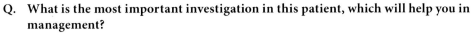
Q. What is the most important investigation in this patient, which will help you in management?

A. Video-urodynamic studies.

Q. What are your indications for urodynamics in general?

A. These include the following:

- Patients with persistent LUTs after appropriate therapy
- *Patients with previous failed incontinence surgery
- Patients with mixed urinary symptoms ± incontinence
- Any patient with suspicion of neurological disease and urinary symptoms
- Patients in whom potential therapy may be hazardous
- Children with complex voiding dysfunction

Q. What do Figure 11.6a and b show?

A. Figure 11.6a demonstrates a classical DSD trace with a saw-toothed appearance on the P_{det} line (also sustained detrusor contraction lasting for more than 5 minutes, with P_{det} pressures of 80–90 cm H_2O).

Figure 11.6b is cystography performed during a VCMG investigation. It shows a hold-up of contrast at the level of the external urethral sphincter, typical of DSD.

Q. How would you treat this patient?

A. The aim is to achieve low-pressure storage and complete bladder emptying while promoting continence.

I would be guided by the urodynamics result but assuming that this patient with T6 SCI has NDO and DSD, I would start him on anticholinergic medication and institute a program of clean intermittent self-catheterisation (CISC). He will be closely monitored and will undergo ultrasound scan of the kidneys and repeat urodynamics in 3–6 months' time to ensure the bladder pressures have come down. Assuming that there are no problems, i.e. UTIs or problems with CISC, he will be reviewed on an annual basis.

Q. The previously discussed patient returns and states he does not like performing CISC and would like to know about other options. Could you explain these to him?

A. Aside from CISC and the Credé manoeuvre (that he was practicing) the other options include

- *Behavioural and timed voiding* – This is not suitable for him.
- *Intradetrusor botulinum toxin injections* – This would, however, be unsuitable as he would continue to have to perform CISC.
- *Indwelling catheter (suprapubic or urethral)* – Not a good option for him as he is very young and mobile.
- *Urethral stents or external sphincterotomy (with a subsequent convene sheath)* – Both of these treat DSD (the urethral stent is placed across the external urethral sphincter thus holding it open) but the patient will be completely incontinent afterwards. Thus as he is young and mobile these are not a good option for him.
- *Augmentation cystoplasty (see preceding section on Overactive Bladder) with or without a Mitrofanoff (catheterisable channel)* – However, following this procedure he will almost certainly need to perform CISC.
- *Sacral anterior nerve root stimulator (SARS) with dorsal rhizotomy* – Not suitable for him as he is walking and has an incomplete SCI. This is an option for wheelchair-bound patients with a complete SCI.

---

* A video-urodynamic study (videocystometrogram [VCMG] – synchronous cystography and cystometry recordings) rather than a CMG is more appropriate in these cases, as this allows a combined evaluation of the anatomy and function of the lower urinary tract.

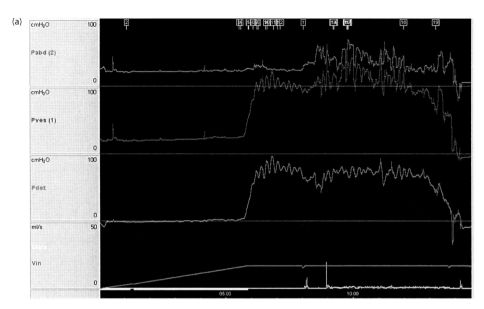

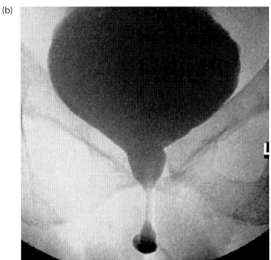

Figure 11.6 (a) Urodynamics trace. The 'saw-tooth' appearance on the detrusor pressure line is classically seen with detrusor-sphincter-dyssynergia (DSD). (b) Cystography at the same time as the VCMG demonstrates a hold up of contrast at the level of the external urethral sphincter, typical of DSD.

Q. What are the advantages and disadvantages of a SARS? (This is currently combined with a sacral dorsal rhizotomy.)

A. The benefits include the following:

- Abolition of reflex bladder
- Increased bladder capacity
- Abolition of autonomic dysreflexia
- Improved bowel management

However the disadvantages are as follows:

- Stress incontinence
- Loss of reflex erections

- Loss of reflex ejaculation
- Loss of reflex defaecation

Q. What are the complications of long-term catheters?

A.

- Recurrent UTIs
- Blockages
- Need for regular changes
- Stones
- Risk of cancer

Q. What are the complications of urethral stents to treat DSD in his case?

A. He will be completely incontinent (as the urethral stent is placed across the external urethral sphincter to hold it open) and will have to wear a sheath with risk of detachment. The urethral stents can migrate, block or become encrusted. They are generally reserved for immobile patients as is external sphincterotomy, which is irreversible.

Q. What is the success rate of botulinum toxin injections in NDO?

A. It is 70%–90% with effects lasting an average of 9 months.

Q. What is autonomic dysreflexia (AD)?

A. This is a medical emergency. It occurs only in patients with a SCI above T6 level (the sympathetic outflow). It is more common in cervical injuries compared to thoracic. It is a result of acute massive disordered autonomic (primarily sympathetic) response to specific stimuli. If left untreated it can lead to convulsions, cerebral haemorrhage and death.

Q. What are the causes of AD?

A. Autonomic dysreflexia can be triggered by many potential causes. Essentially any noxious stimuli below the level of SCI can cause AD. Bladder distension/irritation is responsible in 75%–85% of cases. The second most common cause is bowel distension, usually due to faecal impaction which accounts for 13%–19% of cases [12]. Other causes may include urological interventions (e.g. catheterisation, urodynamics, cystoscopy), UTI and urinary calculi. Non-urological causes include constipation, pressure sores, fractures, ingrown toenails and distal skin infections.

Q. What is the mechanism of AD?

A. Any of the above trigger conditions can cause sympathetic discharges, these results in reflex vasoconstriction leading to systemic hypertension. The carotid body detects this rise in blood pressure, reflex vagal discharges cause vasodilatation and bradycardia as a normal homeostatic response to try to lower blood pressure. However this neural signal cannot cross the level of the injury, vasoconstriction persists below the level of the lesion. The hypertension persists as the compensatory mechanisms are ineffective. Vasodilatation above the SCI level causes profuse sweating and flushing. Vasoconstriction below the level of the injury causes pale clammy skin.

Q. What are the symptoms and signs of AD?

A. A patient with autonomic dysreflexia may complain of headaches, blurred vision, nasal congestion and blotchy skin above the level of spinal cord injury.

Patients during an episode of autonomic dysreflexia may have

- A significant rise in systolic and diastolic blood pressure
- Profuse sweating above the level of the lesion, usually seen in the face, neck and shoulders
- Flushing of the skin above the level of the lesion

- Pale skin and goosebumps below the level of the lesion
- In advanced untreated cases – this can result in convulsions, intracranial bleeds, hypertensive encephalopathy and ultimately death

Q. What is the treatment of AD?

A. AD is a life-threatening condition. Management includes

- Prompt recognition of the condition
- Identification and treatment of the precipitating cause (e.g. drainage of the bladder, evacuation of the bowel)
- Sitting the patient upright (this induces an orthostatic hypotension allowing gravitational pooling of blood in the lower extremities causing a resultant drop in blood pressure)
- Loosening the patient's clothing and any constrictive devices
- Administering sublingual glyceryl trinitrate (GTN)
- Consider immediate-release nifedipine
- Administering IV labetalol/phentolamine
- Continuing to monitor the patient's blood pressure after the episode to make sure that it has truly settled and not just dropped as a result of antihypertensive medication

Q. How would you manage a patient with a conus (S1–S5) SCI?

A. He has a generally safe bladder (see previous discussion) and the options include the following:

- Behavioural and timed voiding
- Emptying by straining if bladder has good capacity
- CISC if incomplete voiding or complains of UTIs

If he complains of (stress) urinary incontinence then

- Sheaths
- Bulking agents
- Tapes/slings
- Artificial urinary sphincter (AUS)

POST-PROSTATECTOMY INCONTINENCE

Q. A 68-year-old man is seen in your clinic. He is 12 months post-robotic-assisted laparoscopic prostatectomy and complains of significant urinary leakage which is affecting his daily life. How would you assess him?

A. I would want details of his histology, margin status and current prostate-specific antigen as well as to know if any further treatment was planned such as radiotherapy. I would want to know about the amount of urinary leakage (pad use, etc.), type of urinary leakage, i.e. stress, urgency and degree of bother these symptoms cause. I would want to know about his current erectile function prior to offering any intervention. I would want to know his overall fitness for further surgery/co-morbidities and hand function.

Q. What investigations would you arrange?

A. To confirm the diagnosis of urinary incontinence after prostatectomy, an initial clinical assessment should include

- Physical examination
- A bladder diary
- An incontinence questionnaire such as the ICIQ-short form (ICIQ-SF for Urinary Incontinence)

- Consider ultrasound scan to assess for residual urine
- Urine analysis
- Pad tests

Q. What is the key investigation?

A. Video-urodynamics.

Q. His video-urodynamics confirm a stable compliant bladder during filling with evidence of large volume stress urinary incontinence. What are his current treatment options?

A. Following radical prostatectomy, patients are often offered a trial of conservative therapy for their incontinence. This often takes the form of pelvic floor muscle training and generalised lifestyle advice. For those men who have severe incontinence in the early stages after surgery containment with absorbent pads or indwelling or sheath catheters are the mainstay of conservative treatment. After failure of conservative methods and sufficient time for natural continence recovery, men with post-prostatectomy incontinence (PPI) should be counselled on the wide range of treatment options available to them.

Male sling: Analogous to the successful use of sling surgery in women (e.g. tension-free vaginal tape) slings have been developed for use in men with urinary incontinence. For example, the AdVance sling is placed suburethrally via the obturator route, to reposition the lax and descended supporting structures of the sphincter to their preoperative position without causing obstruction.

Q. What does Figure 11.7 show?

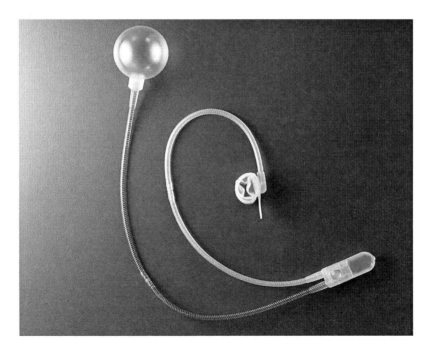

Figure 11.7 An artifical urinary sphincter (AMS 800).

A. Figure 11.7 shows an artificial urinary sphincter (AMS 800).

Q. How many components does an AUS have?

A. It has three components: a urethral cuff, a scrotal control pump and a reservoir (usually implanted in the pre-peritoneal space).

Q. What is the success rate of the AUS?

A. The AUS (AMS 800) allows >75% of patients to be completely continent and >90% to be socially dry. Satisfactory long-term continence is present in approximately 61% of patients between 10 and 15 years after implantation. However, success is less in SCI patients, especially if they are wheelchair bound.

Q. What are the complications of AUS?

A. These include

- Infection
- Cuff erosion
- Urethral atrophy (in up to 33%–39%: Has been reported as the most common cause of surgical revision)
- Persistent leakage
- Mechanical failure
- Upper urinary tract damage (particularly in children with neuropathic bladders)

Q. Are you aware of any trials comparing the male sling to AUS that are currently being recruited to?

A. The MASTER trial (Male synthetic sling versus Artificial urinary Sphincter Trial: Evaluation by Randomised controlled trial) will be the first trial to compare these two PPI treatments and provide evidence for men with PPI in the future.

REFERENCES

1. Abrams P et al. The standardisation of terminology of lower urinary tract function: Report from the standardisation sub-committee of the International Continence Society. *Am J Obstet Gynecol* 2002; 187(1): 116–126.
2. Gray SL et al. Cumulative use of strong anticholinergics and incident dementia. *JAMA Intern Med* 2015; 175(3): 401–407.
3. Greenwell TJ et al. Augmentation cystoplasty. *BJUI* 2001; 88(6): 511–525.
4. Hamid R et al. Routine surveillance cystoscopy for patients with augmentation and substitution cystoplasty for benign urological conditions: Is it necessary? *BJUI* 2009; 104: 392–395.
5. NICE guidelines [CG171]. Urinary incontinence in women 2013.
6. Nilsson CG et al. Eleven years prospective follow-up of the tension-free vaginal tape procedure for treatment of stress urinary incontinence. *Int Urogynecol J Pelvic Floor Dysfunct* 2008; 19: 1043–1047.
7. Liapis A et al. Long-term efficacy of tension-free vaginal tape in the management of stress urinary incontinence in women: Efficacy at 5- and 7-year follow-up. *Int Urogynecol J Pelvic Floor Dysfunct* 2008; 19: 1509–1512.
8. Novara G et al. Tension-free midurethral slings in the treatment of female stress urinary incontinence: A systematic review and meta-analysis of randomized controlled trials of effectiveness. *Eur Urol* 2007; 52: 663–678.
9. Ockrim JL, Allen DJ, Shah PJ, Greenwell TJ. A tertiary experience of urethral diverticulectomy: Diagnosis, imaging and surgical outcomes. *BJU Int* 2009 Jun; 103(11): 1550–1554.
10. Bennett SJ. Urethral diverticula. *Eur J Obstet Gynecol Reprod Biol* 2000 Apr; 89(2): 135–139.
11. McGuire EJ et al. Prognostic value of urodynamic testing in myelodysplastic patients. *J Urol* 1981; 126: 205.
12. Lindan R, Joiner F, Freechafer A, Hazel C. Incidence and clinical features of autonomic dysreflexia in patients with spinal cord injury. *Paraplegia* 1980; 18: 285–292.

FURTHER READING

Arya M, Shergill IS, Silhi N, Grange P, Bott S (eds). 2008. *Essential Urology in General Practice.* London: Quay Books.

Wein AJ, Kavoussi LR, Novick AC, Partin AW, Peters CA (eds). 2016. *Campbell-Walsh Urology,* 11th edn. Philadelphia, PA: Saunders Elsevier.

CHAPTER 12
BENIGN PROSTATIC HYPERPLASIA

*Iqbal S Shergill, Ananda K Dhanasekaran, Jas S Kalsi
and William J McAllister*

Contents

ANATOMY, EMBRYOLOGY AND PATHOPHYSIOLOGY

Q. What is the embryological basis of prostate development?

A. The prostate develops between the 10th and 16th weeks of gestation from epithelial buds which branch out from the posterior aspect of the urogenital sinus to invade the mesenchyme.

Stromal-epithelial interaction is important through production of dihydrotestosterone by epithelial cells acting on mesenchymal androgen receptors.

Q. What is the blood supply to the prostate?

A. The arterial blood supply is from the branches of the inferior vesical artery. This provides the prostatic artery which divides into urethral and capsular groups of arteries. From the urethral group arise Flock's and Badenoch's arteries (both supply the transition zone). Flock's arteries approach the bladder neck at 1 and 11 o'clock and Badenoch's at 5 and 7 o'clock. The capsular branches of the prostatic artery run with the cavernosal nerves.

The venous drainage is via the periprostatic venous plexus. This also receives the deep dorsal vein of the penis and numerous vesical veins. The periprostatic venous plexus eventually drains into the internal iliac vein.

Q. Describe the lymph drainage from the prostate.
A. The lymph drainage is mainly to the obturator nodes and then the internal iliac chain.

Q. Can you describe and draw the zonal anatomy of the prostate?
A. The zonal anatomy is described using McNeal's zones (Figure 12.1).

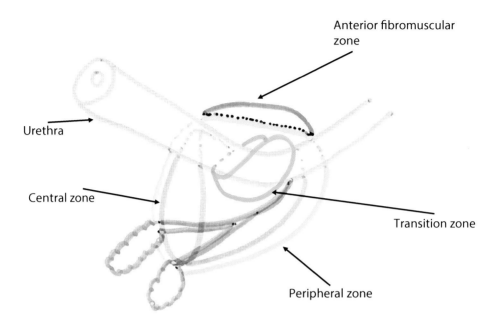

Figure 12.1 McNeal's zones of the prostate.

- Transition zone (comprises 10% glandular tissue of prostate – site of origin of benign prostatic hyperplasia)
- Central zone (comprises 25% glandular tissue of prostate)
- Peripheral zone (comprises 65% glandular tissue of prostate)
- Anterior fibromuscular stroma

LOWER URINARY TRACT SYMPTOMS

Q. A 67-year-old man is referred to you by his GP with 'mild prostatism'. What is 'prostatism'?
A. Prostatism is an outdated term for lower urinary tract symptoms (LUTS) due to benign prostatic enlargement (BPE).

Q. What is BPE?
A. BPE is the clinical finding of an enlarged prostate due to the histological process of benign prostatic hyperplasia (BPH).

Q. What is LUTS?
A. LUTS is a non-specific term for symptoms which may be attributable to lower urinary tract dysfunction. There are two main groups of LUTS – storage and voiding. BPO

(benign prostatic obstruction) is bladder outlet obstruction (urodynamic evidence of blockage of passage of urine) caused by BPE [1].

Q. How would you assess the patient in your clinic?

A. I would take a history, examine the patient and arrange further investigation.

Q. What features would you seek to elicit in your history?

A.

Symptoms	Duration
	Extent
Lifestyle	Impact/bother
	Fluid intake
Drugs	Adjustments already tried by the patient
	Trial of medication in primary care and outcome
	Drugs with sympathomimetic and anticholinergic effects
Past medical history	Urethral injury/instrumentation
	Pelvic surgery
	Neurological disorders

Q. Are you aware of any standardised instruments for the measurement of LUTS in male patients?

A. There have been a number of different questionnaires which have been used in the study of symptomatic BPE. These questionnaires include the International Prostate Symptom Score (IPSS), American Urological Association (AUA) Symptom Score, Danish (DAN) Prostatic Symptom Score and Bristol male LUTS. The IPSS questionnaire, derived from the AUA questionnaire [2] is the most commonly used instrument and has been shown to be valid, reliable and reproducible.

Q. Can you describe the AUA/IPSS questionnaire?

A. The IPSS consists of seven questions based on the extent of symptoms and a single quality-of-life question to assess symptom bother (Table 12.1). On the basis of the answers to the individual questions a total score is derived which can be used to divide patients into three groups – mild (0–7), moderate (8–19) and severe (20–35).

Q. What would you look for on examination?

A.

Specific features	Palpable bladder
	Enlarged (ballotable) kidneys
	Prostate – size, consistency, presence of nodules
	Note: Assess anal tone and sensation during digital rectal examination (DRE)
General features	Renal failure, e.g. fluid overload, signs of uraemia
	Neurological disorders, e.g. tremor, gait disturbance

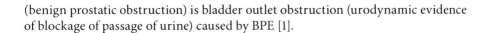

Table 12.1 The IPSS score with supplementary quality of life question

Over the past month, how often have you:	Not at all	Less than 1 time in 5	Less than half the time	About half the time	More than half the time	Almost always
1....had a sensation of not emptying your bladder completely after you finished urinating?	0	1	2	3	4	5
2....had to urinate again less than 2 hours after you finished urinating?	0	1	2	3	4	5
3....stopped and started again several times when you urinated?	0	1	2	3	4	5
4....found it difficult to postpone urination?	0	1	2	3	4	5
5....had a weak urinary stream?	0	1	2	3	4	5
6....had to push or strain to begin urination?	0	1	2	3	4	5
	None	Once	Twice	3 times	4 times	5 times or more
7. Over the past month, how many times did you most typically get up to urinate from the time you went to bed at night until the time you got up in the morning?	0	1	2	3	4	5

Supplementary question – Quality of life due to urinary symptoms.
If you were to spend the rest of your life with your urinary condition the way it is now, how would you feel about that?
  0. Delighted
  1. Pleased
  2. Mostly satisfied
  3. Mixed – about equally satisfied and dissatisfied
  4. Mostly dissatisfied
  5. Unhappy
  6. Terrible

Note: The IPSS scores seven questions on a scale from 0 to 5. Mild LUTS is defined as a score of 0–7, moderate LUTS scores 8–19, and severe LUTS scores 20–35. The quality of life question is scored from 0–6.

Q. **Your history indicates that the patient has an IPSS of 14 with no other relevant medical conditions. Clinical examination confirms a moderately enlarged benign prostate with no other significant findings. How would you investigate the patient?**

A.

I would arrange the following tests:	Frequency-volume chart
	Urinalysis
	Serum creatinine and estimated glomerular filtration rate (eGFR) (if I suspect renal impairment, i.e. if patient has a palpable bladder, nocturnal enuresis, recurrent urinary tract infections or a history of renal stones)
	Prostate-specific antigen (PSA) (I would offer men with LUTS information, advice and time to decide if they wish to have PSA testing if: their LUTS were suggestive of bladder outlet obstruction secondary to BPE, if their prostate felt abnormal on DRE or if they were concerned about prostate cancer)
	Uroflowmetry
	Ultrasound measurement of post-void residual (PVR) urine

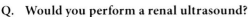

Q. **Would you perform a renal ultrasound?**

A. No. A renal ultrasound would only be indicated in the following situations:

- Chronic retention
- Haematuria
- Recurrent infection
- Sterile pyuria
- Profound symptoms
- Pain

Q. **Would you perform a cystoscopy on this patient?**

A. No. I would only offer cystoscopy when clinically indicated, e.g. if there is a history of any of the following:

- Recurrent infection
- Sterile pyuria
- Haematuria
- Profound symptoms
- Pain

Q. **Is transrectal ultrasound indicated in the investigation of this patient?**

A. No. It would be indicated if there was an elevated PSA, an abnormal DRE or if planning surgical treatment (i.e. transurethral resection of the prostate [TURP], Holmium laser enucleation of the prostate or Millin's prostatectomy – latter if transrectal ultrasound volume >100 mL).

Q. **Which patients should be considered for urodynamics evaluation before surgical intervention?**

A. Invasive urodynamics (pressure flow study) should be performed only in individual patients for specific indications prior to surgery or when evaluation of the underlying pathophysiology of LUTS is warranted.

The EAU guidelines recommend it in the following patients:

1. Men who have had previous unsuccessful (invasive) treatment for LUTS
2. Patients who cannot void >150 mL
3. When considering surgery in men with bothersome, predominantly voiding LUTS men with a PVR >300 mL
4. When considering surgery in men with bothersome, predominantly voiding LUTS men who are aged >80 years and <50 years

I would also consider it in men with equivocal flow rates, e.g. Q_{max} >10 mL/s and those with co-existing neurological disease.

Q. **What do you tell a patient in preparation for a flow rate?**

A. Patient will need to attend for 2–3 hours. I tell the patient to wait until he has a comfortably full bladder before performing the test (usually asked to attend having drank 500–1000 mL of fluid). Drinks are provided so that the patient can continue to drink while providing 2 or 3 flow rates when bladder volumes are at least 150 mL. When he passes urine into the flowmeter he should avoid compressing the penis as this may lead to squeeze artefact. Similarly he should not allow the urinary stream to wander around the funnel as this may also lead to abnormal recordings. I tell him that he should aim to pass at least 150 mL and if it is less than this then I ask him to repeat it. If it is persistently difficult to obtain an adequate voided volume then I ask him whether the flow is representative. If I have any doubts about the veracity of the recordings then I arrange for pressure-flow urodynamics.

Q. What factors affect the flow rate?

A. Flow rates are affected by

- Age
- Sex
- Voided volumes (VV) (should be >150 mL and <500 mL)
- Bladder outflow obstruction/hypocontractility

Q. What are the normal age-specific flow rates (Q_{max}) in males?

A. Normal age-specific flow rates (Q_{max}) in males are

- <40 years = >21 mL/s
- 40–60 years = >18 mL/s
- >60 years = >13 mL/s

Note: Age-specific flow rates (Q_{max}) in females are

- <50 years = >25 mL/s
- >50 years = 18 mL/s

Q. What factors do you analyse when interpreting the flow tracing?

A. Voided volume – adequate, i.e. >150 mL

Overdistention	VV >500 mL	
Maximum flow	Normal >15 mL/s	
	Suggestive of obstruction if <10 mL/s	
Overall pattern	Box-like curve (plateau curve) suggestive of stricture (for trace see Chapter 8)	
	Hyperflow suggestive of overactive bladder	
	Prolonged time to Q_{max} suggestive of BPH	

Q. What is the significance of a reduced urinary flow rate?

A. A reduced Q_{max} is usually taken to be evidence of bladder outflow obstruction (BOO). Approximately 90% of men with a flow rate of less than 10 mL/s will be obstructed on pressure-flow urodynamic criteria. The remaining 10% will have reduced detrusor contractility – low pressure, low flow situation. Similarly 75% of men with a flow rate of more than 15 mL/s will not have BOO. The remainder of men with a good flow rate may have high-pressure, high-flow situations where flow is maintained at the expense of increased detrusor work. (As an approximate guide there is a 90% probability of obstruction with a Q_{max} <10 mL/s, 60% probability of obstruction with a Q_{max} between 10 mL/s–15 mL/s, and 30% probability of obstruction with a Q_{max} >15 mL/s.) In the clinical setting, a reduced flow rate is a risk factor for acute urinary retention [3] and symptomatic progression [4].

Q. If the principal significance of a reduced Q_{max} is that it indicates the likelihood of BOO, then what is the significance of BOO?

A. The main significance of BOO is that it underpins the rationale behind dis-obstructing operations, e.g. TURP, in men with BPH. It allows more accurate prediction of symptomatic outcome after surgical intervention. Studies suggest that men with BOO who undergo TURP have a 90% chance of symptomatic improvement as compared to men without BOO who have a 60% chance of benefit [5].

Q. How can you accurately measure BOO?

A. BOO is an urodynamic diagnosis. It represents a high-pressure, low-flow situation. It can only be defined through the simultaneous measurement of detrusor pressure and urinary flow. There are a number of different ways of categorising the presence or absence of obstruction.

Q. Can you draw the ICS nomogram?

A. The ICS nomogram (Figure 12.2) categorises patients as obstructed, equivocal or unobstructed. The Abrams–Griffith number (Bladder Outlet Obstruction Index) gives a single numeric value through the equation $P_{det}Q_{max} - 2 \times Q_{max} =$ Abrams–Griffith number. Values over 40 are indicative of obstruction, values less than 20 represent unobstructed voiding with values between 20 and 40 being equivocal.

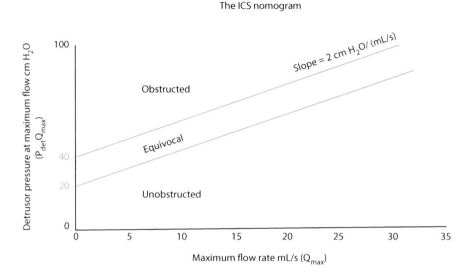

Figure 12.2 Current ICS method for definition of obstruction in patients with BPH.

Q. What is BPH?

A. Benign prostatic hyperplasia (BPH) properly describes the histological basis of a diagnosis of benign prostatic enlargement (BPE) resulting in bladder outflow obstruction (BOO) that gives rise to lower urinary tract symptoms (LUTS).

Q. How would you describe the relationship between BPE, BOO, LUTS and BPH. Can you draw a diagram to illustrate this?

A. The relationship between BOO, BPE, LUTS and BPH is depicted in Figure 12.3.

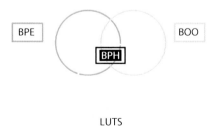

LUTS

Figure 12.3 Relationship between BOO, LUTS, BPE and BPH.

Q. What is BPH?

A. Benign prostatic hyperplasia (BPH) properly describes the histological basis of a diagnosis of benign prostatic enlargement (BPE) resulting in bladder outflow obstruction (BOO) that gives rise to lower urinary tract symptoms (LUTS).

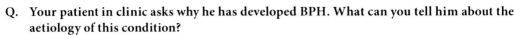

Q. **Your patient in clinic asks why he has developed BPH. What can you tell him about the aetiology of this condition?**

A. We do not understand exactly what the causative agent or agents are in BPH. The following factors are important:

- Age
- Androgens
- Race
- Diet
- Growth factors

Q. **How common is BPH?**

A. The exact prevalence of BPH varies according to the definition used. Data from post-mortem series show that histological evidence of BPH can be detected from the age of 30 and the prevalence increases to 88% of 80-year-olds [6].

Studies which define BPH on the presence of symptoms alone give a higher prevalence than those studies which include reduced urinary flow rates or demonstrable prostatic enlargement. The Olmsted County study (4) showed a prevalence of moderate-to-severe urinary symptoms in 13% of men aged 40–49, rising to 28% of men over the age of 70. A UK series which define BPH as the presence of an enlarged prostate (>20 g) with symptoms or reduced urinary flow (Q_{max} <15 mL/s) give a BPH prevalence of 138/1,000 population age 40–49 (13.8%) rising to 430/1,000 men age 60–69 (43%) [7].

Q. **Your patient asks what will happen if he does not have any treatment. Using the information which you already know about the patient what can you tell him about the likely course of his condition? What other information would you ask for to try to predict the outcome in his particular case?**

A. Information on the natural history of BPH can be obtained from two main sources: cross-sectional studies of community-dwelling men and the placebo arms of drug trials.

The Olmsted County study measured the prevalence of symptoms of BPH in men aged 40–80. An average AUA symptom score deterioration of 0.18/year was observed across the study with the fastest rate of deterioration observed in the 60–69 age group. It seems reasonable to conclude that there is a gradual increase in urinary symptoms with age but that the overall extent of these increases in the population is small.

Some risk factors have been identified which can help predict disease progression in individual patients. Factors which have been shown to be associated with an increased chance of disease progression include age, symptom severity, reduced urinary flow rate and prostate size (Table 12.2). The above patient in clinic has moderate symptoms, a reduced urinary flow and moderate prostate enlargement which would all increase the likelihood of progression but he is under 70 years old which would reduce the overall likelihood of deterioration.

Data from placebo arms of large drug trials have shown that PSA is an independent marker of disease progression. I would therefore ask the patient to have a PSA test performed

Table 12.2 The important risk factors with respect to disease progression and their associated hazard ratio (HR)

Risk factor	Risk of treatment
Moderate to severe symptoms	HR 5.3
Enlarged prostate (Vol >30 cc)	HR 2.3
Reduced flow rate (Q_{max} >12 mL/s)	HR 2.7

in order to try to refine his risk further. A PSA level of 1.4 ng/mL or higher indicates an increased risk of disease progression.

Other potential markers of disease progression include failure to respond to medical therapy [8], symptom deterioration while on treatment, increasing residual urine volume [9] and the presence of inflammation on prostate biopsies [10].

MEDICAL TREATMENT

Q. **A 72-year-old man presents to your outpatient clinic with an IPSS of 18, a PSA of 1.9 and a reduced maximum urinary flow rate of 9 mL/s. Discuss this man's options for non-surgical treatment.**

A. His options are

1. Watchful waiting
2. Lifestyle changes
3. Phytotherapy
4. Medical therapy
   a. Monotherapy
   b. Combination therapy

For many men, the reason for seeking medical attention is a fear regarding cancer. On the basis of his PSA and presuming an unremarkable DRE it is reasonable to reassure him that there are no signs of prostate cancer. If he has minimal bother from his symptoms then no active intervention may be required. I would reassure him that the risk of a significant deterioration in his symptoms or episode of acute urinary retention is low based on data from the placebo arms of randomised controlled trials (RCTs).

Lifestyle changes may have a beneficial effect on some groups of LUTS especially storage LUTS [11]. Advice to maintain a reasonable fluid intake, avoid excess caffeine and restrict fluids before going to bed may help with symptoms of frequency, urgency and nocturia. Double voiding and urethral milking may help to reduce the sensation of incomplete bladder emptying and reduce post-micturition dribble.

Phytotherapy is an increasingly popular therapeutic option in the United Kingdom. Plant extracts, e.g. saw palmetto, rye pollen extract, *Pygeum africanum* and ß-sitosterols may have some benefit in alleviating symptoms and improving urinary flows.

Pharmacological treatment can be with α-adrenergic antagonists, 5-α-reductase inhibitors or a combination of the two. There is a large body of evidence from RCTs to support the efficacy of both these groups of drugs.

Monotherapy with α-blockers is recommended for all men with uncomplicated LUTS. Meta-analysis of α-blocker trials has shown a reduction in symptoms of 30%–40% and an improvement in flow rates of 16%–25%. These effects appear to be durable.

Finasteride appears to be less effective than α-blockers when used as a single agent. The principal advantage of 5-α-reductase inhibitors is their ability to prevent disease progression. Data from the PLESS [12] study shows a reduction in both the need for TURP (55%) and the incidence of acute urinary retention (57%) over 4 years. Similar data are available for dutasteride which blocks both type-1 and type-2 5-α-reductase [13].

Initial trials of combination therapy failed to demonstrate any advantage for combination treatment over monotherapy [14]. The publication of the MTOPS trial [15] and 2-year results from the CombAT [16] study have, however, demonstrated a significant symptomatic benefit from combination therapy. British Association of Urological Surgeons (BAUS) guidelines for the management of men with LUTS suggest combination treatment for those with bothersome LUTS, prostatic obstruction and risk factors for progression [17].

The patient has a number of risk factors for disease progression but we do not know how bothersome his LUTS are. If he has bothersome LUTS then combination treatment would be the best way to alleviate his symptoms and reduce his likelihood of BPH-related adverse events.

SURGICAL TREATMENT

Q. **A fit 64-year-old man is reviewed in your clinic with severe LUTS which have not responded to medical therapy. Investigations confirm benign prostatic obstruction. He is bothered by his LUTS and wants further treatment. What would you offer him?**

A. I would offer him a transurethral resection of prostate (TURP) or a Holmium laser enucleation of the prostate (HoLEP).

Q. **What will you tell him about the likely symptomatic outcome of this operation?**

A. I would advise him that he has a 90% chance of symptom improvement given that he has bladder outlet obstruction. I would also counsel him that voiding symptoms tend to improve much more quickly after surgery than storage symptoms of frequency, urgency and nocturia.

Q. **What other groups of patients may benefit from TURP or HoLEP?**

A. In addition to men with bothersome LUTS who have failed a trial of medical management, the EAU gives the following indications for TURP:

- Refractory urinary retention
- Recurrent urinary retention
- Recurrent haematuria refractory to medical treatment with 5-α-reductase inhibitors
- Renal insufficiency
- Bladder stones
- Recurrent urinary tract infections as a result of BPH resulting in BOO
- Increased post-void residual volume (exact value not defined)
- Also TURP is indicated in those with chronic high-pressure urinary retention

Q. **What complications will you warn him about?**

A. I would use the BAUS procedure specific consent form for TURP or HoLEP. Potential complications of TURP include

- Early
  - Anaesthesia related, ischaemic event, deep vein thrombosis
  - Blood transfusion in 1%–2% (on average 10 mL blood loss per gram of tissue resected)
  - Urinary sepsis in up to 3%
  - Systemic sepsis in up to 1.5%

TUR syndrome	Risk 0.8% if <45 g tissue resected and 1.5% if >45 g tissue resected
	Risk 0.8% if resection time <90 minutes and 2% if resection time >90 minutes (No risk of TUR syndrome in HoLEP)

  - There is a risk of mortality of approximately 0.3% (within 30 days of operation)
- Late
  - Urinary incontinence in <1%
  - Retrograde ejaculation in 80%–100%
  - Erectile dysfunction is reported in approximately 10%
  - Bladder neck stenosis/urethral stricture in 3%–5%

- *Need for re-do surgery* – There is cumulative risk of 2% per year needing re-do surgery (thus 10% at 5 years and 16% at 8 years require re-do TURP)

Q. How do you perform a TURP?

A. I would take an adequately prepared and consented patient to theatre and after the patient has been anaesthetised, I would perform the following steps:

- Place patient in Lloyd–Davies position
- Clean and drape with TUR drape allowing rectal examination to be performed to assess size of prostate
- Perform initial cysto-urethroscopy to exclude other abnormalities of lower urinary tract
- Perform a urethral dilatation or Otis urethrotomy if either urethra is tight or using a 28 Fr resectoscope
- Insert resectoscope and begin by resecting median lobe down to circular fibres of bladder neck
- Resect each lateral lobe in turn by resecting a channel down to capsule at 10 or 2 o'clock and then dislocating lateral lobe to allow efficient resection
- If <10 g resected then perform additional TUIP
- Remove prostate chips using Ellik bladder evacuator
- Achieve haemostasis with rollerball
- Check that all chips have been removed, ureteric orifices are visible and undamaged and that no flaps have been created which might cause obstruction
- Insert three-way urethral catheter using introducer
- Assess catheter drainage and degree of haematuria before endoscopic equipment is removed
- Abdominal palpation to exclude extravasation

Q. What is TUR syndrome?

A. TUR syndrome is the absorption of irrigating fluid during the procedure. The risk of this is 2% in some large series. In the United Kingdom 1.5% glycine solution is the most commonly used irrigating fluid. This fluid is hypotonic with respect to plasma and therefore absorption of irrigating fluid can lead to dilutional hyponatraemia and fluid overload. The clinical manifestations of this may include tachycardia, bradycardia, other cardiac dysrhythmias, hypotension, headache and convulsions. Glycine itself can be metabolised in the GABA pathway to produce a neurotransmitter causing opisthotonus and cerebral irritation (see Chapter 7 for a discussion of TUR syndrome in more detail).

Q. What steps can you take to reduce the likelihood of TUR syndrome?

A. I would keep the height of the irrigating fluid above the patient to the minimum consistent with good vision. I would avoid prolonged resection particularly if there is evidence of capsular perforation or venous haemorrhage. I routinely use a continuous flow resectoscope and examine the patient's abdomen at the end of the operation for any sign of extravasation.

Q. How would you treat a full-blown TUR syndrome?

A. If evidence of TUR syndrome occurred during the procedure then I would act swiftly to obtain haemostasis and bring the operation to a close. I would place a 24 Fr three-way catheter in the bladder and consider traction if there has been venous perforation or in the presence of persistent bleeding. I would ensure that irrigation is kept to an absolute minimum using normal saline solution. I would examine the abdomen for signs of extravasation and if present I would place a retropubic drain. I would ask the anaesthetist to send bloods including full blood count (FBC), urea and electrolytes (U&E) and clotting studies and to give a 40 mg dose of intravenous furosemide. Any dysrhythmias should be treated in accordance with cardiac guidelines and the patient should be carefully monitored post-operatively in an intensive therapy unit (ITU) facility. The serum sodium concentration should be restored slowly through the judicious use of fluid restriction, diuretics and, rarely, hypertonic saline.

Q. **You are called to recovery to see your patient on whom you have just performed a TURP. The nurses are concerned by the extent of the haematuria and inform you that the catheter keeps clotting off. What actions would you take?**

A. I would assess the patient urgently to ensure that he is stable and resuscitate as necessary.

If stable, I would examine the patient's abdomen to see if the bladder is distended. I would then perform a bladder washout with normal saline, also ensuring that the irrigation channel is patent. I would washout any clots and recommence bladder irrigation.

If this failed to control the haematuria, I would then deflate the catheter balloon, push the catheter further into the bladder and then insert 50 mL of water into the catheter balloon and apply traction by strapping the catheter to the patient's thigh. I would reassess the patient's cardiovascular status and the degree of haematuria.

If faced with ongoing haematuria, I would urgently consider returning to theatre, to endoscopically assess the prostate cavity and stop the bleeding. I would ensure that blood was cross-matched and explain to the patient the need to return to theatre to control bleeding. Assuming the patient's condition allows I would take written consent. In theatre, I would re-insert the resectoscope and perform Ellik bladder washouts until no further clots are retrieved, and vision has improved. I would then conduct a thorough inspection of the prostatic bed to look for obvious sources of bleeding. The most common sites of bleeding are from arteries at the bladder neck or from venous perforation. I would attempt to control bleeding with the rollerball accepting that this is usually more successful in arterial bleeding. In the presence of significant venous perforation I would re-insert a catheter, overinflate the balloon and apply traction for 10 minutes by the clock. If none of these measures controlled the bleeding then I would make a lower midline incision, open the bladder between stay sutures, inspect the cavity for bleeding points, diathermise or under-run bleeding vessels as appropriate and ultimately pack the prostatic cavity if none of the aforementioned steps have worked.

Q. **What other conventional operations have been used for the treatment of BPH?**

A. Transvesical prostatectomy was commonly used at the beginning of the twentieth century and is still practised in many developing countries. It can still be indicated if there are large bladder calculi or other bladder abnormalities, e.g. large diverticulae which require simultaneous treatment. Millin's retropubic prostatectomy is the preferred operation if open surgery is indicated as it allows better haemostasis and visualisation of the prostatic cavity.

Open prostatectomy is not commonly performed in the United Kingdom anymore but is indicated with large prostate size (>100 g) or difficulty positioning the patient due to hip contractures. Cancerous prostates or small, fibrous glands in which there is no surgical plane in which to conduct the enucleation should not be treated by a Millin's prostatectomy. In general, the risks of open prostatectomy are greater than those of TURP particularly with respect to bleeding, blood transfusion, incontinence, bladder neck contracture and thromboembolic complications (although need for re-do procedures is decreased).

Small prostate glands (<30 mL) may be treated by transurethral incision of the prostate (TUIP) with good symptomatic results and reduced complications.

Q. **What would you do if you found a stone in the bladder on initial cystoscopy?**

A. Clearly, in an elective setting, one would have anticipated this finding and appropriately counselled the patient pre-operatively, with the preferred treatment strategy. In unforeseen circumstances, the decision making would be based on the size of the stone as well as the size of the prostate gland.

For example, if the stone was small (<3 cm) and the prostate of a reasonable size then I would consider performing a cystolitholapaxy first and then to TURP at the same sitting, if vision was good and patient was clinically stable (not developing sepsis).

If the stone was larger but could still be safely managed endoscopically, then I would deal with the stone and perform a TURP at a later date.

In the situation where the stone was too large to be dealt with endoscopically then open surgery would be necessary, if the patient had consented to it pre-operatively, as an additional procedure. Traditionally this would be an indication for a transvesical prostatectomy and open stone removal. If patient had not consented, then I would stop after cystoscopy and re-evaluate electively. Clearly, if a very large stone had been found on pre-operative assessment, the possible need for open surgery with its attendant complications would have been discussed with the patient.

Q. What other procedures are you aware of as alternatives to conventional monopolar TURP for managing voiding LUTS presumed secondary to BPE?

A. Alternatives to conventional monopolar TURP include that I may offer include Holmium laser enucleation of the prostate (HoLEP). I am aware that I would only perform HoLEP at a centre specialising in the technique, or with mentorship arrangements in place. HoLEP is the endoscopic equivalent of an open prostatectomy in which the plane between the adenoma and the prostatic capsule is developed to dissect the lobes of the prostate out before they are then morcellated to allow extraction. A 10-year follow-up study for HoLEP with 949 patients has shown a significant improvement in IPSS, quality of life, maximum urinary flow rate, and post-void residual urine volume, which was maintained over the 10-year period. Persistent urge and stress incontinence were found in 1% and 0.5% of patients, respectively. Bladder neck contracture, urethral stricture and reoperation due to residual adenoma developed in 0.8%, 1.6% and 0.7% of patients [18]. This may well become the gold standard treatment for BOO in the future as symptomatic outcomes are at least equivalent to, if not better than, conventional TURP but there is a lower risk of bleeding and earlier return to normal activities. The main drawbacks of HoLEP are the expense of the laser, the perceived difficulty of learning the procedure and the inherent risks of bladder damage during the morcellation process.

KTP lasers (greenlight lasers) have been in use for over a decade, but have gradually increased in power with a corresponding increase in vaporisation efficiency (vaporisation creates a cavity by repeated passage of the laser over the surface of the prostate). Currently National Institute for Health and Care Excellence (NICE) suggests that there is insufficient high-quality, comparative evidence to support the routine adoption of the GreenLight XPS in high-risk patients, i.e. those who have an increased risk of bleeding, have prostates greater than 100 mL or have urinary retention.

Recently, NICE guidance has recommended use of Urolift [19] and TURIS (Transurethral Resection in Saline) for BPH surgery [20].

Urolift relieves LUTS while preserving sexual function, with the added advantage of being performed as a day case operation. NICE guidance recommends its use in men who are 50 years or older, with prostate volume less than 100 mL and without an obstructing middle lobe.

NICE recommendations state that TURis, instead of a monopolar system, avoids the risk of TUR syndrome and reduces the need for blood transfusion. It may also reduce the length of hospital stay and hospital readmissions. Using TURis also has some cost savings and there is some evidence of a reduction in readmissions with the TURis system compared with monopolar TURP.

I would offer transurethral incision of the prostate (TUIP) as an alternative to other types of surgery to men with a prostate estimated to be smaller than 30 g. Finally, I am aware that I would only consider offering laser vaporisation techniques, bipolar TUVP or monopolar or bipolar transurethral vaporisation resection of the prostate (TUVRP) as part of a randomised controlled trial that compares these techniques with TURP.

ACUTE URINARY RETENTION

Q. **A 65-year-old man is referred to you by his GP with moderate LUTS. He is primarily concerned that he may develop a 'complete stoppage'. How would you assess and counsel him?**

A. There are a number of risk factors which have been identified for acute urinary retention (AUR) in both community-based observational studies and in RCTs of drug treatment for BPH. These include age, reduced flow rate, prostate volume, PSA and a previous episode of urinary retention (Table 12.3).

Table 12.3 The important risk factors with respect to acute urinary retention (AUR) and their respective relative risk

Risk factor	AUR relative risk
IPSS >7	3.2
Q_{max} <12 mL/s	3.9
Prostate volume >30 mL	3.0
PSA >1.4	2.0
Age >70 versus 40–49	10–11

Q. **A 78-year-old man presents to accident and emergency with a painfully distended bladder and an inability to pass urine. How would you manage this patient?**

A. I would take a concise history, examine the patient and then insert a urinary catheter. Having relieved his discomfort I would then arrange further investigations including urinalysis, FBC, U&E and ultrasound scan.

Q. **Your investigations reveal a serum creatinine of 427 μmol/L and ultrasound demonstrates bilateral hydronephrosis. What is your further management of this patient?**

A. I would arrange for the patient to be admitted. I would ask the nurses to record hourly monitoring of pulse, blood pressure and urine output. I would ask to be informed if the patient produces more than 200 mL of urine per hour for 2 consecutive hours. I would ensure that his admission weight is recorded and request daily weighing to monitor for gross fluid shifts. If there is evidence of post-obstructive diuresis then I would give replacement intravenous *normal saline* equivalent to 90% of the patient's previous hour's urine output (the amount of fluid replacement is variable – some would only replace 50% of the previous hour's urine output). I would recheck the serum U&E to ensure that the creatinine is falling and that potassium levels remain within range. I would expect to continue intravenous fluid support for 24–48 hours.

Q. **What is the mechanism behind post-obstructive diuresis?**

A. There is both a physiological and pathological component to the diuresis. A physiological diuresis occurs because of the accumulation of fluid, electrolytes and waste products in the preceding period of renal failure. Relief of obstruction allows elimination of excess amounts of these substances to occur. Pathological diuresis occurs because of a number of factors which lead to tubular dysfunction and inappropriate salt and water handling by the kidney. These include the following:

1. Defective generation of medullary solute gradient secondary to
   ↓ re-absorption of NaCl by thick ascending LOH
   ↓ reabsorption of urea by collecting tubule
2. Inability to maintain medullary solute gradient secondary to
   ↑ medullary blood flow (solute washout)

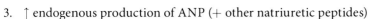

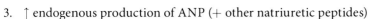

3. ↑ endogenous production of ANP (+ other natriuretic peptides)
4. Poor response of collecting duct to ADH

Q. **Draw a graph to show the recovery of glomerular filtration rate (GFR) following the relief of obstruction.**

A. This is illustrated in Figure 12.4. As the GFR continues to recover for up to 3 months thus plasma creatinine will continue to decrease over this period.

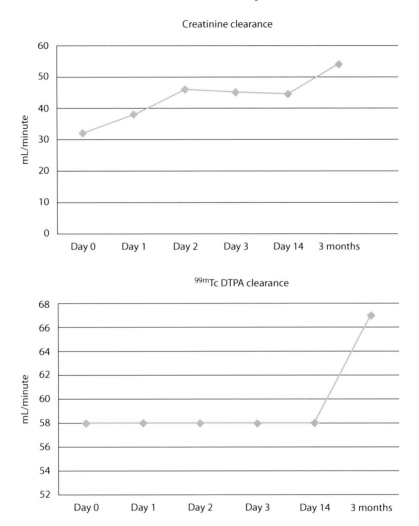

Figure 12.4 Changes in creatinine clearance and ^{99m}Tc DTPA clearance following relief of obstruction. Both are estimates of glomerular filtration rate.

Q. **If creatinine clearance and ^{99m}Tc DTPA (diethylene-triamine-penta-acetic acid) clearance are both indicators of glomerular filtration rate, then why does creatinine clearance improve more quickly?**

A. Creatinine is excreted by the tubules of the kidney as well as through glomerular filtration. Following relief of bilateral ureteric obstruction in this case tubular function recovers in the first 14 days but full recovery of glomerular function may take up to 3 months. The return of tubular function increases creatinine clearance and allows serum creatinine to fall but this does not reflect a real change in GFR.

Note: *Creatinine clearance estimates the GFR and can be measured over 12–24 hours by the equation UV/P where U is the urinary concentration of creatinine, V is volume of urine produced over a timed interval and P is the plasma concentration of creatinine. About 80% of creatinine clearance is due to GFR and 20% is due to renal tubular secretion. Thus creatinine clearance is an overestimate of actual GFR (becomes important in very poor renal function when tubular secretion may be responsible for a relatively greater proportion of the creatinine clearance).*

REFERENCES

1. Abrams P. New words for old: Lower urinary tract symptoms for 'prostatism'. *BMJ* 1994; 308: 929–930.
2. Barry MJ et al. The American Urological Association symptom index for benign prostatic hyperplasia. The Measurement Committee of the American Urological Association. *J Urol* 1992; 148: 1549–1557.
3. Jacobsen SJ et al. Natural history of prostatism: Risk factors for acute urinary retention. *J Urol* 1997; 158: 481–487.
4. Jacobsen SJ et al. Natural history of prostatism: Longitudinal changes in voiding symptoms in community dwelling men. *J Urol* 1996; 155: 595–600.
5. Abrams PH et al. The results of prostatectomy: A symptomatic and urodynamic analysis of 152 patients. *J Urol* 1979; 121: 640–642.
6. Berry SJ et al. The development of human benign prostatic hyperplasia with age. *J Urol* 1984; 132: 474–479.
7. Garraway WM et al. High prevalence of benign prostatic hypertrophy in the community. *Lancet* 1991; 338: 469–471.
8. Emberton M et al. Response to daily 10 mg alfuzosin predicts acute urinary retention and benign prostatic hyperplasia related surgery in men with lower urinary tract symptoms. *J Urol* 2006; 176: 1051–1056.
9. Emberton M. Definition of at-risk patients: Dynamic variables. *BJU Int* 2006; 97(Suppl 2): 12–15.
10. Mishra VC et al. Does intraprostatic inflammation have a role in the pathogenesis and progression of benign prostatic hyperplasia? *BJU Int* 2007; 100: 327–331.
11. Brown CT et al. Self management for men with lower urinary tract symptoms: randomised controlled trial. *BMJ* 2007; 334: 25.
12. Roehrborn CG et al. Serum prostate-specific antigen concentration is a powerful predictor of acute urinary retention and need for surgery in men with clinical benign prostatic hyperplasia. PLESS Study Group. *Urology* 1999; 53: 473–480.
13. Roehrborn CG et al. Efficacy and tolerability of the dual 5-alpha-reductase inhibitor, dutasteride, in the treatment of benign prostatic hyperplasia in African-American men. *Prostate Cancer Prostatic Dis* 2006; 9: 432–438.
14. Lepor H et al. The efficacy of terazosin, finasteride, or both in benign prostatic hyperplasia. Veterans Affairs Cooperative Studies Benign Prostatic Hyperplasia Study Group. *N Engl J Med* 1996; 335: 533–539.
15. McConnell JD et al. The long-term effect of doxazosin, finasteride, and combination therapy on the clinical progression of benign prostatic hyperplasia. *N Engl J Med* 2003; 349: 2387–2398.
16. Roehrborn CG et al. The effects of dutasteride, tamsulosin and combination therapy on lower urinary tract symptoms in men with benign prostatic hyperplasia and prostatic enlargement: 2-year results from the CombAT study. *J Urol* 2008; 179: 616–621.

17. Speakman MJ et al. Guideline for the primary care management of male lower urinary tract symptoms. *BJU Int* 2004; 93: 985–990.
18. Elmansy HM et al. Holmium laser enucleation of the prostate: Long-term durability of clinical outcomes and complication rates during 10 years of followup. *J Urol* 2011; 186: 1972–1976.
19. National Institute for Health and Care Excellence (NICE). UroLift for treating lower urinary tract symptoms of benign prostatic hyperplasia. Medical technologies guidance [MTG26]; September 2015. https://www.nice.org.uk/guidance/mtg26/resources/urolift-for-treating-lower-urinary-tract-symptoms-of-benign-prostatic-hyperplasia-64371938204869.
20. National Institute for Health and Care Excellence (NICE). The TURis system for transurethral resection of the prostate. Medical technologies guidance; February 25, 2015. https://www.nice.org.uk/guidance/mtg23/resources/the-turis-system-for-transurethral-resection-of-the-prostate-64371933166021.

CHAPTER 13
ANDROLOGY

Jas S Kalsi, Suks Minhas and Asif Muneer

Contents

ERECTILE DYSFUNCTION

Q. **A 65-year-old male has noticed a progressive deterioration in his erections over a 1-year period. He is now avoiding sexual relationships with his wife. His wife is very concerned and asks him to see his GP. The GP tells him not to worry as it is a normal part of the ageing process. After a further 6 months as things continue to get worse, he decides to see another partner in the same practice who refers him to see a urologist. How do you define erectile dysfunction?**

A. Erectile dysfunction is defined as the inability to achieve or maintain an erection sufficient for satisfactory sexual performance.

Q. **Can you describe the different phases of a penile erection?**

A. There are five distinct phases of erection that have been demonstrated:

0 – Flaccid
1 – Latent
2 – Tumescence
3 – Full erection
4 – Rigid erection
5 – Detumescence (initial, slow and fast phases)

Q. **Can you explain the physiological process of penile erection?**

A. Penile erection is the result of a complex and delicate interplay between several biochemical, vascular, neurological, physical and psychological pathways. The cavernous smooth muscle and the smooth muscles in the arteriolar and arterial walls, play a key role in erectile function. In the flaccid state, the smooth muscle is tonically contracted, allowing only a small amount of arterial flow into the cavernous spaces. Sexual stimulation triggers the release of neurotransmitters from the cavernous nerve terminals, resulting in smooth muscle relaxation and triggering the following events:

1. Dilatation of the arterioles and arteries by increased blood flow in both the diastolic and the systolic phases
2. Trapping of the incoming blood by the expanding sinusoids
3. Compression of the subtunical venular plexuses between the tunica albuginea and the peripheral sinusoids, which reduces the venous outflow
4. Stretching of the tunica to its capacity, which encloses the emissary veins between the inner circular and the outer longitudinal layers and further decreases the venous outflow to a minimum
5. An increase in intracavernous pressure (maintained at around 100 mm Hg), which raises the penis from the dependent position to the erect state (the full-erection phase)
6. A further pressure increase (to several hundred mm Hg) with contraction of the ischiocavernosus muscles (rigid-erection phase)

Q. What mechanisms allow the penis to achieve a full rigid erection?

A. During the full-erection phase, partial compression of the deep dorsal and circumflex veins between Buck's fascia and the engorged corpora cavernosa contribute to glanular tumescence. In the rigid-erection phase, the ischiocavernosus and bulbocavernosus muscles forcefully compress the spongiosum and penile veins, which results in further engorgement and increased pressure in the glans and spongiosum.

Q. Can you describe the arterial supply of the penis?

A. The main source of blood supply to the penis is from the internal pudendal artery. However, accessory arteries may arise from the external iliac, obturator, vesical and femoral arteries. The internal pudendal artery becomes the common penile artery after giving off a branch to the perineum.

The three branches of the penile artery are the cavernous, dorsal and the bulbourethral:

1. *Cavernous artery* – Involved in tumescence of the corpus cavernosum. Gives off a number of helicine arteries, which supply the trabecular erectile tissue and the sinusoids. These helicine arteries are contracted and tortuous in the flaccid state and become dilated and straight during erection.
2. *Dorsal artery* – Provides engorgement of the glans penis during erection.
3. *Bulbourethral artery* – Blood supply to the bulb and corpus spongiosum.

Distally, the three branches join to form a vascular anastomosis in and around the glans penis.

Q. Can you describe the venous drainage of the penis?

A. The venous drainage from the three corpora originates in tiny venules leading from the peripheral sinusoids immediately beneath the tunica albuginea. These venules travel in the trabeculae between the tunica and the peripheral sinusoids to form the subtunical venular plexus before exiting as the emissary veins.

Outside the tunica albuginea, the venous drainage is dependent on the area of drainage as follows:

- *Skin and subcutaneous tissue* – Multiple superficial veins run subcutaneously and unite near the root of the penis to form the superficial dorsal vein(s), which in turn usually drains into the saphenous veins.
- *Emissary veins from the corpus cavernosum and spongiosum* – These drain dorsally to the deep dorsal vein, laterally to the circumflex vein, and ventrally to the periurethral veins. Beginning at the coronal sulcus, the prominent deep dorsal vein is the main venous drainage of the glans penis, corpus spongiosum and distal two-thirds of the corpora cavernosa. It runs behind the symphysis pubis to join the periprostatic venous plexus.
- *Emissary veins draining the proximal corpora cavernosa* – Form cavernous and crural veins. These veins join the periurethral veins from the urethral bulb to form the internal pudendal veins.

Q. Why should men with erectile dysfunction (ED) be investigated?

A. The correct assessment of men presenting with ED can identify undiagnosed conditions as well as being a risk factor for other disease processes:

- Diabetes (ED may be the first symptom in up to 20%)
- Occult cardiac disease (ED in an otherwise asymptomatic man may be a marker for underlying coronary artery disease). The lead time for this is up to 3 years.
- Dyslipidaemia
- Presence of hypogonadism
- Identifying co-existing lower urinary tract symptoms

Q. What questions will you ask in the history?

A. I would see the patient ideally in a specialist andrology or sexual dysfunction clinic in the presence of the partner if possible. A full sexual history should be taken. First, I would confirm from the history that the problem is genuinely ED (see above definition), as opposed to ejaculatory dysfunction or penile curvature. I would then ascertain the following points in the history:

- Was onset of ED sudden or gradual?
- Are early morning erections still present?
- Is the ED situational (does it vary depending on partner or with masturbation)?
- Severity (objectively assessed using a validated IIEF-5 questionnaire)
- Successful response to any treatment options
- Assessment of the patient's (and partner's) needs and expectations

Q. How would you assess the severity of the condition?

A. I would use a validated questionnaire such as the International Index of Erectile Function (IIEF) or the validated shorter version, the IIEF-5 (SHIM). These are helpful in assessing the domains of sexual function as well as the impact of treatments and interventions. The questionnaire relates to the previous 6 months (see Table 13.1).

The overall score allows the severity to be assessed objectively as follows:

1–7	Severe ED
8–11	Moderate ED
12–16	Mild to moderate ED
17–21	Mild ED
22–25	No ED

Table 13.1 International Index of Erectile Function–5 (IIEF-5) questionnaire

		Very low	Low	Moderate	High	Very high
1. How do you rate your confidence that you could get and keep an erection?		Very low	Low	Moderate	High	Very high
		1	2	3	4	5
2. When you had erections with sexual stimulation, how often were your erections hard enough for penetration (entering your partner)?	No sexual activity	Almost never/ never	A few times (much less than half the time)	Sometimes (about half the time)	Most times (much more than half the time)	Almost always/ always
	0	1	2	3	4	5
3. During sexual intercourse, how often were you able to maintain your erection after you had penetrated (entered) your partner?	Did not attempt intercourse	Almost never/ never	A few times (much less than half the time)	Sometimes (about half the time)	Most times (much more than half the time)	Almost always/ always
	0	1	2	3	4	5
4. During sexual intercourse, how difficult was it to maintain your erection to completion of intercourse?	Did not attempt intercourse	Extremely difficult	Very difficult	Difficult	Slightly difficult	Not difficult
	0	1	2	3	4	5
5. When you attempted sexual intercourse, how often was it satisfactory for you?	Did not attempt intercourse	Almost never/ never	A few times (much less than half the time)	Sometimes (about half the time)	Most times (much more than half the time)	Almost always/ always
	0	1	2	3	4	5

Q. What would you assess on a physical examination?

A. A focused physical examination should be performed on every patient presenting with ED. This should include an emphasis on the neurological, cardiovascular and genital tract. Height, weight, body mass index and blood pressure should be recorded.

In particular it is important to examine for:

- Thyroid evaluation, pulmonary status, and cardiac rhythm
- Abdominal exam with mid waist circumference recorded
- Penile exam (assess for penile plaques, penile lesions and foreskin problems)
- Testis exam (note size, consistencies and irregularities)
- If indicated rectal exam (sphincter tone, prostate size evaluation particularly if co-existent LUTS)

Q. Would you perform any other tests?

A. The routine tests that I would usually perform are:

- Urinalysis
- Fasting blood glucose
- Fasting lipids
- Total testosterone (if low or borderline then perform luteinizing hormone [LH], follicle-stimulating hormone [FSH] and sex hormone binding globulin [SHBG])
- Prostate-specific antigen (if there is an abnormality with the prostate gland and after appropriate counselling especially in age >50)
- Prolactin

Q. This particular patient is a non-insulin-dependent diabetic with a gradual onset of ED and has an IIEF-5 score of 8. All blood tests other than fasting glucose are normal. How would you manage this patient?

A. I would identify and treat any reversible causes of ED such as poorly controlled diabetes. I would also initiate lifestyle changes (including exercise and weight loss) and seek to modify any associated risk factors (stop smoking). If this fails to improve his erections then I would offer him a trial of an oral PDE-5 inhibitor provided that there are no contraindications.

Q. How do PDE-5 inhibitors work? Can you draw a diagram to illustrate this?

A. Nitric oxide (NO) enters the smooth muscle cell, where it activates the soluble form of the enzyme-soluble guanylate cyclase (sGC). Soluble GC catalyses the conversion of guanosine triphosphate (GTP) to the active intracellular second messenger cyclic guanosine monophosphate (cGMP). In turn cGMP leads to activation of a number of intracellular events, which eventually brings about penile smooth muscle relaxation (Figure 13.1) mainly via a reduction in intracellular calcium. The action of cGMP is terminated by its metabolism to GMP by phosphodiesterase type 5 (PDE-5). Drugs inhibiting the action of PDE-5 (PDE-5 inhibitors) facilitate NO-induced smooth muscle relaxation within the penis by causing an accumulation in intracellular cGMP.

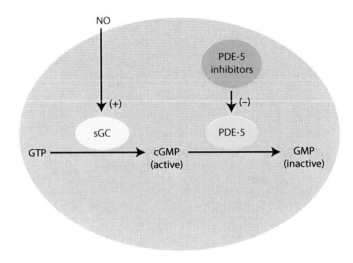

Figure 13.1 The mechanism of action of PDE-5 inhibitors.

Q. Which PDE-5 inhibitors are you aware of?

A. There are a number of PDE-5 inhibitors available including sildenafil (Viagra), tadalafil (Cialis), vardenafil (Levitra) and avanafil (Spedra).

Q. What are the differences between them?

A. The major difference is that sildenafil and vardenafil are relatively short-acting drugs, having a half-life of approximately 4–5 hours, whereas tadalafil has a significantly longer half-life of 17.5 hours. Furthermore, tadalafil is not known to have reduced bioavailability with fatty foods. Tadalafil is also available as a 5 mg daily dose which is the only PDE-5 inhibitor approved for daily dosing and for treating male lower urinary tract symptoms. Avanafil may work within 15 minutes.

Q. How would you counsel a patient and initiate therapy with a PDE-5 inhibitor?

A. First, I would ensure that there are no contraindications to treatment with oral PDE-5 inhibitors. In my practice, the specific choice of which medication is given as first line is patient driven. First, it depends on whether the couple wishes to have more spontaneity in which tadalafil would be the best option. Sometimes patients tolerate a particular PDE-5 inhibitor due to a better side-effect profile. I would then explain that my patient will need to take the medication at least eight times at the maximum dose of the drug, at least 1 hour before sex

(Table 13.2), ideally on an empty stomach together with sexual stimulation before it is deemed a pharmacological failure. A full explanation of the potential side effects is also required (Table 13.2). Having informed him of all these factors, the final choice is made by the patient.

Table 13.2 The characteristics of the different PDE-5 inhibitors

	Sildenafil	Vardenafil	Tadalafil
Onset of action	15 min to 1 hour	15 min to 1 hour	15 min to 2 hours
Half-life	3–5 hours	4–5 hours	17.5 hours
Bioavailability	40%	15%	Not tested
Food effect	Reduced absorption with fatty foods	Reduced absorption with fatty foods	None
Dosages	25, 50, 100 mg	5, 10, 20 mg	5, 10, 20 mg
Side effects	Headache, dyspepsia, facial flushing, blurred/blue vision, rare cases of backache, myalgia	Headache, dyspepsia, facial flushing, rare cases of backache, myalgia, and blurred/blue vision	Headache, dyspepsia, facial flushing, backache, myalgia, rare cases of blurred/blue vision
Contraindications	Nitrates	Nitrates, antiarrhythmics	Nitrates

Q. What are the common side effects associated with PDE-5 inhibitors?

A. All PDE-5 inhibitors produce side effects that are usually associated with peripheral vasodilatation, including nasal congestion, facial flushing, headache and dyspepsia. Tadalafil has been linked to back pain in up to 10% of cases although the side-effect profile is much better for the lower 5 mg dose. Vardenafil has been shown to slightly prolong the QT interval. Optical neuropathies have been reported however, the actual incidence of optical neuropathy is rare.

Q. This same patient has recently been started on antihypertensive medication by his GP. He feels that this has made his ED worse. Which other medications are known to be associated with ED?

A. Diuretics and antihypertensives are known to be associated with ED. Other medications also associated with ED include antidepressants, antianxiety and antiepileptic drugs, antihistamines, non-steroidal anti-inflammatory drugs, medication for Parkinson's disease, antiarrhythmics, histamine H2-receptor antagonists, muscle relaxants, hormone treatment for prostate cancer and chemotherapies.

Q. Unfortunately despite maximum doses of the PDE-5 inhibitor he does not get a satisfactory response. How would you now manage this patient?

A. I would explain to him that approximately 25% of patients do not respond to PDE-5 inhibitors. I would also ensure re-education on the effects of modifiable factors, such as dose, timing of medication, alcohol consumption, adequate sexual arousal and interaction with fatty foods. If he has tried a short-acting PDE-5 inhibitor then it may be worthwhile switching to the longer-acting tadalafil at the maximum dose to enable more spontaneity as a proportion of patients benefit from switching. If the investigations show low or borderline total testosterone, then combination treatment with testosterone replacement and a PDE-5 inhibitor may help some individuals. In patients who are hypogonadal, testosterone replacement may result in a general improvement in sexual function, improved erection and enhanced responsiveness to PDE-5 inhibitors but ensure that they are aware of the risks of testosterone treatment including the effects on spermatogenesis.

Q. Despite trying these options he still does not get satisfactory erections. What alternative treatment options are available?

A. If patients do not benefit from PDE-5 inhibitors or they are contraindicated, then second-line treatment options should be considered which include the following:

- *Alprostadil intraurethral suppositories (MUSE)* – A non-injectable prostaglandin pellet, which improves vascular flow by causing vasodilatation by increasing levels of cyclic AMP; a newer way of delivering Alprostadil is gel formulation (Vitaros) at 300 mcg.
- *Intracavernosal injections* – Local injections of one or a combination of alprostadil, papaverine and phentolamine.
- *Vacuum constriction devices* – Effective in most patients and can be purchased with or without a prescription.
- *Low-intensity shockwave therapy* – This improves endothelial function and allows neovascularisation. Success may be achieved in up to 70% of cases but may need to be repeated.
- If the second-line treatment options fail then third-line therapy includes the following:
- *Penile prostheses* – Surgically placed non-inflatable (semirigid/malleable) or inflatable devices.
- *Penile revascularisation surgery* – Reserved for patients having suffered from pelvic trauma or proven arteriogenic impairment.

Q. Which specialist investigations for ED are you aware of and when are they used?

A. Specialist investigations include nocturnal penile tumescence studies, cavernosometry or cavernosography and Duplex ultrasound. Most patients do not need further investigations. However, some patients wish to know the aetiology of the ED and in others specialist investigations are required. These include the following:

- Young patients who have always had difficulty in obtaining and/or sustaining an erection
- Patients with a history of trauma
- Where an abnormality of the testes or penis is found on examination
- Patients unresponsive to medical therapies who may desire surgical treatment for ED

Q. What is shown in Figure 13.2? How does it work and what is it used for?

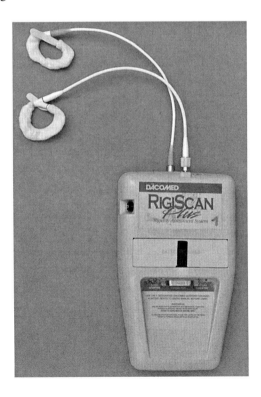

Figure 13.2

A. Figure 13.2 is a Rigiscan device (used to provide a nocturnal penile tumescence [NPT] trace). It comprises two transducer rings which are placed around the tip and base of the penis, respectively. They are used to measure the number, duration and rigidity of nocturnal erections. Nocturnal and early morning erections are a normal physiological event in all men and are associated with the REM pattern of sleep. This test is used to differentiate organic from psychogenic causes of ED.

Q. **What does Figure 13.3 show?**

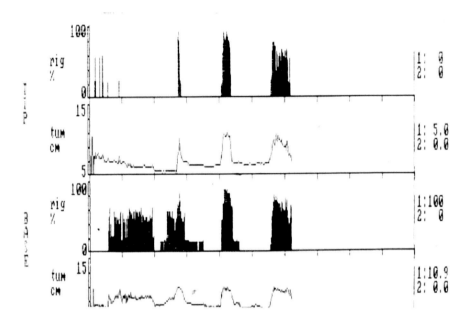

Figure 13.3

A. Figure 13.3 demonstrates a normal NPT trace. A normal trace shows greater than 60% rigidity at the tip for >10 minutes.

Q. **What is the role for penile Doppler as an investigation for ED? What are the normal blood flow parameters?**

A. This radiological investigation is used if there is a suspicion of a vasculogenic cause for ED. It requires an intracavernosal injection of a prostaglandin (PGE1) to induce an erection. The blood flow is then measured and a diagnosis of arteriogenic or veno-occlusive dysfunction or mixed vasculogenic ED can be made. The normal values for the peak systolic velocity are >25–30 cm/s. A peak systolic velocity lower than this is compatible with arteriogenic ED. If the end diastolic velocity >5 cm/s then this may indicate veno-occlusive dysfunction as the normal end diastolic velocity should be <10 cm/s.

Q. **What is the test shown in Figure 13.4 and how is it performed?**

A. Figure 13.4 is a cavernosogram. Cavernosography requires an artificial erection followed by the injection of contrast into the penis. Simultaneous imaging and blood flow parameters are measured and the flow required to maintain the erection is measured to identify any venous leaks. This particular image demonstrates a venous leak although the clinical entity of venous leak is still controversial.

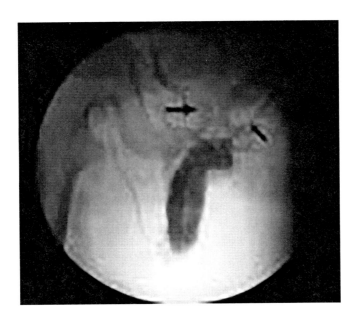

Q. What is shown in Figure 13.5? Explain how it works.

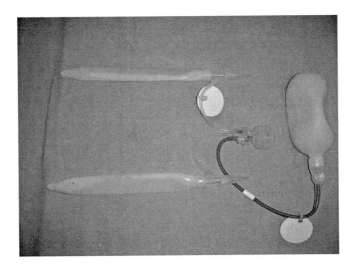

A. Figure 13.5 is a three-piece inflatable penile implant. This consists of a reservoir which is placed in the retropubic space and is filled with saline, a pump placed in the scrotum and a pair of cylinders which are placed within the corpora of the penis. The pump in the scrotum allows fluid to flow from the reservoir to the cylinders which increase in girth and become rigid (inflation). A small release button on the pump is pressed to allow deflation of the cylinders by allowing fluid to pass back from the cylinders to the reservoir. Penile prostheses should be offered to all patients who are unwilling or unable to consider, fail to respond to, or are unable to continue with pharmacological treatment or vacuum erection devices.

All patients and their partners should be fully counselled pre-operatively and shown the different types of implants and how to handle the pump. It often helps to speak to a patient advocate. Penile prostheses are particularly suitable for those patients with severe end-stage organic ED, especially if the cause is Peyronie's disease (severe curvature with erectile dysfunction or significant 'hour-glass' deformity) or those with post-priapism fibrosis.

Q. **What are the possible complications of penile prosthesis surgery?**
A. The long-term risks include infection (<4%), erosion (<5%) and mechanical failure (4%) which may need re-operation. A small number of patients may develop a glans droop which can be corrected at a later date by performing a glanspexy. The initial cost is high but manufacturers do offer a 10 year or lifetime guarantee for mechanical failure. The risks of surgery are higher in patients who are diabetic, have spinal cord injury or are on corticosteroids or immunosuppressives.

Q. **What are the long-term success rates?**
A. The long-term success and satisfaction rates are reported to be over 90% for both the patient and the partner. These high success rates are due to the improved mechanical reliability of the newer prostheses and careful pre-operative counselling and patient selection [1]. The advantages of penile prosthesis surgery include long-term efficacy with a high satisfaction rate, no need for pharmacotherapy and the improved ability to lead a normal sexual life.

INFERTILITY

Q. **You are referred a man who is 32 years old and presents with infertility. He has never fathered a child, but has been married for 5 years. His wife is 37 years old. They have been trying to start a family for 15 months. How do you define infertility?**
A. The inability of a sexually active couple to achieve a pregnancy within 12 months following regular unprotected sexual intercourse.

Q. **What is the baseline fertility rate?**
A. The chance of a normal couple conceiving is estimated to be 20%–25% per month, 75% by 6 months, and 90% by 1 year. The baseline pregnancy rate is 1%–3% per month (in non-azoospermic couples).

Q. **What proportion of infertility cases are due to female or male causes?**
A. Approximately 20% of cases of infertility are caused entirely by a male factor, with an additional 30% of cases due to both male and female factors. Therefore, a male factor is present in one-half of infertile couples. The remaining 50% are due to female factors only.

Q. **When would you begin investigations of this couple if at all?**
A. Of infertile couples without treatment, 25%–35% will conceive at some point by intercourse alone. In the past it was recommended not to investigate patients until 12 months of attempted conception. However, with the advancing age of infertile couples at presentation, a basic, simple, cost-effective evaluation of both the male and the female may be initiated at the time of presentation.

Q. **How would you assess this man with infertility?**
A. I would ensure that his wife is also investigated and this is often best done in a joint infertility clinic, with a female fertility specialist. First, I would establish whether the period of unprotected intercourse has been regular and long enough to meet the criteria for infertility

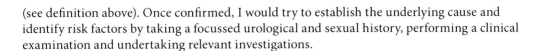

(see definition above). Once confirmed, I would try to establish the underlying cause and identify risk factors by taking a focussed urological and sexual history, performing a clinical examination and undertaking relevant investigations.

Q. What would you ask in the history?

A. In the history, I would ask about the duration of infertility, details of any previous pregnancies, contraceptive use in the past, the couple's frequency of sexual intercourse, as well as the timing of coitus. Both erectile and ejaculatory function should be assessed, and the use of any vaginal lubricants during intercourse should be noted as they may affect sperm quality.

The developmental history of the patient should be noted such as any history of cryptorchidism, age at puberty, and development of secondary sexual characteristics. The patient's past surgical history may be of particular importance such as previous history of orchidopexy, testicular torsion or inguino-scrotal surgery particularly hernia repairs and epididymal cyst excision.

The patient should be questioned for a history of urinary tract infections or sexually transmitted diseases as well as a history of mumps orchitis.

A history of previous chemotherapy, radiation therapy or gonadotoxic treatment should also be ascertained.

A history of chronic upper respiratory tract infections should be actively sought (may indicate cystic fibrosis).

Anabolic steroid abuse and recreational drugs such as marijuana are also risk factors.

Q. What would you be looking for in the physical examination of this man?

A. On examination, the patient's body habitus (obesity) as well as the pattern of virilization should be recorded. After this a focused urogenital examination is performed. The scrotal contents should be examined with the patient standing and lying down in a warm room to allow for relaxation of the cremasteric muscle. The testes should be carefully palpated to determine consistency and to exclude the presence of an intratesticular mass. The dimensions of the testes should be measured and documented. Palpation of the epididymis should determine the presence of the head, body and tail. The possibility of epididymal obstruction is suggested by the presence of a dilated epididymal head and body. Palpation of the vas deferens is performed to ensure its presence bilaterally. The scrotum should be examined with the patient standing up to check for the presence of a varicocele. (Use Valsalva if not obviously palpable.)

Q. What initial tests would you perform on this patient?

A. A semen analysis and hormone profile comprising serum FSH, LH and testosterone will diagnose the cause of infertility in the majority of men. All patients should have at least two semen analyses performed to confirm an abnormal result.

Q. How would you counsel this patient to perform a semen analysis?

A. An accurate semen analysis is an important investigation for the evaluation of the infertile male. To compare different semen samples from the same patient with accuracy, it is important to maintain consistency in the duration of sexual abstinence before collection of the specimen. It is recommended that the patient abstains from ejaculation for 2–5 days before providing the sample. The sample should be provided into a clean, wide-mouthed container at either the laboratory (ideal scenario) or at the patient's home but must be delivered to the laboratory within 1 hour. It is recommended that specimens produced at home should be brought to the lab by placing the container in a shirt pocket next to the body to keep it warm during transit.

I would inform the patient that the specimen should be produced by masturbation without the use of latex condoms as these may interfere with the viability of sperm due to the presence of spermicides. The specimen should be examined in the laboratory within 1 to 2 hours of collection. A label on the container should state the patient's name, the date, the time of collection and the abstinence period.

Q. Can the specimen be produced using coitus interruptus?

A. Although interrupted coitus may be used as an alternative method for obtaining specimens, this is not recommended because the initial portion of the ejaculate may be lost and bacteria and acidic vaginal secretions may contaminate the specimen which can result in inaccurate results.

Q. What are the normal characteristics of the semen analysis?

A. The World Health Organization (2010) defines the following reference values:

Volume:	>1.5 mL
pH:	>7.2
Sperm concentration:	$>15 \times 10^6$/mL
Total sperm number:	$>39 \times 10^6$ or more spermatozoa per ejaculate
Motility:	$>32\%$ with progressive motility
Morphology:	$>4\%$ of normal forms
Vitality:	$>58\%$
White blood cells:	<1 million/mL

Q. This particular patient in question has a semen analysis performed. His results are as follows on two occasions:

Volume:	**2.4 mL**
pH:	**7.5**
Sperm concentration:	**6×10^6 sperm/mL**
Total sperm number:	**14.4×10^6 spermatozoa**
Motility:	**20% with $>$ grade 2 and 11% with grade 4**
Morphology:	**2% of normal forms**
White blood cells:	**<1 million/mL**

His hormone profile is normal. What is this man's diagnosis?

A. Combined defects in sperm density, motility and morphology are known as oligoasthenoteratospermia or OAT syndrome.

Q. What are the potential causes of the OAT syndrome?

A. The OAT syndrome can be associated with a varicocele. Other causes include cryptorchidism, temporary insults to spermatogenesis such as heat, drugs or environmental toxins, or idiopathic causes. A heat effect may be either environmental or endogenous, such as a systemic illness resulting in fever.

Q. Physical examination in this patient's scrotum revealed a large left varicocele. What is a varicocele and how are these graded?

A. A varicocele is defined as an abnormal dilatation of the pampiniform plexus of spermatic veins, and is graded (Hudson classification) according to physical characteristics:

Grade III	Palpable and visible
Grade II	Palpable on standing only, but not visible
Grade I	Palpable on Valsalva manoeuvre, not visible
Grade 0	Subclinical (ultrasound scan diagnosis only)

Q. How common are varicoceles?

A. The prevalence is about 15% in the healthy general population. However in men presenting with infertility they are present in 20%–40%.

Q. Why do patients develop varicoceles?

A. Approximately 90% of varicoceles are on the left side. Differences in the venous drainage patterns of the right and left testicular veins may account for this left-sided predominance. The left testicular vein normally drains directly into the left renal vein, whereas the right testicular vein drains into the inferior vena cava. In addition, an absence of the venous valves is more commonly found on the left side than on the right. Finally, the left renal vein may be compressed between the superior mesenteric artery and the aorta. This 'nutcracker phenomenon' may result in impaired venous drainage in the left testicular venous system.

Q. Are varicoceles associated with infertility?

A. There does appear to be an association with impaired semen parameters. Semen samples from infertile men with varicoceles demonstrate decreased motility in 90% of patients and reduced sperm concentrations in 65% of patients.

Q. Why are varicoceles associated with infertility?

A. It is possible that the countercurrent exchange mechanism which normally maintains a lower intrascrotal temperature is impaired in the presence of a varicocele. Oligospermic patients with varicoceles have a higher intrascrotal temperature (0.6°C higher). Other causes may include reflux of renal and adrenal metabolites from the renal vein, decreased blood flow and hypoxia and impaired sperm DNA quality.

Q. When should varicoceles be treated in the context of fertility?

A. Adolescent patients with grade II/III varicoceles with a reduced ipsilateral testicular volume should undergo treatment. Sub-fertile males with impaired semen parameters can also be offered treatment as there is likely to be an improvement in the semen parameters. This may be enough to allow a natural pregnancy or improve the parameters prior to assisted reproduction which may either be intrauterine insemination (IUI), *in vitro* fertilisation (IVF) or intracytoplasmic sperm injection (ICSI).

Q. How would you manage the varicocele in this patient?

A. Improvement in semen parameters is demonstrated in approximately 70% of patients after a varicocele repair. Improvements in motility are most common, occurring in 70% of patients, with improved sperm densities in 51% and improved morphology in 44% of patients. Semen characteristics usually improve between 3 months to 1 year following surgery or embolisation.

There have been a number of studies reviewing the effects of a varicocele on fertility with conflicting results as the majority of the studies are uncontrolled with heterogenous patient and partner subgroups.

The widely quoted Evers meta-analysis suggested that varicocele treatment does not improve pregnancy rates [2]. However, this meta-analysis included patients with sub-clinical varicoceles and also patients with normal semen parameters. When these are excluded a further meta-analysis reported pregnancy rates of 36.4% versus 20% in the treated versus the untreated group. The recommendations of the Joint Committee of the American Urological

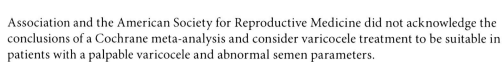

Association and the American Society for Reproductive Medicine did not acknowledge the conclusions of a Cochrane meta-analysis and consider varicocele treatment to be suitable in patients with a palpable varicocele and abnormal semen parameters.

National Institute for Health and Care Excellence (NICE) guidelines recommend that men should not be offered surgical treatment for a varicocele because it does not improve pregnancy rates.

Q. What would you recommend to this couple?

A. I would recommend that they be seen by a urologist and also a fertility specialist. They should be appropriately counselled on the relative success rates of all the available options which would include either a varicocele ligation or IUI/ICSI/IVF depending upon their personal circumstances.

Q. Which assisted reproduction techniques (ARTs) are you aware of?

A. ARTs involve the manipulation of sperm or ova or both in an attempt to improve the chance of conception and resultant live birth rates. These are as follows:

- Intrauterine insemination (IUI)
- *In vitro* fertilization (IVF)
- Intracytoplasmic sperm injection (ICSI)
- Intracytoplasmic morphologically selected sperm injection (IMSI)

Q. Which sperm retrieval techniques are you aware of?

A. Surgical techniques to retrieve sperm include the following:

- Percutaneous sperm aspiration (PESA)
- Microsurgical epididymal sperm aspiration (MESA)
- Testicular sperm aspiration (TESA)
- Testicular sperm extraction (TESE)
- Microdissection TESE (mTESE)

Q. What is a TESE?

A. This refers to the technique of testicular exploration and sperm extraction. The optimal technique of sperm extraction should be minimally invasive and avoid impairment of testicular function while maximising the chance of retrieving enough mature sperm to perform ICSI. Conventional TESE uses single or multiple open testicular biopsies to retrieve seminiferous tubules which are then dissected to retrieve mature sperm which can then be used for ART. MicroTESE utilises high magnification of the seminiferous tubules and more extensive dissection of the testicular tissue to retrieve sperm from the seminiferous tubules. A smaller amount of tissue is removed with targeting of the best seminiferous tubules which are generally of a better calibre and colour. The tubules are then examined within the theatre setting under a light microscope to confirm the presence of mature sperm following which the tissue can either be frozen for future ICSI or sperm harvested for a same-day ICSI cycle.

The conventional TESE technique requires multiple, blind testicular biopsies with excision of a larger volume (>500 mg) of testicular tissue. The microTESE technique of sequential excision of microdissected seminiferous tubules (10–15 mg, or 2 mm in length, of seminiferous tubule) has been shown to be more successful, compared with the results achieved by conventional TESE, or random biopsies of testicular tissue.

Q. What is IVF and how is it performed?

A. IVF refers to *in vitro* fertilisation. Gonadotropins are used to stimulate multiple oocytes during each cycle of treatment. Follicular development is then monitored ultrasonically, and the ova are harvested before ovulation with the use of ultrasound-guided needle aspiration.

IVF is performed by mixing processed sperm with retrieved oocytes. In standard IVF, when fertilization occurs, the developing embryos are incubated for 2–3 days in culture and then placed trans-cervically into the uterus. Using this technique, 20%–30% of transferred embryos will implant and produce clinical pregnancies. More than 90% of inseminated oocytes are routinely fertilized when sperm function is normal. However, fertilization rates are reduced significantly when a male factor for infertility is present.

Q. **What is the ICSI and when is it used?**

A. ICSI refers to intracytoplasmic sperm injection whereby a single sperm is injected into the ovum. This allows for fertilization with extremely low numbers of sperm or sperm retrieved from testicular tissue. ICSI is indicated in cases of severe male factor infertility, in couples with prior failed or poor fertilization during regular IVF cycles, or in cases in which the sperm demonstrate significant fertilizing ability defects. In 2006, ICSI represented 47% of all IVF treatments in the United Kingdom.

Q. **What are the success rates of ICSI?**

A. The clinical pregnancy rates using ICSI average 20%–37% per initiated cycle. Pregnancy rates are affected by the age of the female when undergoing IVF or ICSI. The reported pregnancy rates are 36.9% in women <35 years and 10.7% in women >40 years. In the United Kingdom the HFEA reports a mean take-home baby rate of 23.1% with a rate of 31% for women under the age of 35.

Q. **Is there a difference in congenital malformation rates between IVF and ICSI?**

A. Children born as a result of ICSI (6.2%), compared to IVF (4.1%), may have an increased risk of malformations. Only the difference in the rates between ICSI children and the control group was statistically significant. Furthermore, a recent meta-analysis has suggested a small significant increase in malformations in children born following ARTs versus controls. More recently a malformation rate of 6.2% has been shown with ART versus 4.4% in normal pregnancies.

Q. **Are there any specific concerns when treating patients with severe male factor infertility with ART?**

A. Patients who are considered candidates for the ARTs with either severe oligospermia or azoospermia may have associated chromosomal defects which can be abnormal karyotypes (47XXY), Y microdeletions or carriers of the cystic fibrosis gene. As there is a risk for the offspring patients should undergo these tests and appropriate genetic counselling before treatment.

Q. **Another patient is referred to see you. He is aged 26 and has recently married. This is his first sexual relationship. He has already been to a private laboratory and performed two semen analyses 3 months apart. The results of the latest one are below and are the same as the first one:**

Volume:	2.7 mL
pH:	7.4
Sperm concentration:	None seen
Total sperm number:	Nil
Motility:	Not assessed
Morphology:	Not assessed
White blood cells:	<1 million/mL

Which other tests would you perform?

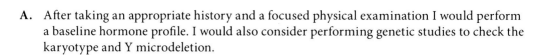

A. After taking an appropriate history and a focused physical examination I would perform a baseline hormone profile. I would also consider performing genetic studies to check the karyotype and Y microdeletion.

Q. His testosterone is 7 and both his FSH and LH are significantly elevated, the FSH is more than three times normal. What is his differential diagnosis?

A. This man is likely to have non-obstructive azoospermia indicating abnormal spermatogenesis. This may be secondary to hypogonadotrophic hypogonadism (Kallmann's syndrome, pituitary tumour) or abnormalities of spermatogenesis (chromosomal abnormalities, toxins, orchitis, previous torsion).

Q. What are you specifically looking for on examination?

A. I am looking specifically for secondary sexual characteristics, body habitus, the presence of gynaecomastia, the size and consistency of the testis and whether the vas are palpable.

Q. This patient has bilateral small soft testes. This is the biopsy from his testis (Figure 13.6). What does it show? What is a possible diagnosis if this was a chromosomal disorder?

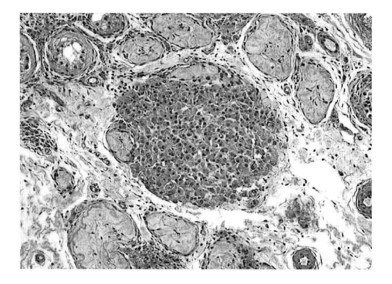

Figure 13.6

A. The testicular biopsy presented in Figure 13.6 shows small hyalinised seminiferous tubules and pseudo-adenomatous clusters of Leydig cells. The likely diagnosis here is Klinefelter's syndrome where patients present with non-obstructive azoospermia, a high FSH with a low testosterone and small volume soft testicles. Although phenotypically they are normal looking males, genetic tests confirm that the karyotype is 47XXY.

Q. Assuming that the genetic testing shows a normal karyotype but the genetic tests report that a Y microdeletion has been detected, can you explain the significance of a Y microdeletion in the context of male infertility?

A. Patients with these microdeletions are usually phenotypically normal, with the only apparent abnormality being a defect in spermatogenesis. The defect occurs in one of three non-overlapping regions of the long arm of the Y chromosome referred to as AZFa (proximal), AZFb (middle) and AZFc (distal). Although there is no strict correlation between these microdeletions and the testis biopsy histology, the following are associated:

- Microdeletion AZFa – Sertoli only
- Microdeletion AZFb – Maturation arrest
- Microdeletion AZFc – Severe oligzoospemia (no histological pattern)

Men with an AZFa or AZFb microdeletion will not have sperm within the testicle and a sperm retrieval is not indicated. However there is a small probability (10%–15%) of finding sperm in the presence of an AZFc microdeletion.

Q. Why is it important to test patients for microdeletions?

A. It is important because these gene deletions will be transmitted to male offspring. Couples in whom the husband has Y chromosome microdeletions should be offered genetic counselling before embarking on ART.

Q. Another 26-year-old man with azoospermia has a normal hormone profile (LH, FSH, testosterone) and a normal testicular volume when examined on his first visit. What do you suspect is the underlying diagnosis?

A. He is likely to have an obstructive cause for his azoospermia, however maturation arrest cannot be excluded without a testicular biopsy.

Q. What would have been an important finding in his clinical examination?

A. It is important to establish the presence of the vas deferens. If there are no palpable vasa bilaterally, the patient may have congenital bilateral absence of vas deferens (CBAVD). CBAVD is a clinical diagnosis and is due to an abnormality in the *CFTR* gene. This may occur in the absence of any respiratory symptoms.

A dilated vas or epididymis is usually indicative of obstruction which can be at the level of the ejaculatory ducts, vas or epididymis.

Q. What is the level of spermatogenesis in patients with obstructive azoospermia and how would you manage them?

A. Most of these patients have normal spermatogenesis within the testicles. A scrotal exploration is reserved for cases where a reconstruction is planned to bypass the obstruction at which time sperm retrieval can ensure that tissue is cryopreserved for future ART. Patients with ejaculatory duct obstruction (EDO) can be offered endoscopic resection, transurethral resection of ejaculatory ducts (TURED).

Q. What is the role of testicular biopsy in azoospermic patients?

A. Isolated diagnostic testicular biopsies are now seldom performed in azoospermic patients as most will be undergoing sperm retrieval for ICSI at which point a biopsy can be performed if no sperm is found. Testicular biopsy is not indicated in patients with oligospermia, because the results will not change the treatment options unless it is required to exclude the presence of ITGCN.

Q. The patient has a testicular biopsy performed at the time of sperm retrieval. How is it evaluated?

A. The most common system used to classify spermatogenesis on a testicular biopsy is the Johnsen score (Table 13.3).

Table 13.3 Johnsen score count

Score	Description
10	Complete spermatogenesis – organised epithelium
9	Many spermatozoa – disorganised epithelium
8	<10 spermatozoa
7	No spermatozoa, but many spermatids
6	No spermatozoa, but <10 spermatids
5	No spermatozoa, spermatids, but many spermatocytes
4	<10 spermatocytes
3	Spermatogonia
2	Sertoli cells only
1	No cells, tubular fibrosis

Q. Figure 13.7 is a slide showing a testicular biopsy. What does it show?

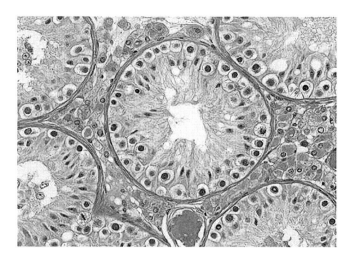

Figure 13.7

A. Figure 13.7 shows maturation arrest.

Q. If the biopsy showed normal spermatogenesis, what would you do next?

A. If reconstruction is contemplated I would perform a vasogram to determine the site of obstruction in azoospermic patients who have active spermatogenesis documented by testis biopsy. Vasography should be ideally performed in conjunction with reconstructive surgery because this procedure carries an inherent risk of vasal injury that could complicate future reconstructive surgery, if performed separately.

Vasography is performed at the level of the straight portion of the scrotal vas deferens by needle puncture with an orange needle on a 2.5 mL syringe containing injection of nonionic contrast agent.

Q. What is a normal vasogram?

A. A normal vasogram is documented when contrast agent is visualized throughout the length of the vas deferens, seminal vesicles, ejaculatory duct and bladder. Proximal patency of the epididymis is documented by microscopic (×400) visualization of sperm in the intravasal fluid.

VASECTOMY AND REVERSAL

Q. You are referred a 29-year-old man by his GP for consideration of a vasectomy. How will you assess him?

A. I will see him in my routine urology outpatients clinic. Before I see him I would send him a patient information sheet about vasectomy. I would recommend that he attends the clinic with his partner.

The important points in the history relate to his age, marital status, number of previous children and the age of the youngest child, previous contraceptive history and previous surgery in the inguino-scrotal region. Also document whether both he and his partner have considered other contraceptive measures.

Q. What are you looking for specifically on examination?

A. As well as a general examination, the specific important points on examination will relate to the laxity of the scrotum, whether the vasa are easily palpable and whether there is any other scrotal pathology present (varicocele, tumour). This also helps to decide on whether to perform the procedure under a local or general anaesthetic.

Q. How would you counsel him for a vasectomy?

A. I would provide written information on the procedure and invite the partner to be involved in the decision-making process. I will explain why the procedure is being performed, what the alternatives are, what the success rate is and what complications may occur. Specifically I would warn the patient that the procedure is irreversible. Importantly, they must continue some form of contraception until the patient produces an azoospermic semen sample (see later discussion). I would explain that failure may occur early (1 in 300 due to surgical error) or late (1 in 2000 due to recanalisation). I would counsel the patient that no one technique ensures 100% success and the early side effects include bruising and swelling (common), haematoma (2%) and infection (3%–4%). Long-term effects include chronic testicular or epididymal pain (1%–10%) and sperm granuloma (10%–15%). Approximately 60%–80% of patients have detectable levels of serum antisperm antibodies.

Q. You find out that he is not married, has no partner and has no children. What will you do?

A. He fits one of the criteria where patients often change their mind or are dissatisfied. These patients require careful counselling and an operation should only be performed after a full discussion with their GP and an undertaking that the patient does not want children in the future. Other groups which require careful attention are young couples, couples with two or less children, patients from lower socio-economic classes and where there is the possibility that the operation is being requested for financial or emotional reasons or that the male may be ambivalent about it. I would also ensure that there is an adequate 'cooling off' period before proceeding with the surgery.

Q. He is adamant that he wants a vasectomy. What is your recommendation?

A. I would make sure that the case is fully discussed with the patient's GP. I would provide a written patient information sheet and a copy of the written consent. I would ask for a period of time between the consent and the operation so that there is sufficient time for the patient to make a fully informed choice. If after all this he is still convinced that this is what he wants and he is supported by his GP then he would be eligible for a vasectomy.

Q. What techniques are you aware of?

A. Single scrotal incision, bilateral scrotal incisions or no-scalpel technique.

Q. What methods of vasal occlusion are you aware of and do they have different success rates?

A. Suture ligation is still the most common method employed worldwide but may result in necrosis and sloughing of the cut end. If both ends slough, recanalization may occur. Vasectomy failure occurs in 1%–5% when ligatures alone are used for occlusion. Recent evidence suggests the use of Vicryl is associated with a higher rate of failure as compared to catgut.

Vasal occlusion using two medium haemoclips on each end results in failure rates of less than 1%.

Intraluminal occlusion with needle electrocautery, or battery-driven thermal cautery set at a power sufficient to destroy mucosa but not high enough to cause transmural destruction of the vas, reduces recanalization rates to less than 0.5%. Using this technique it is recommended that at least 1 cm of the lumen should be cauterized in each direction.

Q. How do you perform a vasectomy under local anaesthesia?

A. Following informed consent and with the patient supine I would perform a vasectomy using a mixture of 1% plain Lidocaine and 0.5% Bupivacaine in a 1:1 ratio. I would perform the procedure in a warm room and with warm preparation solution to relax the scrotum. I prefer bilateral small scrotal incisions. Each vas is isolated from the spermatic cord vessels and manipulated to a superficial position under the scrotal skin. The vas is then firmly trapped between the middle finger, the index finger and the thumb of the left hand (the middle finger can be behind the vas with the thumb and index finger in front thus providing a 'three finger fixation'). The local anaesthetic is injected into the skin (in some patients a cord block at the start of the procedure can be performed) and then advanced into the peri-vasal sheath. Small bilateral transverse incisions through the dartos are performed until the vas sheath is seen and pulled though the incision. A longitudinal incision through the sheath is performed and the bare vas isolated using a vasectomy ring forcep. The vasal artery, veins and accompanying nerves are dissected free of the vas and spared. A 1 cm segment is removed between two haemostats from the straight part of the vas and sent for pathological confirmation. The ends are occluded by using intra-luminal cautery and the ends sutured in different fascial planes (fascial interposition). I then close the skin with interrupted 4-0 Vicryl Rapide. Simple gauze dressings are held in place using a scrotal support.

Q. Please explain why you use this technique?

A. I use a bilateral incision technique as this reduces the chance of dividing the same vas twice and it is also easier to divide the vas on the straight segment with bilateral incisions. I use intra-luminal cautery and fascial interposition to reduce the incidence of vasectomy failure by re-canalisation.

Q. When will you ask him to perform a semen analysis and why?

A. The 2016 Joint Association of Biomedical Andrologists (ABA), British Andrological Society (BAS) and British Association of Urological Surgeons recommend that patients should be instructed to ensure that they have had at least 20 ejaculations and preferably wait at least 12 weeks before submitting a semen sample for examination. This reduces the number of false-positive samples and thus minimises both patient inconvenience and repeat laboratory assessment [3]. A single azoospermic sample in an accredited laboratory is now acceptable.

Q. What is special clearance?

A. A successful vasectomy is based on the production of an azoospermic sample. However, persistent non-motile spermatozoa in the initial ejaculates is not uncommon, with studies reporting up to 33% non-azoospermic samples at 3 months, and 10% of ejaculates containing non-motile sperm at 6 months.

Special clearance is based on the finding of two consecutive sperm counts <100,000/mL with no motile sperm with a minimum of 7 months after vasectomy. Discussion in the literature has suggested that the risk of pregnancy occurring from these non-motile sperm is small, and probably no more than the risk of pregnancy after two azoospermic semen samples, as a result of spontaneous recanalization.

These men with low numbers of persistent non-motile spermatozoa in their ejaculates (that is, after 7 months) may be given 'special clearance' by their clinician to discontinue other contraceptive precautions following appropriate oral counselling and written advice regarding the risk of pregnancy.

Using these criteria only 1 of 50 men examined at least 3 years after vasectomy had sperm in their analysis, the others being azoospermic. Furthermore no pregnancies occurred within the 3 years of follow-up.

Q. He returns 3 years later and is furious as his wife is now pregnant. What do you think has happened and how common is this?

A. It is likely that he has had a late failure of vasectomy which is caused by re-canalisation. It is defined as the re-appearance of sperm after a documented semen analysis showing azoospermia. The quoted incidence is around 1 in 2000.

He needs to give a further semen analysis to make sure that this is the correct diagnosis. If late failure has occurred he should be offered a scrotal exploration, identification of the vasa and further occlusion bilaterally under a general anaesthetic. The patient should use alternate forms of contraception until he has had a further exploration and documented azoospermia.

If the repeat sample shows azoospermia then they should be referred for a paternity test. However, there have been documented pregnancies despite the test showing azoospermia where the patient is the biological father.

Q. A 55-year-old man is referred by his GP with secondary infertility. He had a vasectomy performed 22 years ago. He now wants a reversal. How will you assess him?

A. In the initial consultation, I would want to assess both the male and female partner with respect to their previous health and reproductive histories. I would examine the patient and assess the size and consistency of the testis and epididymis as well as whether the vasa and gap between the two cut ends are easily palpable. I would ask the patient to perform a semen analysis if it has not already been performed. I would explain to the patient that the chances of success (patency or pregnancy) are based on the surgical expertise of the surgeon, the method used to perform the original vasectomy, the patient's health history, and the age and reproductive potential of his partner.

Q. Is it common for patients to ask for a reversal?

A. Approximately 6% of men who have undergone a vasectomy will subsequently request a reversal. The reason most frequently given by men requesting a vasectomy reversal is divorce and remarriage with a desire to have children with their new spouse.

Q. What techniques can be used for the vasectomy reversal?

A. Techniques vary according to the type of magnification used. This can be micro-surgical using an operating microscope, magnified vision using loupes or some will just use a macroscopic technique.

The anastomosis can be one of the following:

- *Multilayer vasovasostomy* – Using inner mucosal sutures as well as sutures through the muscularis layer
- *Modified single-layer vasovasostomy* – Easier technique; may be equivalent in outcome

- *Inguinal vasovasostomy* – If obstruction of the vas is within the inguinal canal, i.e. after hernia repair
- *Epididymo-vasostomy* – Is required in 20%–30%

Q. What are the important surgical principles required for a successful reversal?

A. There should be sufficient mobilization of both ends of the vas deferens to prevent any tension on the anastomosis.

The perivasal adventitia must remain intact as stripping of the adventitia surrounding the cut ends of the vas risks excising an important blood supply to the vas and may lead to ischemia and ultimately stenosis of the anastomosis.

Precise approximation of the cut lumens is mandatory to avoid sperm leakage with formation of a sperm granuloma that may disrupt the lumen and result in a failed procedure. Patients can be offered a sperm retrieval at the same time so that if the reversal is unsuccessful, then the patients have sperm stored for ICSI use.

Q. How would you perform the procedure?

A. I prefer a microsurgical technique under a general anaesthetic. With the patient supine, the cut ends of the vas deferens are brought through two bilateral scrotal incisions or a midline raphe incision. The vas is mobilised both proximally and distally allowing sufficient length for the freshly cut ends of the vas to slightly overlap one another once they are positioned for the anastomosis. The opposite side is then isolated in a similar fashion. When both vasa have been dissected free, the vasa are held in a vasectomy reversal clamp above skin level.

The vas above and below the vasectomy site is then transected until a patent lumen is seen both proximally and distally.

A few drops of fluid from the testicular end of the vas lumen are placed on a sterile glass slide and examined using a light microscope. If there are sperm or sperm parts (sperm heads, sperm with partial tails) with clear copious fluid then a vasovasostomy can be performed.

The cut ends of the vas deferens are positioned next to one another. A modified double-layer technique is used with four to six interrupted 9-0/10-0 sutures passed through the lumen and mucosal layer followed by six interrupted 9-0 sutures through the muscularis and the adventitial layers. The technique is then repeated on the other side.

Q. Can all patients be treated with a vasovasostomy?

A. Unfortunately some patients will require a vasoepididymostomy rather than a vasovasostomy because of a secondary obstruction at the level of the epididymis. This appears to be a time-related phenomenon; the longer the time interval is from the original vasectomy, the greater the chances of an epididymal obstruction. More recently a model to pre-operatively identify patients who may require vasoepididymostomy was created which is based on time since vasectomy and patient age. The predictive model provides 84% sensitivity for detecting patients who may require vasoepididymostomy during vasectomy reversal (58% specificity). This model more accurately predicts the need for vasoepididymostomy than using a specific duration from vasectomy cut-off alone.

Q. How will you decide which patients need a vasoepididymostomy?

A. The decision to perform a vasoepididymostomy is based on the quality of fluid found in the proximal vas deferens at the time of surgery. Fluid obtained from the proximal vas lumen should be examined under 400× magnification using a light microscope. I would consider performing a vasoepididymostomy:

1. When the material coming from the proximal vas lumen is thick and devoid of sperm
2. If the fluid is creamy, containing only debris
3. If there is no fluid whatsoever when the vas is milked toward the cut end

4. If irrigation of the proximal vas with 0.1 to 0.2 mL of saline with a plastic angiocatheter attached to a tuberculin syringe fails to wash out any sperm.

Q. What are the success rates of the reversal?

A. If a vasovasostomy is performed then the success rates (patency rate and pregnancy rate) varies depending on the interval from the vasectomy until its reversal (Table 13.4). This is based upon a large series of 1469 men who underwent microsurgical vasectomy reversal procedures who were studied at five institutions [4].

Table 13.4 Patency and pregnancy rates according to interval from the vasectomy until its reversal

Interval from the vasectomy until its reversal (years)	Patency rate	Pregnancy rate
<3	97%	76%
3–8	88%	53%
9–14	79%	44%
≥15	71%	30%

Q. Are there any other factors which are important with respect to success?

A. More recently, pre-operative factors have been associated with a successful outcome including the same female partner as well as a short obstructive interval. Intraoperative factors included the use of surgical clips rather than suture at vasectomy, the presence of sperm granuloma and the presence and quality of the vasal fluid.

Q. Does the age of the female partner matter?

A. In a recent study using the microsurgical vasovasostomy technique it was reported that the pregnancy rate for couples with a female partner aged 40 or older was significantly lower than for those with the female partner aged 39 or younger (14% versus 56%). The age of the female partner is therefore important in the counselling process and it may not be cost-effective to perform vasectomy reversals in couples with a female partner older than age 40.

Q. Does it matter which technique you use?

A. There is controversy as to whether the outcomes using microsurgery, loupes or macroscopic techniques are equally effective or not. However, most experts believe that the results of microsurgical vasectomy reversal are superior to results of non-microsurgical techniques in terms of patency and pregnancy. However, microsurgery requires more training and experience to obtain the best results. Patency and pregnancy rates do not appear to be significantly different if a multilayer anastomosis is performed as opposed to a modified single-layer technique but the success is physician dependent.

Q. The patient returns 1 year after the reversal. He is upset that despite the post-operative tests showing sperm in the semen, his new partner has not been able to conceive. Does he have any other options?

A. It is important to establish whether he does indeed have sperm in his semen or not and what the fertility potential of his partner is. His other option if he still wishes to have his own biologically related children is to either use his sperm (if there is enough in the semen) or have a surgical sperm retrieval in conjunction with ICSI. He also still has the option of donor sperm and adoption.

Q. The couple now decide that they would like to be referred for IVF on the National Health Service (NHS). They ask whether they have to pay for IVF treatment.

A. Some NHS-operated fertility clinics offer free *in vitro* (IVF) fertilisation treatment to people who have been sponsored by their primary care trust (PCT). They need to contact their local PCT to find out how to qualify for sponsorship.

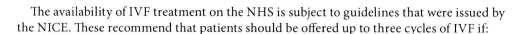

The availability of IVF treatment on the NHS is subject to guidelines that were issued by the NICE. These recommend that patients should be offered up to three cycles of IVF if:

- They are between 23 and 39 years of age at the time of treatment.
- One, or both, of them has been diagnosed with a fertility problem.
- They have been infertile for at least 3 years.

Some PCTs also have additional criteria that may affect their eligibility for funding. For example, some PCTs will not provide funding for couples where one partner already has a child.

EJACULATORY DYSFUNCTION

Q. **A 36-year-old man is referred as an urgent 2-week wait referral with a 3-month history of haematospermia. He is otherwise fit and well. He is now abstaining from sexual contact as his partner is suspicious that he may have a sexually transmitted infection. Does he need urological evaluation?**

A. Haematospermia is commonly seen after a prolonged period of sexual abstinence. It almost always resolves spontaneously. However, if it persists beyond several weeks patients should undergo further urologic evaluation as it can occasionally be a result of an underlying significant urological pathology.

Q. **How would you investigate the patient?**

A. A careful history should be taken to exclude the presence of haematuria, a past history of tuberculosis (TB) and a family history of prostate cancer. Other important features in the history include recent trauma, infection and a history of bleeding disorders. A careful examination should also include a blood pressure measurement, genital and rectal examination to exclude the presence of tuberculosis and a prostate-specific antigen (PSA) and a rectal examination performed in men >50 years to exclude an underlying prostate carcinoma. The penis needs to be examined to exclude any lesions that may bleed and contribute to the ejaculate and a thorough palpation along the course of the vas is required to ensure their presence and assess for dilatation (signifies distal obstruction). Furthermore, a midstream specimen of urine (MSU) and urinary cytology are sent to exclude the possibility of transitional cell carcinoma at the level of the verumontanum or prostatic urethra and the presence of sterile pyuria. In younger men, urethritis should be considered in the differential diagnosis and urethral swabs should be obtained.

Q. **Are there any features in the history which would suggest that the patient may require further evaluation?**

A. The three factors that dictate the extent of the evaluation and treatment are patients' age, the duration and recurrence of the haematospermia, and the presence of any associated haematuria.

Q. **What are the common urological causes of haematospermia?**

A. The common urological causes include:
- Infections and inflammatory disorders (up to 40% of cases)
  - Infectious causes include TB, HIV and cytomegalovirus (CMV).
  - Patients with symptoms of a sexually transmitted infection are commonly found to have titres positive for herpes simplex, *Chlamydia*, *Enterococcus* or *Ureaplasma* allowing appropriate treatment to be initiated.
- Prostatitis (up to 30% of cases)
- Post-transrectal ultrasound (TRUS) biopsy of the prostate (9%–45%)

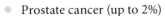

- Prostate cancer (up to 2%)
- Urethritis/urethral stricture in younger men
- Acquired and congenital cysts of the seminal vesicles or prostate
- Systemic disorders (hypertension, chronic liver disease, amyloidosis, lymphoma and bleeding disorders)

Q. **All his investigations are negative. He continues to have haematospermia. How would you investigate him further?**

A. I would request a TRUS. TRUS may reveal the presence of abnormalities in up to 95% of patients. Commonly seen abnormalities include prostatic calcifications (42%), ejaculatory duct calculi (39%), dilated ejaculatory ducts (33%), benign prostatic hyperplasia (33%), dilated seminal vesicles (22%), calcifications in seminal vesicles (20%), ejaculatory duct cysts (11%) and Müllerian duct remnants (7%).

Q. **Are any further investigations warranted?**

A. If there is persisting haematospermia in a patient over the age of 40 especially if associated with haematuria, a cysto-urethroscopy is required.

Q. **TRUS and cystoscopy do not reveal any abnormalities. The haematospermia continues. What is your management plan?**

A. The most important goal in the management of these patients is reassurance if they have been fully investigated and no cause can be identified. In younger patients it is important to exclude infective causes and a referral to a genitourinary clinic is useful.

Q. **A 37-year-old male attended the clinic along with his 34-year-old wife. They have been trying to conceive for 3 years without success. He has already performed two semen analyses which show the following:**

Volume: 0.4 mL
pH: 8.3
Sperm concentration: $<1 \times 10^6$/mL
Motility: Non-motile

How would you investigate him further?

A. Standard workup including focused history and examination. I would request baseline blood tests including hormone profile.

Q. **In the history he says that he has a normal orgasm but complains that when he passes urine the first time after he ejaculates the urine is cloudy. What do you think is the underlying diagnosis?**

A. I suspect he is suffering from retrograde ejaculation.

Q. **How would you confirm this?**

A. A post-orgasm urine examination should be performed to look for the presence of sperm in the urine on light microscopy.

Q. **What are the known causes?**

A. The most common cause is retroperitoneal lymph node dissection, followed by diabetes mellitus, bladder neck surgery, trauma, medications such as α-blockers, urethral strictures, spinal cord injury and post-TURP.

Q. **What treatment options does he have?**

A. Medical treatments can be used to try to close the bladder neck and prevent retrograde ejaculation. Sympathomimetics, such as pseudoephedrine and ephedrine, can help close the bladder neck and enhance antegrade ejaculation. Imipramine, a tricyclic antidepressant that has mixed anticholinergic and sympathomimetic properties may also be used. At best medical treatments are successful in 50%–60% of patients.

Q. What other options are there?
A. If medical therapy fails, sperm can be retrieved from an alkalinized post-ejaculate urine specimen and used for intrauterine insemination or IVF.

Q. How would you organise for the patient to provide an alkalinised post-ejaculate urine specimen?
A. The normally acidic urine is considered to be spermicidal. Patients are instructed to alkalinise their urine by the ingestion of 1 g of sodium bicarbonate the night before and a further 1 g on the morning of the collection. They are then asked to empty their bladders before masturbation. They are then instructed to obtain the post-ejaculatory urine as quickly as possible after orgasm and deliver the sample immediately to the laboratory. More recently a solution of sodium bicarbonate and sodium chloride (the Liverpool solution) has been shown to be safe to be used in units treating couples with retrograde ejaculation (RE). It is a noninvasive and inexpensive regimen that may optimize urine pH and osmolarity for sperm survival after RE.

Q. Can alkalinized urine be used in combination IVF?
A. Yes, ICSI can be performed with spermatozoa retrieved from post-ejaculatory urine. Using this technique, the fertilization rate has been reported to be as high as 51% with 7 of 16 couples achieving clinical pregnancies and three live offspring delivered.

Q. A 42-year-old male is referred by his GP with erectile dysfunction. However, when you see him in the clinic you find that his main complaint is that he ejaculates within a minute of sexual intercourse. He is very embarrassed about the problem and he has just broken up with his girlfriend. He has never had this problem before. What is his diagnosis?
A. He is suffering from premature ejaculation.

Q. What is the definition of *premature ejaculation*?
A. There is no absolute definition. However, most physicians use the American Psychiatric Association's *Diagnostic and Statistical Manual of Mental Disorders* (*DSM-IV-R*). They define it as 'persistent or recurrent ejaculation with minimal stimulation before, on, or shortly after penetration and before the person wishes it'.

Q. He asks you how long he should be able to last before ejaculation?
A. The ejaculatory latency has been measured by the intravaginal ejaculatory latency time (IVELT), which is defined as the time between vaginal intromission and ejaculation. The International Society for Sexual Medicine (ISSM) defines it as a male sexual dysfunction characterized by ejaculation which always or nearly always occurs before or within about 1 minute of vaginal penetration.

Q. He is concerned that there is something anatomically wrong with him.
A. Premature ejaculation is classified as being either lifelong or acquired. Usually lifelong PE is very unlikely to have biological or anatomical cause. His history suggests the need to address relationship issues and it is unlikely to be secondary to a biologic cause.

Q. What are the key points in the history?
A. The essential components in the history for a diagnosis of PE include a short ejaculatory latency time, a lack of control and sexual dissatisfaction.

Q. How will you investigate him?

A. I would take a detailed medical and sexual history, perform a physical examination and order appropriate investigations. The key to the investigations is to establish the true presenting complaint (differentiate between early penile detumescence), identify obvious biologic causes such as medication or recent pelvic surgery so that an optimal treatment plan can be instituted.

Q. What is premature ejaculation caused by?

A. A number of theories have been proposed regarding the causes of PE.
They are divided into psychogenic and biologic causes:

- *Psychogenic* – Anxiety, early sexual experience, infrequent sexual intercourse, poor ejaculatory control techniques, evolutional
- *Biogenic* – Penile hypersensitivity, hyperexcitable ejaculatory reflex, hyperarousability, endocrinopathy, genetic predisposition, 5-HT-receptor dysfunction

Q. What can be done to help this young man?

A. He can be treated with either behavioural therapy or pharmacological therapy or a combination of the two.

- Psychological/behavioural methods:
  - *Advantage* – Neither harmful nor painful, with few side effects and encourages open communication.
  - *Disadvantage* – Is time consuming and may be expensive. It requires the partner's co-operation and produces mixed results.
- Two main techniques:
  - Stop-squeeze method
  - Stop-pause method
  Both suppress the urge to ejaculate by stopping sexual stimulation.
- Pharmacological treatments:
  - *Selective serotonin reuptake inhibitors (SSRIs)* – Citalopram, fluoxetine, fluvoxamine, paroxetine and sertraline and dapoxetine.
    Daily treatment can be undertaken with paroxetine (20–40 mg), clomipramine (10–50 mg), sertraline (50–100 mg) and fluoxetine (20–40 mg). On-demand treatment using dapoxetine (30–60 mg) 2 hours before intercourse. A meta-analysis of drug treatment studies has demonstrated that paroxetine exerts the strongest ejaculation delay. Ejaculation delay with daily treatment usually manifests itself at the end of the first or second week. This is the only NICE-approved treatment for premature ejaculation. With the exception of fluoxetine, SSRIs should not be withdrawn acutely, but gradually within 3 to 4 weeks. It has been reported that clomipramine (25 mg) taken about 5 hours before intercourse can delay ejaculation in men with lifelong PE when given in an on-demand basis.
  - *Topical local anaesthetics* – The use of topical local anaesthetics such as lidocaine and/or prilocaine as a cream, gel or spray is well established. However, a side effect is significant penile hypoanesthesia and possible transvaginal absorption and vaginal numbness.
    More recently, it has been reported that the application of SS cream results in a significant improvement in up to 89% of patients. SS cream is a natural compound made with extracts from nine herbs, some of which have a local anaesthetic property.
  - *PDE-5 inhibitors* – Several authors have reported their experience with sildenafil (Viagra) as a treatment for PE. However, its major role appears to be in the treatment of acquired PE secondary to ED rather than lifelong or acquired PE without ED.

It may however be used successfully as an adjunct to other therapies in the treatment of premature ejaculation.

ANEJACULATION

Q. **A 22-year-old male attends clinic with a 1-year history of worsening inability to ejaculate. He is otherwise well other than having had a road traffic accident 3 years ago. How would you investigate him?**

A. After taking a full history and examining him I would like to know how severe his spinal injuries are and whether he has a spinal level injury. In particular I would like to ask him specifically about his bowel and bladder function.

Q. **What do you think is wrong with him?**

A. I suspect that he has anejaculation. I would confirm this with a semen analysis which would show complete absence of antegrade ejaculation and the absence of fructose and sperm in a post-orgasmic urine analysis.

Q. **What are the most common causes of this problem?**

A. The most common causes are spinal cord injury, followed by retroperitoneal lymph node dissection. Some patients have psychological causes for their problem and this should be suspected in patients who are suddenly unable to ejaculate, those who can still masturbate to completion and if no other causes of ejaculatory dysfunction can be identified.

Q. **What is this instrument? And what is it used for?**

A. Figure 13.8 shows a Seager electro-ejaculator. It may be used to perform electro-ejaculation on spinal cord injured patients.

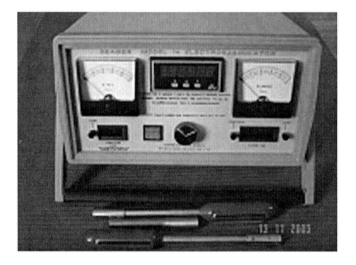

Figure 13.8

Q. **How is electro-ejaculation performed? What precautions should be taken?**

A. Electro-ejaculation involves the use of a rectal probe to stimulate the perirectal, periprostatic sympathetic nerves electrically. Patients without a spinal cord injury or those with low or incomplete spinal cord lesions require general anesthesia. During electro-ejaculation, spinal cord–injured patients with lesions above T6 or a history of autonomic dysreflexia should have blood pressure monitored frequently for signs of autonomic dysreflexia and severe hypertension.

Q. **When electro-ejaculation is performed, what is the quality of the sperm retrieved?**

A. Sperm obtained from electro-ejaculation has been shown to be of a poorer quality with poor motility and impaired fertilizing capacity. As a result, low pregnancy rates have been reported in patients undergoing electro-ejaculation and subsequent intrauterine insemination.

Q. **Are there any other available options for patients who do not wish to have electro-ejaculation?**

A. In infertile men with anejaculation, sperm retrieval can be performing using a PESA technique. The sperm can then be used for either intrauterine insemination (pregnancy rate of 73.1%) or IVF (pregnancy rate of 71.4%).

PEYRONIE'S DISEASE

Q. **A 43-year-old man is referred by his GP with a 2-month history of penile pain, penile deviation and a subcutaneous lump on the dorsum of the penis. How will you assess him?**

A. I would take a detailed subjective history, including the duration of symptoms, the presence or absence of pain, degree of erectile function, amount of curvature (degree and direction), ability to penetrate and any previous treatment modalities. I would use a validated questionnaire such as the IIEF, to assess erectile function. I would ask specifically about any risk factors for ED, such as diabetes, hypertension and hyperlipidaemia and for a past history of penile trauma.

In the physical examination, I would note the size and location of the plaque/mass, the presence or absence of a foreskin and whether there were any signs of previous trauma. I would specifically measure the penile length in both the stretched and flaccid state. Unless the patient has brought in a good-quality digital photograph showing the degree and direction of the curvature, I would perform an artificial erection using an intracavernosal injection of PGE-1. I would then perform an examination of the extremities to identify any co-existing Dupuytren's contracture.

Q. **What is the diagnosis in Figure 13.9?**

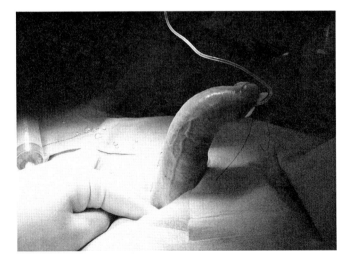

Figure 13.9

A. Figure 13.9 shows an image of a penile curvature due to Peyronie's disease.

Q. What are the cardinal features of this disease?

A. It is characterized by the development of a fibrous plaque or scar tissue within the tunica albuginea of the penis. It can present with one or a combination of symptoms, such as penile curvature, indentation, buckling, penile pain and penile shortening. It can also result in erectile dysfunction (ED) due to the altered hemodynamics of cavernosal blood flow.

Q. What is it caused by?

A. It is not known as to the exact underlying cause. However, the most common hypothesis is that recurrent micro-trauma of the tunica albuginea during sexual intercourse leads to a small subtunical bleed that activates the processes of wound healing and the eventual development of a fibrotic plaque. Transforming growth factor beta (TGF-β1) seems to have an important role in this process as it is overexpressed in the plaque.

Q. Is Peyronie's known to be associated with any other diseases?

A. Up to 30%–40% of men with Peyronie's disease will also have a Dupuytren's contracture. Also associated with Peyronie's disease are plantar fascial contracture (Ledderhose's disease), tympanosclerosis and post-penile trauma.

Q. Which cytokines are implicated in the pathogenesis of Peyronie's disease?

A. There appears to be an imbalance between pro- and antifibrotic cytokines. Research suggests an overexpression of TGF-β1 in penile plaques. Furthermore, fibrin and plasminogen activator inhibitor-1 (PAI-1) levels have also been shown to be increased in these plaques.

Q. How common is this condition and what is the natural history?

A. It has a prevalence of 0.4%–3.2% and usually occurs in men between 40 and 70 years of age. Managed conservatively 14% of patients have complete, spontaneous resolution and 40% of patients experience progression of the disease within 1 year.

Q. What disease stages are you aware of?

A. There are two stages of the disease. Initially, a third of patients present with painful erections during the acute phase. This period can also be characterized by worsening deformity of the penis. The second stage of PD is characterized by a stabilization of the deformity. Pains with erections generally subside as the chronic phase begins.

Q. Does the patient require any further evaluation?

A. If the history and examination are characteristic then no further evaluation is required. However, objective evaluation may include penile Doppler ultrasonography after the administration of an intracavernosal injection of a vasoactive agent to stimulate an erection. This test is also useful in cases where patients have erectile dysfunction with Peyronie's disease and also if surgery using grafts is to be performed. A magnetic resonance imaging (MRI) scan of the penis with an artificial erection can also demonstrate the presence of hourglass deformities and any hinge defects that may lead to buckling with axial loading and allows visualisation of the amount of muscle within the corpus cavernosum.

Q. Are there any medical treatments available?

A. There are several options available for the medical management of Peyronie's disease including oral medical therapy, topical and intralesional injection therapy, extracorporeal shockwave therapy (ESWL) and iontophoresis. Many of these therapies have not undergone rigorous evaluation in controlled clinical trials with most of the relevant studies being retrospective and provide little more than anecdotal evidence to support the use of the agents studied.

The oral medical therapies that have been investigated include vitamin E, tamoxifen, para-aminobenzoate (POTABA), colchicines, L-arginine and pentoxifylline. Intralesional

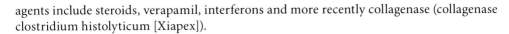

agents include steroids, verapamil, interferons and more recently collagenase (collagenase clostridium histolyticum [Xiapex]).

Q. The patient says that he has already had ESWL for renal stones in the past. He was impressed with the results of this. He would like to have ESWL for Peyronie's. Why was ESWL used for Peyronie's and what are the success rates?

A. ESWL was used because it was thought that initiating an inflammatory reaction through direct damage to the plaque would result in plaque resorption. However, multiple randomized studies designed to evaluate the efficacy of shockwave therapy have failed to show any improvements in curvature or plaque size. Furthermore NICE guidelines in the United Kingdom do not recommend it unless the patient has been informed of the low success rate and appropriate arrangements for audit and research are in place.

Q. He decides on no treatment for the present time. The patient returns 9 months later. The pain has settled. The curvature is stable at 45° dorsally. What is important in the history?

A. Whether the patient has ED and whether he can have penetrative sexual intercourse.

Q. He is unable to penetrate and has no ED. What are his options?

A. His options are either to treat conservatively by trying a vacuum erection device or traction therapy, injection therapy with Xiapex or undergoing a surgical penile straightening procedure.

Q. Which patients should undergo surgery for Peyronie's disease (PD)?

A. Surgical treatment is indicated in patients with stable PD and erections which allow penetrative intercourse with or without pharmacological agents. Problematic angulations or a hinge deformity causing difficult penetration are indications for surgery.

Q. Which surgical straightening procedures are you aware of?

A. The surgical treatment involves either penile shortening or potentially penile lengthening procedures. Penile shortening procedures involve plication techniques, such as the Nesbit procedure or the 16 dot plication. Penile lengthening procedures involve excision or incision of the Peyronie's plaque with the subsequent defect being filled by a graft.

Q. Which patients are candidates for a plication technique?

A. Penile plication procedures are typically employed in patients with normal erectile function and a mild-to-moderate curvature (<60°). Also, these patients should have no hourglass deformities or destabilizing hinge effect.

Q. What types of plication technique are you aware of?

A. Penile plication involves shortening the convex side of the penis. Patients need to be thoroughly counselled regarding the expected postoperative penile shortening.
There are several methods for performing the plication.

1. *Nesbit* – Involves excising an elliptical portion of the tunica albuginea on the convex side. Success rate – 82% penis straight, all had penile shortening and 1.2% developed postoperative ED [5].
2. *Yachia procedure* – No excision of tunica, multiple longitudinal incisions in the tunica closed horizontally straightening the penis.
3. *Essed and Schroeder* – No excision or incision of the tunica albuginea. Plicating sutures are simply placed on the convex side of the curvature.

Q. He is concerned about penile shortening. What else is available?

A. An alternative to plication procedures involves extending or lengthening the concave side of the curvature. This is generally performed by incising the plaque with placement of graft over the defect in the tunica albuginea. Regardless of the shape of the incision, the goal is to completely relax the tunica and to cover the tunical defect with graft material.

Q. Should the plaque be incised or excised?

A. It is not recommended that the plaque be completely excised as this may compromise the veno-occlusive mechanism and increase the risk for postoperative ED.

Q. How would you counsel them with respect to a plaque incision and grafting procedure?

A. After making sure that the operation is appropriate for them I would inform the patient of the success rate (straight penis 86%) and of any important potential risks (bleeding, bruising, infection, need for a circumcision, loss of length >1 cm in 26%, erectile dysfunction 15%, glans hypoaesthesia). Some surgeons recommend penile traction devices postoperatively, as well as penile rehabilitation with PDE-5 inhibitors.

Q. What types of graft have been used?

A. They can be divided into autografts (tunica vaginalis, fascia lata), allografts (cadaveric pericardium), xenografts (porcine small intestine submucosa) and synthetic grafts (Dacron mesh, polytetrafluoroethylene). No graft has been shown to be superior. For example the results using fascia lata graft are similar to that with autologous vein.

Q. By the time he returns for surgery he now complains of severe ED. Will you still go ahead with surgery?

A. After counselling, I would cancel his operation and then discuss alternative options. If he responds to pharmacotherapies (oral or intracavernosal) then a plication procedure can be performed provided that the patient accepts that pharmacotherapy is likely to be required post-operatively. However in the presence of severe ED unresponsive to pharmacotherapy then the option of a penile prosthesis insertion should be discussed. This is indicated for patients with Peyronie's and concomitant severe ED.

Q. Do you know how to straighten the penis with severe angulations of a patient who is undergoing inflatable penile prosthesis insertion?

A. After insertion and inflation of the penile prosthesis the angulation is checked. If this is mild (<30°) then the curvature will resolve as the device is cycled over a 6-month period. For more severe dorsal angulations a modelling technique can be used which involves bending the penis in the opposite direction to the curvature. If this fails then the Peyronie's plaque can be excised and a graft sutured into the defect or multiple relaxing incisions into the plaque can be performed without grafting.

HYPOGONADISM

Q. A 52-year-old man is referred by his GP complaining of increasing fatigue, mood changes and decreased libido. How would you assess him?

A. I would take a full medical history and perform a full physical examination including height, weight and waist circumference. I would then ask for baseline blood tests including a fasting glucose, lipids and early morning hormone profile.

Q. You find that he has no previous medical problems and takes no medication currently. He stopped smoking 10 years ago. There is a family history of hypertension and a father who died of a myocardial infarction at age 62. His body mass index is 30.8 kg/m²; waist circumference is 41 inches; blood pressure is 143/87 mm, cardio-respiratory examination is unremarkable. Which hormone tests would you request and when?

A. Hypogonadism can be confirmed by checking a testosterone level; morning values (between 8 a.m. and 11 a.m.) are preferred to afternoon blood samples because testosterone levels peak in the morning. This should include total testosterone, SHBG, LH, and FSH.

Q. Would you request an oestradiol level?

A. Not routinely. Oestradiol is useful when the patient has a higher body mass index as in this case. Prolactin and a thyroid profile can also be useful in diagnosing secondary causes in selected cases.

Q. His laboratory test results are fasting plasma glucose 6.2; HbA1c 6.2%; total cholesterol 6.7 nmol/L; triglycerides 3.1 nmol/L; creatinine 78 umol/L. His total testosterone level in an early morning sample is 7.2 nmol/L. How would you manage this patient?

A. The European Atherosclerosis Society suggests levels of total cholesterol between 5.2 and 6.5 require dietary advice and correction of other risk factors. As his level is greater than 6.5, I would counsel the patient on starting regular exercise and would consider initiation of therapy with a statin by notifying his GP. As his morning testosterone level is below 8 nmol/L I would also consider starting testosterone replacement therapy.

Q. What is your diagnosis?

A. This man is suffering from late-onset male hypogonadism. This is defined as a symptom complex resulting from the age-related decline in testosterone levels in men.

Q. What are the common causes of this condition?

A. Hypogonadism is a failure of the testes to produce normal levels of testosterone and/or sperm. Primary causes of hypogonadism are commonly due to testicular failure, while secondary causes are due to pituitary or hypothalamic causes (Kallman's syndrome), and combined hypogonadism is due to the combinations of the decreased pulsatile release of the pituitary gonadotropins coupled with the decreased response of the testicular Leydig cells. Hypogonadism is more common in aging males who have passed through their reproductive stage.

Q. What are the common signs and symptoms of this condition?

A. Hypogonadism in the adult commonly results in changes in sexual function, behaviour, muscle mass and loss of secondary sexual characteristics. The patient may also report changes in mood and behavioural symptoms (depression, irritability, loss of motivation) in addition to complaints of lethargy or loss of energy. Physical examination may demonstrate some regression of secondary sexual characteristics such as hair loss and possible loss of muscle bulk in addition to the findings of softer small volume testes.

Q. On examination you find he has bilateral gynaecomastia. How do you explain this?

A. Obesity can lead to the peripheral aromatization of testosterone in adipose tissue to oestradiol, leaving less bioavailable testosterone for maintenance and virilization functions. As a result of lowered free testosterone, a clinically obese male may demonstrate evidence of feminization such as gynecomastia.

Q. How would you treat this?

A. The most definitive treatment is weight loss, but some patients may also respond well to treatment with clomiphene citrate, a synthetic non-steroidal anti-oestrogen or tamoxifen.

Q. How common is late-onset hypogonadism?

A. It may occur in up to 18.4% of men older than 70 years of age regardless of ethnic background.

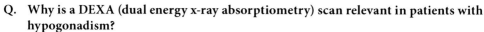

Q. **Why is a DEXA (dual energy x-ray absorptiometry) scan relevant in patients with hypogonadism?**

A. Height loss, low-trauma fractures and lowered bone-mineral density are more common in the aging male. Testosterone deficiency is more common in men who have experienced a hip fracture. Therefore it is important to check the bone mineral density in men who are recognized to be hypogonadal with a DEXA scan.

Q. **On further questioning he also admits to suffering from ED for 2 years. What percentage of patients with ED also have hypogonadism?**

A. Overall, fewer than 10% of men who present with ED are found to have testosterone deficiency.

Q. **What is the relationship between ageing and testosterone levels?**

A. Several population-based studies have demonstrated that serum testosterone levels fall with advancing age.

Q. **What is the relationship between testosterone levels and sex hormone binding globulin?**

A. Free and albumin-bound testosterone make up the circulating bioavailable testosterone. Testosterone that is bound to sex hormone binding globulin (SHBG) is tightly bound and not available to tissues; this portion constitutes approximately 45% of the total circulating testosterone in healthy young men. Numerous factors can alter SHBG and thus total testosterone without affecting the bioavailable testosterone.

Q. **What factors may increase the level of the SHBG?**

A. SHBG levels are increased by ageing, hepatic cirrhosis, hyperthyroidism, use of anticonvulsants, use of oestrogens and HIV infection.

Q. **Should the SHBG be measured in all patients?**

A. No – it should only be measured in cases where there is a low total testosterone level or conditions known to affect the SHBG concentration such as ageing. The age-related fall in serum testosterone levels may underestimate the fall in free and bioavailable testosterone levels because SHBG increases with age.

Q. **How would you manage the patient?**

A. After I have fully evaluated the patient and ensured there are no contraindications and the patient is aware of the side effects of testosterone replacement therapy, I would commence testosterone replacement initially using a short-acting agent.

Q. **Are there any contraindications to testosterone treatment?**

A. The presence of active prostate or breast cancer is an absolute contraindication to treatment.

Polycythaemia, or an excessive increase in the number of red blood cells, may be seen in some men over age 50 years who have been treated with testosterone replacement. Therefore pre-existing polycythaemia is a contraindication as an increase in the haematocrit above 54% or 55% is associated with increased blood viscosity and decreased blood flow.

Hypogonadal men who are treated with testosterone may develop or may have an exacerbation of sleep apnoea. Sleep apnoea should be treated and testosterone levels evaluated again before considering testosterone replacement.

Testosterone is an anabolic agent that increases retention of nitrogen, sodium, potassium and water. Men who have diseases such as congestive heart failure, liver failure or renal failure, which cause fluid retention, may experience a worsening of these conditions when treated with testosterone. Thus, testosterone replacement therapy is to be avoided in men with stage III or IV heart failure or severe renal or liver failure.

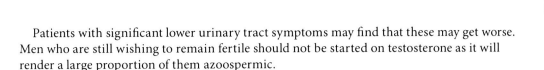

Patients with significant lower urinary tract symptoms may find that these may get worse. Men who are still wishing to remain fertile should not be started on testosterone as it will render a large proportion of them azoospermic.

Q. What delivery methods for testosterone are you aware of?

A. When testosterone is administered orally, it is metabolized by the liver on the first pass, too rapidly for it to have an effect. In order to render it clinically useful, the chemical structure of testosterone has been modified or reformulated for alternate routes of administration (Table 13.5).

Formulations of testosterone are now available for oral administration, intramuscular injection and transdermal administration by gel or patch, subcutaneous implantation of testosterone pellets or intramuscular injections.

Table 13.5 Formulations available for testosterone therapy

Route	Dose
Oral	
Testosterone undecanoate	120–160 mg once daily during first 2–3 weeks, then 40–120 mg daily
Buccal T system	30 mg every 12 hours
Intramuscular injections	
Testosterone cypionate/enanthate	100–200 mg every 2 weeks
Testosterone undecanoate	1000 mg every 6 weeks during first 12 weeks, then 1000 mg every 3 months
Transdermal	
T gel	5–10 g daily (5–10 mg testosterone)
T patch	5–10 mg daily
Subdermal	
T pellets	4 (200 mg) pellets every 5–7 months

Q. How would you monitor the testosterone replacement therapy?

A. It is important to measure serum testosterone in patients receiving replacement therapy to determine whether the treatment is raising the level to the desired range. Furthermore, the clinical signs and symptoms that initially caused the patient to be diagnosed and treated for testosterone deficiency should be monitored. Additionally, it is useful to assess bone mineral density prior to treatment and this may require re-evaluation at regular intervals.

In the older man it is very important to monitor for potential adverse effects of testosterone treatment and for delivery system-specific adverse effects. The most common adverse effect is an excessive rise in the hematocrit (>54%). When this occurs, treatment should be stopped to allow the hematocrit to normalize, after which treatment should be resumed at a lower dose.

The most serious safety concern is the potential for stimulating an occult prostate cancer to become a clinically significant prostate cancer. One should also consider using shorter-acting delivery systems when initiating testosterone treatment in older men. Should a patient develop a significant rise in hematocrit or PSA, or an abnormal DRE, it would be easier to stop this treatment while further evaluation is being conducted. This usually is of less concern after a patient has been on testosterone replacement therapy for at least 3 months whereupon a longer-acting depot form can be used.

Q. What is the relationship between testosterone levels, testosterone replacement and prostate cancer?

A. Prospective epidemiological studies have found no positive correlation with both total or bioavailable testosterone levels and prostate cancer. However, there are reports that men with low testosterone levels are more likely to have prostate cancer and perhaps a higher grade of prostate cancer than men who are eugonadal. These findings have not been duplicated in population-based studies. There is also some evidence that low testosterone levels may cause some reduction in PSA levels and that replacement therapy will consequently be associated with some increase in PSA levels. The relatively small clinical trials that have been conducted have not shown an increase in clinical prostate cancer in the testosterone groups compared with the placebo groups, but the small size of these trials and the short follow-up do not provide enough data for definitive conclusions concerning the safety of testosterone replacement therapy in regard to prostate cancer.

Q. What are the common side effects of testosterone treatment?

A. Younger men receiving testosterone replacement therapy may experience acne, increased oiliness of the skin, gynaecomastia, suppression of fertility, and some testicular atrophy. These changes may also be seen in the older male, but they rarely limit therapy.

ANDROLOGICAL EMERGENCIES

Q. A 20-year-old man attends casualty with a 7-hour history of a painful erection. How would you assess him?

A. A prolonged erection of this duration is due to priapism which is a urological emergency. I would see the patient immediately in the emergency department. I would ensure that he has adequate analgesia including a local anaesthetic penile block, intravenous access and then perform baseline blood tests which would include a full blood count (FBC) and sickle cell screen if indicated, renal function and electrolytes. I would then enquire as to whether this is the first or recurrent episode of the problem. An accurate history is required in order to establish as to whether this is an ischaemic or non-ischaemic priapism.

Q. What is important in the history?

A. In the history the important features are whether the erection is related to sexual stimulation or not (unlikely if it is 7 hours), the onset and duration of the erection and whether it is painful. It is then important to ask about any specific risk factors such as pelvic, genital or perineal trauma which may precede this episode by several weeks, any pharmacotherapy for erectile dysfunction, both oral and intracavernous injections, other medications particularly antipsychotics, a history of haematological disease such as sickle cell disease or leukaemia. This may be a first episode in which case document the pre-existing erectile function. However, in a proportion of patients a priapism episode is preceded by recurrent short self-limiting erections termed *stuttering priapism*.

Q. What is important in the examination?

A. It is important to ensure that analgesia is given before examining the patient. The baseline blood pressure and pulse must be recorded. A focused urological examination is performed to assess for any signs of trauma or which may have precipitated the event. The genitalia, perineum and abdomen should be carefully examined to assess for evidence of trauma and to ensure that there is no obvious intra-abdominal or pelvic lesion. Older patients should have a careful PR examination to exclude an underlying advanced pelvic malignancy. The degree of rigidity of the corpus cavernosum and glans may indicate the of priapism subtype.

Q. What types of priapism are you aware of?

A. The two common types of priapism are either ischaemic (low-flow) or non-ischaemic (high-low). A more uncommon subtype is stuttering priapism or recurrent priapism.

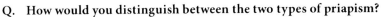

Q. How would you distinguish between the two types of priapism?

A. On the basis of the history, examination and with the aid of diagnostic investigations such as a cavernous blood analysis and radiological investigations such as penile Doppler ultrasound.

Q. How would you manage him in casualty?

A. After ensuring adequate analgesia and taking a focused history and examining the patient, I would send off baseline blood tests including a full blood count and sickle cell screen or haemoglobin electrophoresis, renal function and electrolytes. I would then perform a penile block and aspirate blood from the corpus cavernosum using a large 19-gauge butterfly needle inserted through the glans penis and into the distal corporal tip or inserted into the side of the penis. Following aspiration of blood, a sample is sent for blood gas analysis and if possible glucose analysis. I would then continue aspirating blood (up to 100 mL) from the corpus cavernosum until the penis is flaccid.

Q. The blood gas analysis is shown as follows. The blood was dark when aspirated. What is the likely priapism subtype of priapism?

$_pO_2$ 12 mm Hg
$_pCO_2$ 72 mm Hg
pH 7.1
Glucose 0.2 mmol/L

A. The blood gas analysis is consistent with ischaemia as there is evidence of hypoxia and acidosis and glucopenia. Therefore this is an ischaemic (low flow) priapism.

Q. What is the success rate of cavernosal aspiration in low flow priapism?

A. Reported success rates are 24%–36% but this is dependent on the duration of the priapism at presentation.

Q. When is aspiration alone successful in the management of priapism?

A. When it is done at an early stage generally within 12 hours.

Q. Are there any alternate ways of differentiating low and high flow priapism without cavernosal aspiration?

A. Yes, penile Doppler ultrasound may be utilised as an alternative to differentiate between ischaemic and non-ischaemic priapism. Patients with ischaemic priapism have little or no flow in the cavernosal arteries and corpus cavernosum on duplex ultrasound, whereas non ischaemic priapism shows high peak systolic velocities and a possible fistula.

Q. The priapism responds to cavernosal aspiration but then 2 hours later re-occurs. Now what would you do?

A. A step-wise approach is recommended. I would move the patient to an area where he can be monitored haemodynamically. I would repeat the aspiration using a large-gauge butterfly needle in 50 mL portions and also wash out the corpus cavernosum. If the priapism persists I would inject an α-agonist such as phenylephrine into the corpus cavernosum. I would also ensure that the Hb level is normal and that this is not a manifestation of an acute sickle cell crisis.

Q. How would you administer the phenylephrine?

A. Phenylephrine is available as 10 mg in 1 mL aliquots. I would dilute the phenylephrine in 19 mL of saline such that the concentration becomes 0.5 mg/mL. I would then inject 0.5 mL aliquots (250 µg) every 10–15 minutes until detumescence occurs. Careful monitoring of the blood pressure (BP) and pulse is required.

Q. Assuming he presents with an ischaemic priapism beyond 24 hours' duration which has not responded to corporal blood aspiration and α-agonists. Now what will you do?

A. I would then proceed to consenting the patient for shunt surgery.

Q. What types of shunts are you aware of?

A. Proximal and distal shunts.

Q. What types of distal shunts are you aware of?

A. I am aware of the Winter shunt (large biopsy needle) or Ebbehoj shunt (scalpel) where a fistula is created between the glans and corpus cavernosum through the glans. There is also a T-shunt described by Lue again using a scalpel through the glans and into the corporal tip followed by a 90° rotation.

Q. What is the shunt in Figure 13.10?

A. Figure 13.10 is a picture of an Al-Ghorab shunt where a piece of the tunica albuginea is excised at the tips of the corpora cavernosa via a dorsal transverse incision (on each side) distal to the coronal ridge.

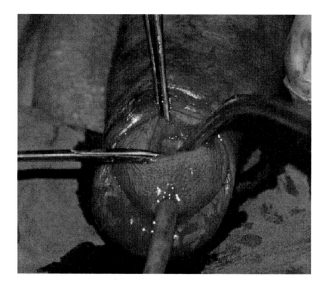

Figure 13.10

Q. A Winter shunt is performed bilaterally. However, this again fails to resolve the priapism. What is your next step of management?

A. The easiest shunt to perform is the T-shunt. If this fails despite being performed on both sides, I would proceed to a tunnelling procedure using a narrow size 8 Hegar dilator and inserting this into the glans and corpus cavernosum and repeating this on the opposite side.

Q. What types of proximal shunt are you aware of?

A. I am aware of the Quackels (corporo-spongiosal) and the Grayhack (corporo-saphenous) procedures.

Q. What are the success rates of shunt procedures and are there long-term problems?

A. The literature suggests success rates of 73%–77% for the shunt procedures, but this depends on the duration of the priapism. Although they may succeed in detumescence there is a high rate of long-term erectile dysfunction (over 90%).

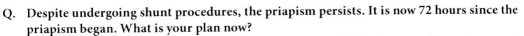

Q. Despite undergoing shunt procedures, the priapism persists. It is now 72 hours since the priapism began. What is your plan now?

A. I would again discuss the case with a specialist centre. It is likely that he will require transfer to a tertiary centre.

Q. He is transferred to a tertiary centre. What do you think they will plan for him and why?

A. It is likely that they will undertake a penile MRI and explore the patient surgically and undertake a cavernosal muscle biopsy to determine whether necrosis has already occurred. This would allow patients with prolonged ischemic priapism with non-viable tissue to be treated with the immediate insertion of a malleable penile prosthesis. This minimises penile shortening and deformity and allows adequate rigidity for sexual function.

Q. What is the role of penile prosthesis insertion?

A. Prolonged ischaemic priapism using conservative measures or shunt surgery may result in cavernosal fibrosis, penile induration and shortening. Unfortunately the resulting erectile dysfunction is usually severe and unresponsive to pharmacotherapy and the subsequent placement of a penile prosthesis into a fibrotic penis can be extremely difficult and is associated with a higher complication rate. It is now recommended that in cases of severe prolonged low-flow priapism, a (malleable) penile prosthesis is inserted early to maintain penile length and allow for an exchange to an inflatable prosthesis at a later date.

Q. Another 36-year-old patient attends casualty with a persistent erection for >8 hours. What is important in the history?

A. In the history the important features are whether the erection is related to sexual stimulation or not, the onset and duration of the erection and whether it is painful or not. It is then important to ask about any relevant risk factors such as pelvic, genital or perineal trauma, therapy for erectile dysfunction or other medications, a history of haematological disease such as sickle cell or leukaemia and any previous history of neurological disease. This may be the first or a recurrent episode. It is imperative to ask about the previous erectile function as priapism may result in erectile dysfunction.

Q. The patient is in pain but the pain is in his perineum. What is important in his examination?

A. It is important to ensure that analgesia is given before examining the patient. The baseline blood pressure and pulse must be recorded. A focused urological examination is performed to assess for any signs of trauma or infection which may have precipitated the event. In this case it is important to assess the genitalia, perineum and abdomen carefully for evidence of trauma. Again the degree of rigidity of the corpus cavernosum and glans may indicate the type of priapism present.

Q. He has severe bruising of his genitalia. He was involved in a motorbike accident earlier in the evening but did not attend casualty as he was not seriously injured. How would you manage him?

A. I would make sure he is comfortable. I would send off baseline blood tests and ensure intravenous access. It is important to exclude any other co-existing injuries. Once this has been done, I would ask a radiologist to perform a penile duplex ultrasound on him.

Q. Would you aspirate the corpus cavernosum?

A. As the history and examination are highly suggestive of a high-flow priapism I would aspirate a small amount of blood to confirm the diagnosis but only after the penile duplex has been performed to prevent aberrant blood flow.

Q. The duplex ultrasound confirmed high-flow priapism. How would you manage this patient?

A. This is not a urological emergency and can be managed conservatively. If a fistula is demonstrated on the Duplex ultrasound, compression with the probe can be applied.

Q. The patient is discharged home after undergoing investigations and confirming the diagnosis. His priapism persists and he returns after 1 week. He requests treatment. How would you manage him?

A. The site of the vascular injury may be diagnosed by pudendal angiography with super-selective embolisation of any fistula that is seen.

Q. What type of material would you recommend he is embolised with?

A. Non-absorbable materials (39%) used during embolisation pose a greater risk of erectile dysfunction than absorbable (5%) materials. It is therefore recommended that autologous clots and absorbable gels are preferable to coils and permanent chemicals.

Q. How successful is embolisation for high-flow priapism?

A. The literature suggests the success rate is 74%–78% regardless of whether absorbable or non-absorbable materials are used.

Q. Unfortunately the embolisation fails. He has had persisting priapism for 6 weeks. What would you do?

A. I would ask for a further colour duplex ultrasound and consider repeating the embolisation. If imaging demonstrates a thick-walled cystic mass, I would counsel the patient for an open penile exploration and direct ligation. However, this only occurs rarely.

Q. What is the success rate and risk of complications?

A. The literature suggests that open exploration and ligation is successful in 63% of cases but has a very high risk of ED (up to 50%).

Q. You are asked to see an 86-year-old man in casualty. He has a long-term catheter *in situ* and is from a nursing home. You are told that he has scrotal swelling (Figure 13.11). What are you concerned about the most?

A. Figure 13.11 shows Fournier's gangrene, which is a form of necrotizing fasciitis affecting the perineum and male genitalia.

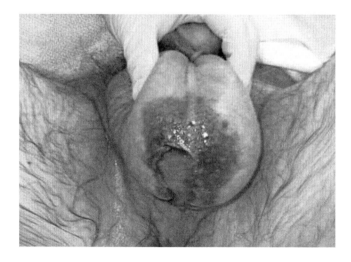

Figure 13.11

Q. What are the important aspects in the history?

A. It is important to ascertain the age of the patient, whether this has appeared suddenly or insidiously and since when. It is also important to enquire about risk factors such as:

- Any recent instrumentation of the urinary tract?
- Any recent surgery in the ano-genital area or gynaecological procedures if a female?
- Is a long-term catheter present?
- Is there reduced mobility? In particular wheelchair bound/paraplegic/bed bound?
- Is the patient normally continent?
- Are there any co-morbidities which may result in immunosuppression, i.e. diabetes, alcohol abuse or steroid treatment?

Q. What is important in the clinical examination?

A. It is important to first resuscitate these patients aggressively as they are often very sick.

It is important to record the vital observations such as the temperature, BP, O_2 saturations, pulse, peripheral circulation, sensorium and urine output to exclude signs of signs of shock.

A focused uro-genital examination is required including an evaluation of the perineum, perianal region and the genitals. Specifically one is looking for any areas of skin necrosis and the presence or absence of crepitus in the anterior abdominal wall. Perianal involvement signifies an anorectal source and the presence of skip lesions suggests more extensive involvement.

Q. Where does the infection normally arise from?

A. Infection most commonly arises from the skin, urethra or anorectal regions. There is an association between stricture disease and urethral instrumentation and the development of Fournier's gangrene. Predisposing factors include diabetes mellitus, local trauma, paraphimosis, periurethral extravasation or urine, perirectal or perianal infections, and surgery such as circumcision or hernia repair.

Q. How are you going to manage him?

A. Prompt diagnosis is critical because of the rapidity with which the process can progress. It may initially be difficult to differentiate the necrotizing fasciitis from cellulitis but the presence of marked systemic toxicity out of proportion to the local finding is often found.

I would then make sure he is transferred urgently to a urological ward or intensive therapy unit/high-dependency unit (ITU/HDU) depending on his clinical severity. There I would ensure he is resuscitated with adequate intravenous hydration and antimicrobial therapy so that he may be suitably prepared for surgical debridement.

Q. What investigations are required?

A. I would ensure baseline bloods tests are performed (FBC, urea and electrolytes [U&E], liver function test [LFT] Group and Save (G+S) and Glucose) as well as blood gases to exclude a metabolic acidosis. I would send cultures of the blood and urine as well as culture of any obvious pus from the affected region. In severe cases, I would ask the anaesthetist to insert appropriate arterial and intravenous lines for monitoring before surgery. If possible a computed tomography (CT) scan is useful pre-operatively to identify the possible source of infection.

Q. Which organisms are usually responsible?

A. There is a synergistic action so normally multiple organisms are present. The most common organism is *Escherichia coli,* however they are often mixed containing facultative organisms

(*E. coli*, *Klebsiella*, enterococci) along with anaerobes (*Bacteroides*, *Fusobacterium*, *Clostridium*, microaerophilic streptococci).

Q. Which antibiotic do you plan to use?

A. I would use an antimicrobial regimen recommended following discussion with the microbiologist. It would commonly include triple therapy such as co-amoxiclav or a parenteral third-generation cephalosporin such as ceftriaxone, along with gentamicin, and metronidazole.

Q. How would you consent the patient?

A. The patients are often gravely ill and unable to give consent. It is therefore important to involve the family early and explain that the patient needs an operation as a matter of extreme urgency. I would explain the gravity of the situation and that more than one procedure is likely to be required. I would explain that we need to remove the subcutaneous gangrenous tissue and that a urinary diversion with a supra-pubic catheter is likely. In the longer term I would explain that large skin and subcutaneous tissue defects are likely which may require plastic surgery for functional and cosmetic results. I would explain that the patient would be required to stay in ITU/HDU depending on his clinical condition for optimal support.

Q. Explain what you will do in the theatre?

A. An incision should be made through the skin and subcutaneous tissues, going beyond the areas of involvement which show end arteritis until normal fascia is found and the subcutaneous tissue is bleeding. Necrotic fat and fascia should be excised, and the wound should be left open. A second procedure 24 hours later is always indicated. A suprapubic diversion should be performed in cases in which urethral trauma or extravasation is suspected. Colostomy should be performed if there is colonic or rectal perforation.

Q. Do these patients normally require an orchidectomy?

A. Orchidectomy is almost never required, because the testes have their own blood supply independent of the compromised fascial and cutaneous circulation to the scrotum.

Q. What is his long-term outlook?

A. The literature suggests that the mortality rate averages approximately 20%. Higher mortality rates are found in diabetics, alcoholics and those with colorectal sources of infection who often have a less typical presentation, greater delay in diagnosis, and more widespread extension.

Q. Are there any scoring systems which can predict mortality and outcome in these patients?

A. The mortality risk can be assessed using the Laor scoring system (Fournier's gangrene severity index) which looks at parameters on admission including the temperature, heart rate, respiratory rate, sodium, potassium, creatinine, packed cell volume and whole blood cell count. A score of over 9 predicts mortality in 75%.

Q. Are there any adjunctive therapies which may be helpful in wound healing?

A. Using hyperbaric oxygen therapy in patients with Fournier's gangrene has reported favourable results. Hyperbaric oxygen therapy has shown some promise in shortening hospital stays, increasing wound healing, and decreasing the gangrenous spread when used in conjunction with debridement and antimicrobials.

A small recent study suggests that vacuum-assisted closure (VAC) is equally effective in healing the wounds as compared to conventional management. However with the use of VAC, patients had fewer dressing changes, less pain, fewer skipped meals and greater mobility resulting in greater patient and physician satisfaction.

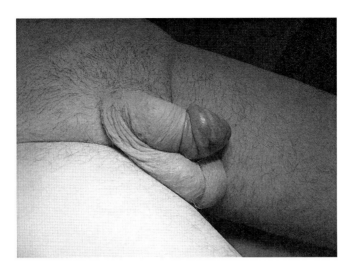

Figure 13.12

Q. **You are asked to see a patient on the ward who had a TURP 2 days ago. He has been complaining of penile pain. The nurse is asked to remove the catheter. What is the diagnosis (Figure 13.12)?**

A. Figure 13.12 shows a paraphimosis.

Q. **How does it commonly occur?**

A. It is often iatrogenic and frequently occurs after a well-meaning healthcare professional has examined the penis or inserted a urethral catheter and forgotten to replace the foreskin in its natural position. It develops when the tip of the foreskin retracts proximal to the coronal sulcus and becomes fixed in position and develops a constriction ring. Severe oedema of the foreskin occurs within several hours, depending on the tightness of the ring of the foreskin.

Q. **What is your management plan?**

A. In most cases, manual compression of the glans with placement of distal traction on the oedematous foreskin allows reduction of the paraphimotic ring.

Q. **What is different about the dorsal band traction technique and how is it performed?**

A. Most methods of reduction of paraphimosis focus on decreasing the oedema before reduction. This technique uses the basic surgical principles of traction and countertraction by applying a pair of Adson forceps directly to the band formed by the retracted preputial opening.

Q. **What is the Dundee technique?**

A. This is a technique in which the oedematous prepuce is first cleaned with an antiseptic cream and then a 26-gauge needle (outer diameter 0.45 mm) is used to make ≈20 puncture holes in the oedematous prepuce. Using gentle but firm pressure, the oedema fluid is then expressed from the foreskin until it had been completely decompressed, allowing easy reduction of the prepuce.

Q. **What will you do once the foreskin is reduced?**

A. If the tip of the foreskin is tight, then there is a risk of recurrence. I would then list the patient for an elective circumcision. However as the tissue planes can be difficult it is advisable to wait until the oedema has settled completely. If all procedures fail it is possible to perform a dorsal slit under a local anaesthetic.

REFERENCES

1. Mulcahy JJ. Penile implant infections: Prevention and treatment. *Curr Urol Rep* 2008; 9: 487–491.

2. Evers JL et al. Surgery or embolisation for varicocele in subfertile men. *Cochrane Database Syst Rev* 2004; (3): CD000479.

3. Hancock P, Woodward BJ, Muneer A, Kirkman-Brown JC. Laboratory guidelines for post-vasectomy semen analysis: Association of Biomedical Andrologists, the British Andrology Society and the British Association of Urological Surgeons. *J Clin Pathol* 2016; 69(7): 655–660.

4. Belker AM et al. Results of 1,469 microsurgical vasectomy reversals by the Vasovasostomy Study Group. *J Urol* 1991; 145: 505–511.

5. Ralph DJ et al. The Nesbit operation for Peyronie's disease: 16-year experience. *J Urol* 1995; 154: 1362–1363.

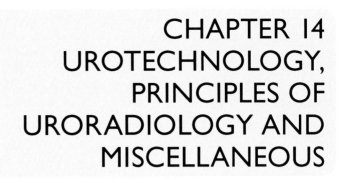

CHAPTER 14
UROTECHNOLOGY, PRINCIPLES OF URORADIOLOGY AND MISCELLANEOUS

Gidon Ellis, Daniel Cohen, John A Bycroft and Jim Adshead

Contents

ENDOUROLOGY TECHNOLOGY

Q. **What are the characteristics of the 'ideal' stent?**

A. The ideal stent would have the following characteristics [1]:

- Have good memory, with a configuration that prevents migration
- Have excellent flow characteristics
- Be radio-opaque
- Be biologically inert (biocompatible)
- Resist biofilm formation, encrustation and infection
- Be made of a flexible material with a high tensile strength
- Be easy to insert
- Be easy to remove or exchange
- Have a reasonable price
- Be used with minimal complications

Q. **What are the indications for stent insertion?**

A. The indications can be divided into elective and emergency. Elective indications include protection of anastomosis (pyeloplasty, ureteric reimplantation), to overcome extrinsic ureteric compression, prior to chemotherapy to optimise renal function in obstructive uropathy and pre-operatively (gynaecological or colorectal surgery) to aid identification of the ureter. Emergency indications include relief of ureteric obstruction and management of ureteric trauma.

Q. What are the complications of ureteric stent placement?

A. As well as those of actual insertion, complications can be divided into common and rare, as described in Table 14.1 [1].

Table 14.1 Common and rare problems of ureteric stent

Common	Rare
Trigonal irritation	Obstruction
Haematuria	Kinking
Fever	Ureteric injury/ureteric perforation
Infection	Stent misplacement
Inflammation	Stent migration
Encrustation	'Missed'/forgotten stent
Biofilm formation	Tissue hyperplasia

Q. What are ureteric stents made of? Why are they radio-opaque?

A. Ureteric stents are manufactured from a variety of polymers, such as polyurethane and styrene-ethylene-butylene (C-flex). The radio-opacity of stents is increased by coating them in metals such as bismuth and barium.

Silicone stents are also manufactured – these are stiffer and thus may cause more mucosal irritation but can be left *in situ* for up to 1 year (cf conventional polyurethane stents, which need to be changed every 6 months).

Stents are generally between 22 and 30 cm in length and are usually of the 'double-pigtail' variety. Sizes are generally 4.7 to 8 Fr.

Metallic ureteric stents are variably used for benign or malignant ureteric strictures, e.g. Memokath ureteric stent made of nickel-titanium memory-shape alloy (Nitinol).

Q. What are the different types of ureteric guidewires available?

A. Many forms of ureteric guidewires have evolved over the years. Most guidewires are in the order of 0.035–0.038 inches in diameter, and approximately 150 cm long. Various configurations exist, and commonly wires may be coated with PTFE (polytetrafluoroethylene) and have flexible tips of various lengths. Variations include hydrophilic wires (such as the Terumo wire), guidewires with a hydrophilic tip (e.g. the sensor wire) and stiff wires (e.g. the Amplatz Super Stiff).

Q. What are the various baskets available for ureteroscopic surgery?

A. A large number of ureteroscopic baskets are commercially available. They may either be 'tipped' or 'flat wire', as used in semi-rigid ureteroscopy, or 'tipless', as used in flexible ureterorenoscopy. The tipless variety may allow easier access using the flexible scope, and avoid trauma to the collecting system (easily inserted into renal calyx if necessary). Baskets are commonly made of nickel-titanium memory-shape alloy (Nitinol), and range in size, from about 2 to 3.2 Fr. Baskets are available that open in different ways, such as 'parachute' and 'helical'. (You should be prepared to talk about the baskets that you use in your practice.)

Q. Describe how a modern telescope, as used in cystoscopy, works.

A. Originally, before the work of Prof. Harold Hopkins, telescopes consisted of fine lenses cemented into long metal cylinders separated by long airspaces. This was replaced by the

'Hopkins Rod-Lens System' in the 1960s. This system is still in place today, and involves a series of long glass rods in a metal cylinder separated by shorter 'lenses' of air. The advantages of this are as follows: durability, superior light passage and image quality, reduced diameter of instrument (permitting parallel access channels), colour reproduction and the ability to 'document' images with photography or video.

Light is transmitted by optic fibre bundles running from an external light source (note this is usually a halogen external light source, which emits 'yellowish' light – thus the need for white balancing; neon light sources are expensive but do not need white balancing).

Q. How does an optic fibre work? What are the two main applications in urology and how do they differ?

A. Optic fibres are flexible glass (or plastic) fibres that allow light to pass through them via a process termed *total internal reflection*. Optic fibres are grouped together in a parallel fashion and protected by external plastic sleeves.

The two main uses in urology are for

- *Transmission of a light source.* 'Light leads' transmit light from an external source to endoscopes. These leads consist of *non-coherent* fibres, and are relatively inexpensive to produce.
- *Transmission of images.* Image transmission (e.g. from a camera) relies upon *coherent* bundles of optic fibres. In this case, the orientation of the fibres at the proximal end must be the same as the orientation at the distal end to prevent image distortion.

Flexible cystoscopes and both semi-rigid and flexible ureterorenoscopes have traditionally used a fibre-optic system, although some newer scopes utilise a digital system. As well as a non-coherent bundle of fibres to transmit light from the external light source, a fibre-optic endoscope utilises a coherent glass fibre bundle, which transmits light back to the eye-piece of the scope in an ordered fashion. Light is transmitted via a process known as total internal reflection through many thousands of fibres and the resultant image can be visualised directly or via a camera-stack system.

In common with rigid scopes, a working channel allows the passage of irrigation and instruments into the patient, although this channel is often of a smaller calibre. A flexible endoscope has a deflecting tip, which moves in response to the deflecting lever controlled by the surgeon. These are connected by two control wires. Flexible scopes are expensive to purchase and maintain and susceptible to damage. As many of the elements of the flexible scope are not heat resistant these scopes cannot be sterilised but rather decontaminated only.

Semi-rigid ureteroscopes utilise fibre-optics encased in a metal sheath, and not a rod-lens system. This provides the surgeon with a rigid instrument while permitting certain flexibility and is ideal for operating in the ureter.

Digital endoscope systems utilise a chip at the distal end of the scope which captures and transmits a digital image. The image tends to be of a much higher quality and the light cable and camera are integrated within the system, removing the need for extra cables and a heavy camera-piece to be attached to the hand-piece of the scope. These instruments are more expensive and at the present time tend to be slightly larger diameter than fibre-optic devices but will no doubt play an important role in the future of endo-urology. The development of disposable flexible ureterorenoscopes is currently being evaluated.

Q. How do we express the size/diameter of surgical instruments (e.g. cystoscopes, catheters etc.)?

A. The 'French gauge' is used (Fr). This was developed by Charrière in the nineteenth century. The French gauge corresponds to three times the diameter (in mm). For example, a 21 Fr cystoscope sheath has an external diameter of 7 mm.

Q. What are the approximate lengths, diameters and working channel configurations of the major endo-urological instruments? (You should be prepared to draw the internal configurations of endo-urological instruments.)

A. *Semi-rigid ureteroscopes* vary in size dependent on manufacturer and working channel configuration. It should be remembered that they use fibre-optics for image transmission rather than the rod-lens system of traditional rigid instruments, and hence have a relatively small diameter that usually obviates the need for formal ureteric dilatation. The working element is in the order of 34 cm long, with the tip approximately 7–10 Fr (i.e. about 3 mm diameter). If one working channel is present it is usually about 3.4 Fr; if two are present they are about 2.3 Fr each.

Flexible ureteroscopes (ureterorenoscopes) configurations vary dependent on age and model. The distal end of the instrument is less than 9 Fr, and modern instruments may be even smaller (5.4 Fr, i.e. <2 mm diameter). Lengths vary but are usually around 70–80 cm. Working channels are approximately 3.6 Fr, permitting passage of instruments such as biopsy forceps up to 3 Fr and LASER fibres. The endoscope may be inserted by means of a hydrophilic access sheath, placed over a guidewire. These sheaths are approximately 45 cm and 10–14 Fr. They may have dual lumens to permit parallel instrument passage.

Cystoscopes vary in size. Adult cystoscope sheaths are generally between 17 and 25 Fr, and approximately 30 cm long. The components of the cystoscope are the telescope (rod-lens), bridge, obturator and sheath. The telescopes themselves are angled for various procedures, and are generally 0° (for urethrotomy, etc.), 30° and 70° (for cystoscopy). Telescopes are colour coded with bands around the light-lead connector, for example green, red, yellow for 0°, 30° and 70°, respectively.

Resectoscopes again vary in size dependent on manufacturer and configurations. Common external sheath diameters are 26 and 28 Fr.

STERILISATION AND DISINFECTION

Q. What is the difference between sterilisation, disinfection and cleaning?

A. Sterilisation is defined as the complete destruction of living organisms (including spores and viruses). This differs from disinfection, which is a process used to remove most viable organisms, but one which does not necessarily inactivate some viruses and bacterial spores. Cleaning is a process which physically removes contamination but does not necessarily destroy micro-organisms.

Q. How is autoclaving performed?

A. Autoclaving is a process that combines heat and pressure to sterilise instruments. By combining pressure with heat the temperatures of liquids such as water may be raised above their usual boiling points to facilitate the process. The autoclave is thus a form of 'pressure cooker'. The three variables used in autoclaving are therefore pressure, temperature and time. Typical cycles include 134°C for a 'hold time' of 3 minutes, and 121°C for a 'hold time' of 15 minutes. The actual timing of the whole process is longer than these figures of course, as the machines need to safely heat up and down.

Q. How is disinfection carried out?

A. Flexible instruments (e.g. flexible cystoscope) would generally be unable to withstand the conditions of autoclaving. They are therefore processed by high-level disinfection. They are manually cleaned with brushes and detergent, and then disinfected in an automated manner. Ultrasound is used in some devices to facilitate the cleaning process. Automated machines use a cycle whereby the flexible endoscope is disinfected with solutions of chemical such as chlorine dioxide ('Tristel').

Q. How do you determine the level of disinfection required for reusable medical instruments?

A. Divided into three classes according to Spaulding Classification: critical, semi-critical and non-critical.

Critical instruments are those that penetrate normally sterile tissue (surgical instruments). They generally require sterilisation before and after use. Semi-critical instruments contact mucous membranes or non-intact skin (cystoscopes). Non-critical items are those that come in contact with only intact skin (blood pressure cuffs).

Q. What do you use for scrubbing and skin preparation, prior to surgery?

A.

- Scrubbing
  - 4% Chlorhexidine (Hydrex)
  - 7.5% Povidone iodine (Betadine or Videne)
- Skin preparation
  - Inguinoscrotal: 10% Aqueous povidone iodine (Betadine or Videne)
  - Genital: Chlorhexidine 0.015% Cetrimide 0.15% (Travasept solution)

Q. What are the ideal climate conditions for an operating theatre?

A. 21°C and 55% humidity.

DIATHERMY

Q. What is shown in Figure 14.1?

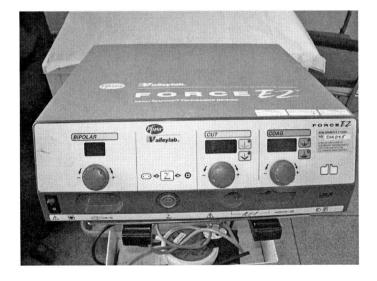

Figure 14.1

A. Figure 14.1 is an image of a diathermy machine.

Q. What is diathermy?

A. The passage of high-frequency alternating current, in the range 400 KHz–10 MHz, through body tissue. Where the current is concentrated, heat up to 1000°C is produced, to allow cutting or coagulation of tissue [2].

Nerves and muscles are not stimulated with such a high-frequency alternating current (400 KHz–10 MHz) as there is no time for the cell membranes of nerve and muscle to become depolarised (they are stimulated at lower frequencies only).

Q. What sort of diathermy do you use in theatres, and how does it work?

A. The main types of diathermy used in an operating theatre are monopolar and bipolar.

Monopolar diathermy involves the delivery of high-frequency current from a diathermy generator, to the active electrode (diathermy forceps or standard resectoscope loop or ball). High current density at the active electrode, which has a small surface area, results in heat at the point of contact with tissue. Current density then spreads from this point, throughout the body, returning to the diathermy generator via the patient electrode plate (Earth Plate), which is the diathermy pad placed on the patient. Low current density at this electrode plate, due to its large surface area (70–150 cm²), results in no heat formation. Importantly, the patient electrode plate should be a well-vascularised area away from any prosthesis and the underlying skin should be free of scarring or hair to allow good contact of the plate with the patient.

With bipolar diathermy, current passes down one limb of forceps (active electrode) and back to the diathermy generator via the other limb (patient electrode plate). The advantages are that there is no need for a plate to be placed on the patient. The disadvantages are that there is no cutting facility, the forceps need to be kept apart and there is less power.

Q. What is the difference between cutting and coagulation?

A. The differences are listed in Table 14.2 and Figure 14.2.

Table 14.2 Differences between cutting and coagulation

Cutting	Coagulation
Continuous output (sine wave) 100% on 0% off (See Figure 14.2)	Pulsed output (interrupted sine wave) 6% on 94% off (See Figure 14.2)
Low voltage	High voltage
Non-contact mode: Vapourises and cuts Contact mode: Dessicates (Coagulum)	Non-contact mode: Fulguration Contact mode: Dessication
Intense heat 1000°C Charring/spread: Low	Less heat Charring/spread: High
Power 125–250 W	Power 10–75 W
Typical diathermy machine setting 150–160 W	Typical diathermy machine setting 40–70 W

Note: Blend only works in cutting mode – pulsed output (50% on and 50% off).

Q. What are the potential complications and precautions with diathermy?

A. The complications and precautions are as follows:

- Burns
  - Due to misapplication of the patient electrode plate
  - Metal prosthesis or implants should not be touched directly with the active electrode or the patient electrode plate
  - Use of inflammable preparatory solution may result in superficial burns on skin or in cavities

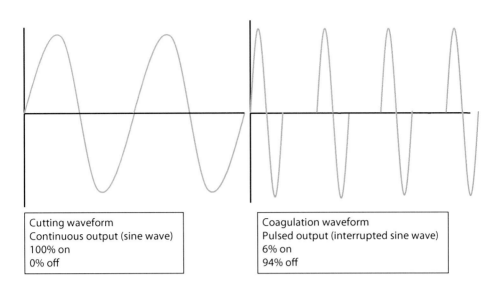

| Cutting waveform
Continuous output (sine wave)
100% on
0% off | Coagulation waveform
Pulsed output (interrupted sine wave)
6% on
94% off |

Figure 14.2 Cutting and coagulation waveforms.

- Explosions
  - In obstructed hollow viscera
  - If inflammable volatile anaesthetic agents are used (ether)
- High-voltage electrocution
  - To the patient or the surgeon because of faulty cables
- Obturator kick
- End artery necrosis
  - Especially with monopolar diathermy, during penile surgery
- Pacemakers
  - Diathermy needs to be used with caution in patients with pacemakers (see following discussion)

Q. How are diathermy burns avoided?

A. Inflammable liquids (e.g. containing alcohol) should be avoided. The patient electrode plate should be of at least 70 cm² in size, and placed appropriately (see previous discussion). The patient should not be in contact with any other metal objects (e.g. drip stands). Additionally, touching other instruments with the diathermy probe (either inadvertently or purposefully) should be avoided (direct coupling).

Q. You are in the middle of a transurethral resection of the prostate (TURP), when the diathermy stops working. How do you resolve the situation to complete the procedure?

A. I perform a series of checks, as follows:

1. Make sure that the machine has not been switched off inadvertently
2. Check that the diathermy cable is still connected to the diathermy machine
3. Ensure that the diathermy cable has not broken
4. Make sure that the diathermy cable is properly connected to the working element of the resectoscope
5. Ensure that the loop is not broken
6. Check that the irrigating fluid is still glycine (1.5%)
7. Make sure that the patient electrode plate is appropriately attached to the patient and that the return cable to the diathermy machine is still connected

Q. You are contacted by your junior colleague regarding a 78-year-old patient who is due to have a TURP in 2 weeks time. The doctor suspects the patient has a pacemaker and wishes to seek advice. What are the potential risks?

A. The main risks with pacemakers and implantable cardioverter defibrillators (ICDs) are pacemaker inhibition, phantom reprogramming and ventricular fibrillation.

Pacemaker inhibition: the high frequency of the diathermy current may simulate cardiac electrical activity, thus inhibiting the pacemaker. If the patient is pacemaker-dependent, the heart may stop beating.

Phantom reprogramming: the high frequency of the diathermy current may simulate the radiofrequency impulse by which pacemakers are reprogrammed. As a result the pacemaker may start to work in an entirely different mode.

Q. What precautions should be taken before, during and after the operation?

A. All information of the pacemaker/ICD should be available, including type of device (pacemaker/ICD), serial numbers, date of implantation, hospital implanting the device, indication and date/result of last check. Patients should have a card displaying this information. The cardiac clinic should be contacted to determine the precise indication for the device, and to determine whether the device is due for replacement.

Generally, diathermy should be avoided in the first instance in such patients, and an alternative treatment strategy should be considered. If the surgical procedure is deemed unavoidable, then the following points should be considered.

Prior to the surgery, carefully consult the cardiologist, pacemaker clinic and cardiac technician in elective cases (see previous discussion). Most devices will not need to be adjusted pre-operatively; however advice should still be sought as the consequences may otherwise be life threatening. ICDs are generally set to 'monitor only' to prevent inadvertent activation, and should of course be switched back after the operation. Consider if procedure can be performed with bipolar diathermy (e.g. TURP).

During the procedure, the patient plate electrode should be sited so that the current path does not go right through the pacemaker. Furthermore, ensure it is properly applied. Avoid inappropriate grounding through ECG leads. The diathermy machine should be well away from the pacemaker (>15 cm). The patient's heart rate should be continuously monitored; a defibrillator should be immediately available, as well as an external pacemaker. Surgically, short bursts of diathermy should be used and the operative time should be as short as possible. Antibiotic prophylaxis should be given and fluid overload should be avoided in these cases.

Clinical magnets may be secured over ICDs to prevent inadvertent shocks and to allow pacemakers to function at a fixed rate. However, they are very rarely used in current practice, because of the risk of phantom reprogramming.

In emergency situations pre-operative checks may not be possible. The device should however be checked post-operatively as soon as practicable [3].

EXTRACORPOREAL SHOCKWAVE LITHOTRIPSY (ESWL)

Q. Describe the various components of the shockwave lithotripter?

A. Whatever the device used, the lithotripter will have four main components: an energy source, a media for transmission of the energy (e.g. water), a focusing device and an imaging modality.

The first machines used were the Dornier lithotripters. These used electrohydraulic lithotripsy (EHL), whereby a spark is produced between two electrodes under water, which results in the rapid expansion and collapse of a gas bubble and subsequent energy transmission. A metal hemi-ellipsoid reflector is used to focus the energy. This modality produces the most effective shocks but can be painful, and the intensity of the shock wave is variable. An example of such a machine used today would be the Dornier Lithotripter S II.

A second form is the electromagnetic lithotripter. This relies on a cylindrical electromagnetic source, and energy is focused by an acoustic lens. An example of this would be the Storz Modulith SLX-F2.

Third, piezoelectric technology may be used to produce the energy. Piezoelectric materials consist of ceramic or crystal elements that produce an electrical discharge under stress or tension (the direct effect). Energy transmission in this lithotripter relies on the 'converse piezoelectric effect', whereby energy is produced via the movement of the source when electricity is passed through it. An example of a piezoelectric lithotripter would be the EDAP LT 02.

The acoustic shockwave produced has two main phases. First a short *positive phase* causes erosion at the entry and exit points of the calculus. The stone also shatters internally due to the compressive effect of this wave. The effect of compression/tension induced cracks is sometimes referred to as 'spallation'. Second, a longer *negative pressure phase* component to the wave results in the formation of microbubbles, and the collapse of these microbubbles causes further erosion of the stone surface via the formation of 'microjets'. The two phases are demonstrated schematically in Figure 14.3.

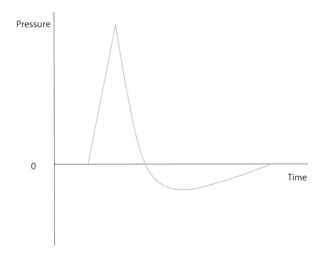

Figure 14.3 The two phases of a shockwave (shockwave pressure profile).

Q. What are the indications for ESWL?

A. In general the indications are

- Renal pelvis stones <20 mm
- Lower pole stones <10 mm, or 10–20 mm if favourable factors (see stone chapter)
- Upper or distal ureteric stones <10 mm
- Sandwich therapy in conjunction with PCNL
- Indications vary according to patient factors and choice.

Q. What are the contra-indications for ESWL?

A. The contra-indications can be divided into absolute and relative:

Absolute
- Uncorrected coagulopathy
- Sepsis or active urinary tract infection (UTI)
- Distal obstruction
- Pregnancy
- Arterial aneurysm in vicinity of stone

Relative

- Hard stones (cystine or Ca oxalate monohydrate)
- Morbid obesity (>135 Kg) or skeletal malformations that prevent targeting of the stone
- Abdominal pacemaker

Q. How would you consent a patient for ESWL?

A. Informed consent for ESWL would involve a description of the procedure, discussion of alternative treatments and an explanation of potential complications [4]. Patients should be warned that repeated ESWL treatments may be required and stones may recur. In addition, the complications below are taken from the BAUS 2016 patient information leaflet.
- *Common complications (greater than 1 in 10):*
    - Haematuria
    - Renal/ureteric colic
    - UTI needing antibiotic treatment
    - Skin bruising
    - Stone will not break as too hard, requiring an alternative treatment
- *Occasional complications (between 1 in 10 and 1 in 50):*
    - Steinstrasse requiring surgical treatment
- *Rare complications*
    - Perinephric haematoma; bleeding may require further treatment
    - Severe infection requiring intravenous antibiotics +/− nephrostomy
    - Adjacent organ damage
    - Hypertension (not on BAUS form but well-described)
    - Arrhythmias

INTRACORPOREAL ENERGY FORMS

Q. A 53-year-old male patient with an 8 mm mid-ureteric stone and JJ stent *in situ* presents for ureteroscopy. Can you tell me what energy source you would use to fragment this stone?

A. I would use a Ho:YAG (Holmium:Yttrium-Aluminium-Garnet) LASER. LASER is an acronym for Light Amplification by Stimulated Emission of Radiation. LASER is formed by applying energy to a lasing medium; a process known as 'pumping'. The energy may be light, chemical or even another LASER, and the medium may be solid, liquid or a gas. The LASER chamber itself is fully reflective apart from an aperture at one end that is able to let light escape when it reaches a certain intensity. A photon is released from an atom within the medium when it is excited by the energy applied, in a process known as spontaneous emission. These photons are reflected internally and collide with atoms already in an excited state, leading to the release of more photons from the medium, a process known as stimulated emission. The light is therefore amplified and a state known as 'population inversion' occurs, whereby more light is released than is absorbed.

LASER light has three characteristics: it is monochromatic (single wavelength and therefore the same colour), collimated (waves are parallel) and coherent (waves are in phase).

The wavelength of Holmium LASER is 2140 nm, and it is therefore invisible. A secondary red aiming beam is utilised. The depth of penetration is 0.4 mm. LASER works primarily via a photoexcitation/photothermal effect (i.e. heat production). Different LASER fibres sizes exist. The 200 μm fibres should be used with the flexible ureterorenoscope and 365 μm fibres (or less) with the semi-rigid ureteroscope.

Q. What alternative forms of energy could you use to fragment a stone?

A. The lithoclast is a contact-type intracorporeal lithotripter and is used in rigid endoscopes. Pneumatically generated energy (compressed air) fires a projectile in the handpiece of the lithoclast into a probe; the kinetic energy is directly transmitted to the calculus (the probe must be in contact with the stone to fragment it). The probe tends to 'bounce' off the wall of the ureter minimising trauma and is considered a safe modality in the ureter (however ureteric perforation may still occur if used without care). A disadvantage of the device is retrograde propulsion of the stone into the renal pelvis. Lithoclast energy may be combined with ultrasonic energy and suction for use in percutaneous nephrolithotomy (PCNL). The Swiss Lithoclast Master is a popular device combining all three modalities (EMS, Switzerland). However, ultrasonic energy should be avoided in the ureter because of thermal side effects (i.e. high temperature at tip of the ultrasound probe). EHL is a further option for stone fragmentation (see next question).

Q. How does EHL work?

A. An underwater spark plug is generated by applying voltage/current to two concentric electrodes with different voltage polarities, which are 1 mm apart and separated by insulation. This electrically generated spark at the tip of the probe results in momentary heat in a localised area and a small amount of fluid surrounding the electrode is vaporised forming a gas bubble. Subsequent expansion and collapse of the gas bubble generates a hydraulic shockwave in 1/800 second, which impacts on the stone. Collapse of the cavitation bubble can be symmetrical ($\gg$1 mm from stone) or asymmetrical ($\gg$3 mm from stone). The symmetrical aspect results in the production of a strong secondary shockwave, while the asymmetrical part results in the formation of high-speed microjets. Both these then result in stone breakage in a similar mechanism to ESWL (see previous discussion).

The probe should be placed on or not more than 1 mm from the stone. EHL is delivered using a flexible probe (via cystoscope) and is generally used to fragment bladder stones. EHL should never be used in the ureter as it may result in ureteric perforation.

Q. How does ultrasound lithotripsy work?

A. Ultrasound waves, produced by an ultrasound generator, are transmitted down a hollow probe resulting in vibration of the probe tip. This vibration, when in contact with the stone, produces a drilling or grinding action leading to stone fragmentation. Ultrasound is used in PCNL, often in combination with lithoclast – the hollow ultrasound probe allows suction of stone fragments. Additionally, this energy form is used for disintegration of bladder stones. As it is a rigid probe it is used with rigid endoscopes only.

Note that ultrasound must not be used in the ureter as vibration of the tip results in high temperatures and thus there is a significant risk of ureteric perforation.

Q. What other types of LASER are used in contemporary urology?

A. LASERs commonly used in contemporary urology include Holmium, Nd:YAG, Greenlight, Thulium and Diode. Their use is determined by the target tissues, which absorb lights of different wavelengths. The properties of the most commonly used LASERs in urology are shown in Table 14.3.

Diode LASERs require a much smaller box size and are more energy efficient than others and can usually be operated from a standard power outlet.

Table 14.3 LASERS in urology

Active crystal	Abbreviation	Wavelength (nm)	Uses
Holmium	Ho:YAG	2140	• Ablation, resection or enucleation of prostate (HoLAP/HoLRP/HoLEP) • Resection or ablation of TCC • Fragmentation of urinary tract calculi
Neodymium	Nd:YAG	1064	• Coagulation of prostate tissue • Ablation of TCC
Kalium titanyl phosphate (Greenlight)	KTP:Nd:YAG	532	• Absorbed by haemoglobin, can be used to vaporise prostate tissue
Lithium borate (Greenlight)	LBO:Nd:YAG	532	
Thulium	Tm:YAG	2013	• Vaporisation or enucleation of prostate • Ablation of TCC
Diode LASERs		830–1470	• Vaporisation of prostate or TCC

Greenlight LASER has a wavelength of 532 nm, which is absorbed by haemoglobin at a penetration of 0.8 mm. It can be used to vaporise prostate tissue.

Nd:YAG has a wavelength of 1064 nm and is absorbed by water and haemoglobin. It penetrates tissue up to 10 mm and can be used to coagulate prostate tissue or ablate TCC.

Holmium:YAG LASER has a wavelength of 2140 nm and is absorbed by water. It penetrates tissue up to 0.4 mm and can be used to ablate, resect or enucleate the prostate (HoLAP/HoLRP/HoLEP), to resect or ablate TCC or to fragment urinary tract calculi.

Thulium has a wavelength of 2000 nm and is absorbed by water with a tissue penetration of 0.25 mm. It can be used to vaporise or enucleate prostate or to ablate TCC.

Diode LASERs have wavelengths ranging from 830 to 1470 nm and are therefore absorbed by both water and haemoglobin. Use of them causes vaporisation, which can be used in both prostate and TCC.

Q. How do you ensure LASER safety in theatre?

A. LASER presents a significant hazard to both the patient and anyone present in the operating theatre. The main risks are of burns to the skin and to the eyes. The various properties of different LASERs mean that they pose slightly different risks, e.g. Nd:YAG has a tissue penetration depth of 10 mm and can cause retinal injuries whereas LASERs that penetrate more superficially may cause corneal injuries. While everyone present should take a degree of responsibility for LASER safety, the LASER operator and the surgeon are chiefly responsible and both should have had up-to-date, certified training in the safe use of LASER. General precautions include minimising the number of staff in theatre and locking and utilising warning signs at the theatre doors. Within the theatre windows must be covered and all surfaces should have non-reflective coatings. All present, including the patient, should wear LASER safety goggles that are specific to the particular wavelength of that LASER and the skin of sedated or anaesthetised patients must be carefully draped. The LASER pedal should have a guard to prevent inadvertent activation and fastidious care should be taken to ensure that the LASER is placed on standby whenever it is not in use. The use of LASER in close proximity to oxygen poses a risk of LASER fire and significant burns and great care must be taken.

Q. What is the device in Figure 14.4a and b and how does it work?

A. The Swiss Lithoclast Master has both a lithoclast and ultrasound probe and is used for PCNLs. During PCNL the lithoclast is combined with the *hollow* ultrasound probe, the latter of which is able to suck up stone fragments.

(a)

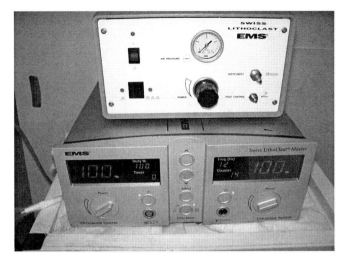

(b)

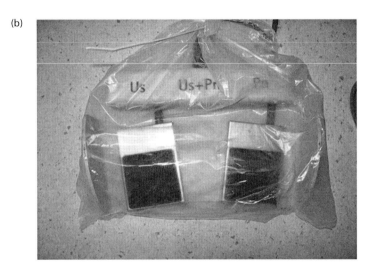

Figure 14.4 (a) The generator for the Swiss Lithoclast Master. (b) The foot pedals used to activate the Swiss Lithoclast Master.

PRINCIPLES OF URORADIOLOGY

Q. **What is the machine shown in Figure 14.5 and how does it work?**

A. Figure 14.5 is a picture of an ultrasound machine. This can be used as either a diagnostic or therapeutic tool in medicine. High-frequency sound waves are produced by the passage of current through a piezoelectric transducer, and subsequently focused. Medical ultrasound waves vary from 2 to 18 MHz. Lower frequencies are used to look at 'deeper' tissues, as the attenuation of sound waves is greater at higher frequencies. For example a transrectal ultrasound (TRUS) probe works at about 7 MHz, and transabdominal ultrasound works at around 3.5 MHz. Ultrasound waves pass into the body via an interface comprising the soft rubber coating on the transducer and gel. The sound waves are deflected back to the transducer, depending on an appropriate density change within the tissues. Large density changes (e.g. fluid and stone) produce a greater 'echo', and the time the waves take to come back to the transducer can determine the depth of the tissue.

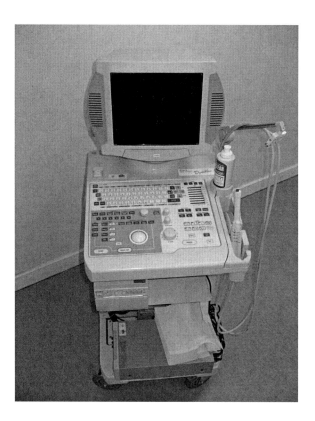

Figure 14.5

Q. What are the main therapeutic applications of ultrasound?

A. The main current therapeutic applications of ultrasound are lithotripsy (extracorporeal, during percutaneous nephrolithotomy and intracorporeal) and high-intensity focused ultrasound (HIFU), which is used in the treatment of prostate cancer. Ultrasound as a modality can guide other therapies such as prostate brachytherapy, cryotherapy and ESWL.

Q. What are the general contraindications to administration of intravenous contrast media?

A. The Royal College of Radiologists state that increased risk of adverse reactions may be seen in patients with a previous contrast reaction, asthma, renal impairment, diabetes mellitus and metformin therapy. In patients with normal renal function, there is no need to stop metformin. If renal function is impaired, metformin may be stopped for 48 hours following contrast administration. Untreated hyperthyroidism and myelomatosis are contraindications to contrast use. Nephrogenic systemic fibrosis is a rare complication seen after administration of gadolinium-based contrast agents in patients with severe renal impairment.

Q. A 64-year-old male is referred for an MRI following the diagnosis of prostate cancer. He has previously had intracranial surgery following a stroke and works as an electrical engineer. What would be your concerns?

A. In this particular case, the concerns would be that the patient has an intracranial clip (for an aneurysm, e.g.), or may have an intra-ocular ferrous foreign body (secondary to his job). Imaging should not be performed on patients with intra-cranial clips, unless one is absolutely certain that they are MRI compatible. Patients who may have metal foreign bodies in their eyes should have radiographs of their orbits performed prior to MRI scanning. Radiographs can pick up objects greater or equal to 0.1 mm in size, and ferrous foreign bodies are thought not to be dangerous below this size.

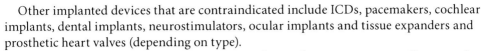

Other implanted devices that are contraindicated include ICDs, pacemakers, cochlear implants, dental implants, neurostimulators, ocular implants and tissue expanders and prosthetic heart valves (depending on type).

Extra-cranial surgical clips, e.g. following abdominal surgery, are generally encased in fibrous tissue, however they may cause artefact, and scanning should be deferred for 6 weeks post-operatively.

Q. **Briefly describe the physics behind MRI. What is the difference between T1 and T2 images?**

A. MRI utilises the nuclei of hydrogen atoms (protons). The protons usually spin in a random fashion, however on entering the MRI scanner they align with the magnetic field in the longitudinal plane (the magnet in an MRI scanner is always 'on'!), and produce a secondary spin (precession) at the same frequency, which will vary according to the strength of the magnet. A radiofrequency (RF) pulse is applied, which gives the nuclei the energy to move out of alignment and into the transverse plane, and to process in phase with one another. When this pulse is removed the atoms release their energy in two ways. First, energy is released back into the surrounding environment causing magnetic movements to relax and realign back into the longitudinal plane, a process referred to as T1 relaxation. Second, nuclei then lose their precessional coherence and dephase, due to energy loss between adjacent nuclei, and this is referred to as T2 decay. The release of energy is picked up in the transverse plane as an electrical voltage by a receiver coil, and this is the MR signal.

T1 relaxation occurs more rapidly in fat, as the size of the molecules enables them to give energy back to the environment more quickly. This means that there is a greater degree of transverse magnetisation following the next RF pulse, resulting in a very bright signal from fat on T1-weighted images, while fluid remains dark. These scans are excellent for viewing anatomy due to the good tissue differentiation.

T2-weighted images rely on the process of T2 decay, which occurs more slowly in water, and therefore maintains transverse magnetisation for longer resulting in a higher signal. Consequently water has a very bright signal on these images, producing a scan which is more useful for demonstrating pathology.

Q. **What is nephrogenic systemic fibrosis? How may this be related to MRI investigations?**

A. Nephrogenic systemic fibrosis (NSF) is a condition of unknown cause that affects patients with renal disease. It causes collagen deposition and tightening of the skin of the extremities and sometimes trunk. It can be fatal, and 5% of patients develop the fulminant form. Causes of death are related to respiratory complications, clotting abnormalities and fractures/falls, among others. There is no consistently successful treatment for NSF, although various strategies such as steroids, plasmapheresis and renal transplant have all been used.

Recent reports have linked the use of gadolinium-containing contrast agents to the development of NSF in patients with renal impairment. Gadolinium-containing contrast is used with great caution in patients with a GFR <60 mL/min/1.73 m^2, including dialysis patients. The Royal College of Radiologists have recommended that if patients must receive these agents they should be specific 'highly stable' agents, and that the use should not be repeated within 7 days. The smallest dose possible should be used. Specific agents (Omniscan, Magnevist and OptiMARK) should *not* be used.

Q. **You have requested a MAG-3 scan on a 29-year-old male you suspect has a pelviureteric junction obstruction. What is MAG-3, how is it handled by the kidney and what should the patient know prior to the test?**

A. MAG-3 stands for mercaptoacetyltriglycine. MAG-3 is attached to the radioactive tracer Technetium-99m, an isotope with a short half-life (approximately 6 hours) that is used for other nuclear medicine scans, such as dimercapto-succinic acid (DMSA). MAG-3 is principally excreted by tubular secretion (90%), although approximately 10% is filtered at the glomerulus. Radioactivity is recorded via a gamma-camera (as with DMSA).

The patient will be asked to attend the nuclear medicine unit, and before the investigation the patient will have to empty his bladder. Usual medications should not be stopped, and the patient should be well hydrated. Children should not be brought along for the scan due to the potential radiation risk. A cannula is inserted, and a diuretic is injected (usually 15 minutes prior to the test, although protocols vary). The patient does not need to undress, although metal objects should be removed. The patient then sits on a chair while the MAG-3 is injected through the cannula. The patient then has to sit still for approximately 20 minutes while images are recorded. The patient is asked to keep well hydrated after the test, with no specific instructions otherwise. (Please also refer to Chapter 6.)

Q. **A 2-year-old girl requires a MAG-3 scan to investigate a unilateral hydronephrosis. The parents are concerned about the process surrounding the scan and the risk of radiation. How would you reassure them?**

A. Although the investigation is associated with radiation exposure, the overall dose is low (approximately 0.7 microSv). This is equivalent to about 4 months of background radiation. As a comparison, air travel (at 26,000 feet) provides approximately 3 microSv per hour at temperate latitudes, and approximately 1 microSv per hour around the equator. Therefore no investigation involving radiation is entirely without risk; however the benefits of the investigation need to be weighed against the risks.

Children should eat and drink as normal before the scan and not stop any regular medications. The child should attend the ward in a well-hydrated state, and the paediatrician will insert a cannula after the application of anaesthetic cream. Occasionally the child may need some sedation. Diuretic may be injected prior to the isotope injection. The child must lie on a bed for approximately 20 minutes. The child does not need to be undressed, but will have to remove metal objects. After the scan the child should be kept well hydrated and empty the bladder regularly. (Please also refer to Chapter 6.)

Q. **You have requested a DMSA scan on a 34-year-old female to look for the presence of renal scarring suggested on an ultrasound scan. What is DMSA, and how is the scan performed?**

A. DMSA stands for dimercapto-succinic acid. It is attached to the radio-tracer Technetium-99m (see previous discussion). DMSA is a cortical-scanning agent that localises in the proximal tubule. It is minimally excreted, and its presence is a reflection of functioning renal tissue and nephrons.

An important difference between the 'patient experience' of DMSA versus MAG-3 is that patients may be in the hospital for many hours (during a DMSA renogram). If females suspect that they may be pregnant they should inform the department before attending, and should not be accompanied by children. A cannula is inserted into the patient, and the isotope injected. The static images are taken after an interval of approximately 2–4 hours post-injection. Patients are not required to undress, but metal objects should be removed. During the scan itself they will have to lie still on a couch. The gamma 'camera' is placed close to the kidneys but not touching the patient. After the scan patients are asked to keep well hydrated and empty their bladders regularly. (Please also refer to Chapter 6.)

Q. **What steps are applied to ensure x-ray safety in theatres?**

A. First, it is important that the surgeon has an understanding of the equipment in use and an up-to-date knowledge of radiation protection issues. The image intensifier should be operated by a trained radiographer and ideally the surgeon should have received specialised training from a medical physicist in protection aspects of fluoroscopy. It is important that all fluoroscopy equipment is periodically tested and maintained to ensure it is functioning correctly.

The main source of radiation to staff is scattered radiation from the x-ray tube, which in urological procedures is usually the end of the C-arm situated under the patient's bed. Keeping the tube as close as possible to the table minimises radiation scatter. Staff should stand as far from the x-ray tube as possible to reduce their radiation exposure. Personal protective equipment should be worn by everyone in the operating theatre, with the exception of the patient. Lead aprons are the most effective and may reduce the dose received by around 90%. A lead apron with 0.35 mm lead thickness equivalence should be sufficient for most fluoroscopic procedures. A 0.25 mm apron may suffice for low work load fluoroscopy. Other equipment, such as thyroid shields and lead glass eyewear should be available and worn, especially when staff are exposed to regular and long fluoroscopy times. A personal radiation dosimeter should be worn at all times that fluoroscopy is in use.

For each individual case, the exposure of patients and staff to radiation must be reviewed and justified. Female patients of childbearing age must have a pregnancy test prior to leaving the ward. While fluoroscopic screening is in progress the theatre doors should be closed and a warning sign displayed. A red light at the theatre entrance indicates that fluoroscopy is in progress. The rationale for each image taken should be considered and rationalised in accordance with the ALARA (as little as is reasonably appropriate) principle. Intermittent screening, as opposed to continuous is preferred. Hands (patient or staff) should be kept out of the primary beam unless unavoidable for clinical reasons as the automatic exposure control system will trigger an increase in exposure to maintain image quality. An alarm can be set on the x-ray machine, which sounds when preset radiation dose limit is reached.

MISCELLANEOUS

Renal failure and transplantation

Q. Outline the main complications of chronic renal failure.

A. The main complications affecting patients symptomatically are fluid overload, anaemia, renal osteodystrophy, pericarditis, anaemia and the effects of cardiovascular disease. Hypertension, dyslipidaemia and the metabolic complications of acidosis and hyperkalaemia are factors that can lead to progression of these complications.

Q. Describe what you see in Figure 14.6. What is the composition of this solution?

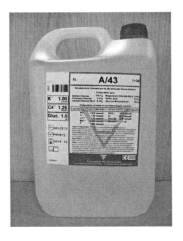

Figure 14.6

A. Figure 14.6 shows a dialysate solution. It consists of water, sodium (132–155 mmol/L), potassium (0–4 mmol/L, i.e. sub-physiological), calcium, magnesium, chloride, bicarbonate (or acetate – as a buffer) and glucose. The pH lies between 7.1 and 7.3.

Q. **What is the device shown in Figure 14.7? What are the principal differences between haemodialysis and haemofiltration?**

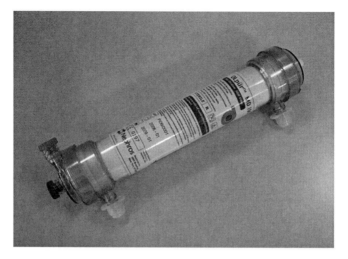

Figure 14.7

A. This device is a haemodiafiltration (HDF) filter. HDF is a process that combines dialysis and haemofiltration.

Haemodialysis works by two main mechanisms, principally the *diffusion* of solutes across a semi-permeable filter (made of modified cellulose or synthetic material) and second the principle of *ultrafiltration*, which is caused by the convective flow of solutes and liquids. The negative pressure to allow this is produced via the outlet pump of the dialysis machine. Haemofiltration does not use a dialysate solution, and relies on a hydrostatic pressure gradient alone to produce ultrafiltration. Fluid is replaced either before or after filtration. Haemodynamic stability of patients is thought to be better maintained by utilising filtration alone rather than diffusion.

Q. **How may permanent venous access be created, and what are the complications?**
A. Permanent access is provided principally via either radial or brachial fistulae. The arteries are anastamosed to the cephalic vein. Brachial fistulae are associated with a higher risk of 'steal' syndrome due to the higher flow rates. Alternatively the arteries and veins may be linked with a 'bridging graft'.

Common complications include thrombosis of the fistula or graft, stenosis (usually occurring at or distal to the fistula or graft), ischaemia of the digits, infection (of grafts), aneurysm/pseudoaneurysm formation, superior vena cava obstruction or extravasation into limbs.

Q. **What are the principles of peritoneal dialysis? What are the different types of peritoneal dialysis? What complications may occur?**
A. Peritoneal dialysis uses the peritoneum as the 'dialysis membrane', and dialysis fluid is instilled into the peritoneal cavity. Solutes move via diffusion down a concentration gradient, and fluid transfers occur via osmosis, 'dragging' some molecules with it.

Peritoneal dialysis can be divided into two main systems: continuous ambulatory peritoneal dialysis (CAPD) and automated peritoneal dialysis (APD). CAPD originally used glass bottles that had to be disconnected and reconnected. This was superseded by a method using plastic bags, the disadvantage of this being that the patient had a plastic bag continuously attached to him or her. Modern methods rely on a 'two-bag' system with a 'Y' connector; this is associated with lower rates of peritonitis and allows the patient to be free from a bag while not performing fluid exchanges. Typically patients exchange 2 litres of solution four times in 24 hours. The solution consists of sodium, potassium, calcium, magnesium, lactate and bicarbonate. The pH is low (approximately 5.5). The tonicity of the fluid is increased by the addition of either dextrose, icodextrin (a glucose polymer produced from the hydrolysis of starch) or amino acids. APD is not dissimilar but facilitates an automated system whereby fast exchanges can be performed overnight.

Access to the peritoneal cavity is via a semi-permanent catheter, such as the Tenckhoff catheter. This uses a 'double-cuff' method to reduce the chance of infection. Catheters are placed using the Seldinger technique under local anaesthesia, or placed surgically either open or laparoscopically.

Complications associated with peritoneal dialysis may occur at the time of insertion of the catheter, and include visceral injury (bladder and bowel), haemorrhage, leak or infection. General complications of peritoneal dialysis include local infections around the catheter (ultimately tunnel infection). One of the most serious complications is peritonitis. Although potentially fatal, this is often treatable by administering antibiotics intraperitoneally. An uncommon complication is sclerosing peritonitis, where the peritoneum becomes sclerosed and fibrosed. Filtration is greatly affected. The aetiology is ultimately unknown but is associated with long-term peritoneal dialysis usage and recurrent infections. An even rarer complication is sclerosing encapsulating peritonitis, which results in bowel obstruction and intestinal failure.

PREGNANCY

Q. Outline the main maternal renal tract changes during pregnancy.

A. Pregnancy results in generalised relaxation of smooth muscle (due to effects of progesterone), which in addition to mechanical factors such as dextro-rotation of the uterus contribute to the hydronephrosis of pregnancy commencing in weeks 6–10. Hydronephrosis is seen particularly on the right, probably due to the uterine dextro-rotation. By 28 weeks of gestation 90% of pregnant women will have hydronephrosis.

Pregnancy is associated with an increase in renal blood flow (up to 75%) and an approximate 50% increase in GFR. Creatinine clearance is therefore increased in pregnancy, and this is reflected in relatively reduced levels of serum creatinine and urea. Proteinuria increases up to 3 g/day and glycosuria is very common.

Q. A 24-year-old female is referred to you by the obstetricians. The patient is 21 weeks pregnant and has acute left loin to groin pain, a normal serum creatinine and no evidence of sepsis either clinically or biochemically. What imaging modalities are available to you diagnostically?

A. Ultrasound is the least invasive investigation, but is not particularly sensitive in the detection of ureteric calculi, and is obviously operator dependent. Hydronephrosis as mentioned above is not a specific marker for obstruction and stones; however a dilated ureter *below* the iliac vessels may be more suggestive of a stone/obstruction. The presence or absence of ureteric jets may also be helpful.

Intravenous urography (IVU) is feasible, but carries an inherent risk of radiation exposure. This modality is not commonly utilised; however the absolute risk of a (limited) IVU is low. The contrast media itself carries no specific risk to the pregnancy.

Regarding cross-sectional imaging, CT is avoided due to the relatively high radiation risk. MRI safety and pregnancy has not been fully elucidated, however an experienced radiologist may be able to detect the stone as a filling defect within the ureter, and this imaging modality is therefore sometimes used.

Q. The patient mentioned previously is found to have a left lower ureteric stone with moderate hydronephrosis on MRI and ultrasound. How should this patient be treated medically?

A. Close consultation with the obstetric team should be undertaken. Additionally, for those who are unfamiliar with prescribing in pregnancy the British National Formulary should be referred to. Simple analgesia such as paracetamol or co-dydramol may be used, but non-steroidal anti-inflammatory drugs should be avoided (particularly in the third trimester) due to the risk of premature closure of the patent ductus arteriosus in the unborn. Maternal use of opiates such as pethidine and morphine are associated with respiratory depression in the newborn.

Q. What are the options for antibiotic usage in pregnant females with urinary tract infection?

A. Again, the British National Formulary should be referred to. Generally, penicillins or cephalosporins are safe in the non-allergic patient. Antibiotics used commonly in non-pregnant patients may have adverse effects. Trimethoprim's mechanism of action is to interfere with bacterial dihydrofolate reductase and the production of folic acid. There is therefore the possibility of teratogenicity, particularly if used in the first trimester. Quinolones, such as ciprofloxacin, are contraindicated in pregnancy due to the risk of arthropathy in the foetus. Finally gentamicin has been found to lead to an increased risk of auditory or vestibular nerve damage in the second and third trimesters.

OTHER TOPICS

Q. How do you ensure correct site surgery, for example in patients undergoing radical inguinal orchidectomy or nephrectomy?

A. I follow the guidelines, as set out by the National Patient Safety Agency (NPSA) [5], which provides a checklist of steps taken at various times before and at the time of surgery and by various members of the operative team, as follows:

1. The operating surgeon or a member of his team should see the patient at the time of consent and prior to transfer to theatres. The patient's identity should be confirmed, imaging and documentation reviewed and, in conjunction with the patient (prior to any anaesthetic premedications being taken), the site should be marked in indelible pen.
2. Prior to transfer to theatre the ward staff should review the documentation and inspect/confirm the presence of the mark.
3. Once in the anaesthetic room, prior to anaesthesia, a member of the operating team should again review the relevant imaging and documentation and should re-inspect the mark made.
4. In the operating theatre, immediately prior to the start of surgery all theatre staff involved in the case should as part of the World Health Organisation (WHO) checklist confirm the patient's identity, the procedure to be performed and the marking of the correct skin site.

The WHO Surgical Safety Checklist, incorporating the Sign In before induction of anaesthesia, the Time Out before skin incision and the Sign Out before the patient leaves the operating room incorporates steps 3 and 4 in the previous list.

There may be certain circumstances where marking may not be appropriate, such as where it may cause a delay to emergency surgery, bilateral procedures, surgery to teeth or mucus membranes and situations where the laterality of the procedure would be confirmed during surgery. If a patient was to refuse preoperative skin marking, it is recommended that this should be carefully documented in the patient's notes. The correct site surgery checklist should still be followed to ensure that staffs are aware at each stage.

Q. What precautions do you take when inserting a prosthesis (e.g. artificial urinary sphincter, penile)?

A. In my practice, steps to reduce the risk of infection begin prior to the surgical procedure itself. The patient is advised to have Hibiscrub/chlorhexidine washes or shower for 24–48 hours and Naseptin cream. Any other focus of infection, detected pre-operatively is also treated, prior to consideration for surgery. At induction of anaesthesia, prophylactic, broad-spectrum, intravenous antibiotics to cover skin commensals are given. Shaving of the surgical site is performed in theatre prior to surgery. During the procedure itself, I ensure that there is the least number of theatre staff in the operating room as possible, and that their movement in and out of theatre is minimised. I ensure meticulous haemostasis at time of surgery. Antibiotic solutions can be applied to the prosthesis (e.g. gentamicin), once removed from the sterile packaging, as well as irrigating the wound with antibiotics prior to placement. When inserting the prosthesis fresh gloves are applied and a no-touch technique is used. Typically, I will use a small swab to handle the prosthesis. After the procedure antibiotic treatment is continued as per local policy.

Q. How would you manage a patient who begins to have difficulty breathing following scrotal injection of lignocaine, prior to vasectomy under local anaesthetic?

A. Treat this as an emergency as the patient is likely to be having an anaphylactic reaction (allergy to lignocaine). Initially assess the patient and confirm the diagnosis and request a nurse/colleague to fast bleep the 'Arrest' team. While waiting for the emergency team, follow advanced life support principles and check airway, breathing and circulation. Oxygenate patient and gain intravenous access. From the resuscitation trolley give 0.5 mL 1 in 1:1000 adrenaline intramuscularly. Give 200 mg intravenous hydrocortisone and 10 mg intravenous chlorpheniramine (Piriton).

Q. An alcoholic 73-year-old man presents with a prostate-specific antigen (PSA) of 120 and bony metastatic disease. He is commenced on androgen deprivation therapy. Your SpR correctly recognises that he has risk factors for osteoporosis and requests a DEXA scan, but he is not sure how it works. Can you explain?

A. Dual energy x-ray absorptiometry (DEXA) is a highly accurate and reproducible diagnostic test used to estimate bone mineral density (BMD), which relates to risks of osteoporosis and fracture. The total radiation dose is similar to that of a chest x-ray. The patient cannot wear any metal, and the scan must take place at least 24 hours after radionuclide, intravenous contrast or barium studies.

An x-ray arm emitting two distinct, low-energy beams is passed over a supine patient. The bone area can be segmented and the difference in attenuation used to calculate estimated density of bone, fat and lean muscle.

The BMD is compared with sex-matched peak density to give WHO-defined 'T'-score based on standard deviations from normal, used to define osteoporosis as less than −2.5; osteopenia between −1 and −2.5; normal greater than −1. The T score is used in older men and post-menopausal women.

'Z'-scores, based on age, sex and ethnicity-matched data are utilised in children and pre-menopausal patients, again based on standard deviations.

NICE currently recommend assessment of osteoporosis risk using algorithms such as WHO-FRAX or QFracture tool prior to obtaining a DEXA scan.

Q. Can you describe how a CT-PET scan works and how it is carried out?

A. Static anatomical images from a CT scan are combined with the functional images of the positron emission tomography (PET) scan; the combination may have a greater diagnostic yield over either modality alone.

PET is a dynamic nuclear medicine technique. A radiolabelled analogue such as 18F-FDG (18 fluorine-fluorodeoxyglucose) is injected; the analogue and radionuclide accumulates in metabolically active tissue. On decay the radionuclide emits a positron – positively charged electron – which reacts with a local electron to produce diametrically opposite 511 keV photons. This process is known as 'annihilation'. The photons are detected by a PET camera. The scan takes around 30 minutes.

Q. What are the indications for a PET scan in urological malignancy? What different types of scan can you describe?

A. An 18F-FDG PET is recommended in advanced seminomatous germ cell tumours of the testis, where a greater than 3 cm nodal mass persists following chemotherapy, to guide surveillance or active treatment. However, PET is not recommended in non-seminomatous germ cell tumours (NSGCTs) due to high false-negative rates (TE22 study). FDG is excreted by the kidneys and accumulates in the urinary tract, limiting its use in urological malignancy.

In prostate cancer, 11C-choline PET is recommended in cases of biochemical failure after radical radiotherapy or prostatectomy, if salvage treatment is being considered. There is no role for PET in primary staging. Prostate-specific membrane antigen (PSMA) is a glycoprotein that has increased expression in high-grade prostate cancer. There is increasing evidence that 68-Gallium labelled PSMA PET-CT may have improved sensitivity in detecting nodal metastasis over CT imaging alone in preoperative high-risk disease, and also in detecting recurrent disease following radical therapy.

PET CT may be used for assessment of nodal disease in advanced penile cancer. There is no recommendation for PET in the European Association of Urology (EAU) guidelines for renal, non-muscle invasive bladder, upper tract urothelial cancers. Small-scale studies have shown some use in muscle-invasive bladder cancer but this is not part of established treatment protocols.

Q. What do you know about SPECT and its use in urology?

A. A single-photon emission computed tomography (SPECT) scan uses similar principles to a bone scan; however the injected radiopharmaceutical, typically ^{99m}Tc, is utilised and detected by a gamma camera that rotates around the patient, rather than just taking anterior and posterior views. The images are reconstructed and combined with CT images which can be taken concurrently. SPECT has demonstrated some promise in differentiation of oncocytomas in recent trials.

RADIOTHERAPY

Q. A 78-year-old man is diagnosed with Gleason 4 + 4 adenocarcinoma of the prostate in 4/12 cores on TRUS biopsies. Imaging suggests organ-confined disease and after MDT discussion the patient opts to have radical radiotherapy. What is radiation? What is radiotherapy? How does it work?

A. Radiation is the emission of energy in the form of waves or particles. Ionising radiation is radiation that carries enough energy to remove electrons from an atom, causing the atom to become charged or ionised. X-rays and gamma rays are the two types of electromagnetic waves that can ionise atoms. Radiotherapy is the therapeutic use of ionising radiation to treat malignancy. The effects of radiation can be direct, whereby an electron interacts directly with DNA, or indirect, whereby an electron interacts with water molecules to produce a hydroxyl radical which in turn causes damage to DNA. The latter of these is the major process in therapeutic radiation.

Q. How is radiation delivered? What kind of machines do you know?

A. Radiation is most commonly delivered either from a linear accelerator or by the insertion of internal radiation sources (brachytherapy). Radiation that is delivered by a linear accelerator is often referred to as external beam radiotherapy. This can be delivered using an individual beam, which is often simple palliative radiotherapy, or from several directions at the target tissue. The ability to deliver high-dose radiation via this technique is limited by damage caused to healthy adjacent tissues. In three-dimensional conformal radiation therapy the profile of each radiation beam is shaped to the target tissue reducing damage to normal surrounding tissue and enabling delivery of higher doses of radiation. Intensity modulated radiation therapy (IMRT) enables delivery of highly conformal radiation doses to specific target tissues. This is achieved by regulating the intensity of the radiation beam and enables improved targeting of tumours with less side effects and better treatment outcomes. By better avoiding normal tissues, higher doses of radiation can be given to the target increasing the chance of cure.

Q. What is fractionation? What is the rationale behind it?

A. Fractionation is the process by which the total dose of radiation is divided into a number of fractions to optimise the desired effects to cancer cells, while sparing adjacent normal tissues. This confers a number of benefits:

1. Repair of sub-lethal damage between dose fractionations which is usually more effective in non-proliferating cells.
2. Repopulation of normal cells that divide rapidly, such as bowel.
3. Fractionation enables reoxygenation; hypoxic cells are relatively radioresistant and tumours may be acutely or chronically hypoxic.
4. Reassortment. The effects of radiotherapy are most effective in cells about to divide (G2 or M phases of the cell cycle). Cells in the S phase are relatively radioresistant. With reapplication of radiotherapy at time intervals, cells redistribute themselves over all phases of the cell cycle.

Q. What other types of radiotherapy can be encountered in urology?

A. Other types of radiotherapy include brachytherapy and systemic radiotherapy.

Brachytherapy is a form of radiotherapy, used to treat organ-confined prostate cancer, although it is not recommended as monotherapy for high-risk prostate cancer. It involves the insertion of targeted radioactive pellets directly into the prostate gland via the perineum. In low-dose brachytherapy (LDR) permanent Iodine-125 or Palladium-103 seeds are inserted under ultrasound guidance, which deliver radiation over weeks or months. Patients should be counselled to avoid close contact with pregnant women or children for 3 months, and to use condoms for intercourse for the first few weeks after implantation.

In HDR brachytherapy iridium-192 seeds are temporarily inserted, delivering radiation in minutes. In contrast with LDR, there are no radiation protection issues. HDR brachytherapy may be given in combination with external beam radiation therapy for men with intermediate- and high-risk organ-confined prostate cancer.

Strontium-99 can be injected systemically to deliver systemic radiation. It is metabolised in a similar fashion to calcium and it therefore preferentially targets metabolically active areas of bone. In patients with metastatic prostate cancer this has been shown to have a benefit in the palliation of painful bony lesions.

REFERENCES

1. Tolley D. Ureteric stents, far from ideal. *The Lancet* 2000; 356: 872–873.
2. Medtronic. http://www.valleylab.com/education/poes/index.html
3. Medicines and Healthcare products Regulatory Agency. http://webarchive.nationalarchives.gov.uk/20141204111618/http://www.mhra.gov.uk/home/groups/dts-bi/documents/websiteresources/con2023451.pdf
4. The British Association of Urological Surgeons. https://www.baus.org.uk/patients/information_leaflets/
5. National Patient Safety Agency and Royal College of Surgeons of England. National Patient Safety Alert 06. Joint Commission on Accreditation of Healthcare Organizations, April 2003; 2. www.npsa.nhs.uk

CHAPTER 15
TNM CLASSIFICATION FOR UROLOGICAL CANCERS

Herman S Fernando

Content

Tables 15.1 through to 15.7 describe the latest TNM staging system for individual urological cancers.

Table 15.1 TNM (8th edition) staging of bladder cancer

Tx	Primary tumour cannot be assessed
Ta	Non-invasive papillary carcinoma
Tis	Carcinoma *in situ*: 'flat tumour'
T1	Tumour invades subepithelial connective tissue
T2	
	T2a: Tumour invades superficial muscularis propria (inner half)
	T2b: Tumour invades deep muscularis propria (outer half)
T3	
	T3a: Tumour invades perivesical tissue microscopically
	T3b: Tumour invades perivesical tissue macroscopically (extravesical mass)
T4	
	T4a: Tumour invades prostate stroma, seminal vesicles, uterus or vagina
	T4b: Tumour invades pelvic wall or abdominal wall
Nx	Regional lymph nodes cannot be assessed
N0	No regional lymph node metastasis
N1	Metastasis in a single lymph node in true pelvis (hypogastric, obturator, external iliac or presacral)
N2	Metastasis in multiple lymph nodes in true pelvis (hypogastric, obturator, external iliac or presacral)
N3	Metastasis in common iliac lymph node(s)
Mx	Distant metastasis cannot be assessed
M0	No distant metastasis
M1	M1a: Non-regional lymph nodes
	M1b: Other distant metastases

Table 15.2 TNM (8th edition) classification for upper tract urothelial carcinoma

Tx	Primary tumour cannot be assessed
T0	No evidence of primary tumour
Ta	Non-invasive papillary carcinoma
Tis	Carcinoma *in situ*
T1	Invades subepithelial connective tissue
T2	Tumour invades muscularis propria
T3	Renal pelvis – Tumour invades beyond muscularis into peripelvic fat or renal parenchyma Ureter – Tumour invades beyond muscularis into periureteric fat
T4	Tumour invades into adjacent organs or through kidney into perinephric fat
Nx	Regional lymph nodes cannot be assessed
N0	No regional lymph node metastasis
N1	Metastasis in a single lymph node 2 cm or less in the greatest dimension
N2	Metastasis in a single lymph node more than 2 cm, or multiple lymph nodes
Mx	Distant metastasis not assessed
M0	No distant metastasis
M1	Distant metastasis

Table 15.3 TNM (8th edition) classification for penile cancer (note that the *pathological* classification is given here as candidates often have difficulty with this)

TX	Primary tumour cannot be assessed
T0	No evidence of primary tumour
Tis	Carcinoma *in situ* (penile intraepithelial neoplasia [PeIN])
Ta	Non-invasive localised squamous cell carcinoma/non-invasive verrucous carcinoma (not associated with destructive invasion)
T1	Tumour invades subepithelial connective tissue (lamina propria)
	T1a: Tumour invades subepithelial connective tissue without perineural or lymphovascular invasion and is not poorly differentiated or undifferentiated (T1G1-2)
	T1b: Tumour invades subepithelial connective tissue with perineural or lymphovascular invasion or is poorly differentiated or undifferentiated (T1G3-4)
T2	Tumour invades corpus spongiosum with or without invasion of the urethra
T3	Tumour invades corpus cavernosum (including tunica albuginea) with or without invasion of the urethra
T4	Tumour invades other adjacent structures (scrotum, prostate, bone)
NX	Regional lymph nodes cannot be assessed
N0	No lymph node metastasis
pN1	Metastasis in one or two unilateral inguinal lymph nodes, but without extra-nodal extension
pN2	Metastasis in three or more *unilateral* inguinal lymph nodes without extra-nodal extension, *or*, any number of *bilateral* positive inguinal lymph nodes without extra-nodal extension
pN3	Metastasis to any number of inguinal lymph nodes with extra-nodal extension, or, metastasis to pelvic lymph nodes
M0	No distant metastases
M1	Distant metastases

Table 15.4 TNM (8th edition) classification for renal cancer

Tx	Primary tumour cannot be assessed
T0	No evidence of primary tumour
T1	Tumour <7 cm in greatest dimension, limited to the kidney
	T1a: Tumour ≤4 cm in greatest dimension, limited to the kidney
	T1b: Tumour >4 cm but ≤7 cm in greatest dimension
T2	Tumour >7 cm in greatest dimension, limited to the kidney
	T2a: Tumour >7 cm but ≤10 cm in greatest dimension
	T2b: Tumour >10 cm limited to the kidney
T3	Tumour extends into major veins or perinephric tissues but not into the ipsilateral adrenal gland and not beyond Gerota's fascia
	T3a: Tumour extends into the renal vein or its segmental branches, or tumour invades the pelvi-calyceal system or tumour invades perirenal and/or renal sinus fat (peripelvic fat) but not beyond Gerota's fascia
	T3b: Tumour extends into the vena cava (VC) below the diaphragm
	T3c: Tumour extends into vena cava above the diaphragm or invades the wall of the vena cava
T4	Tumour invades beyond Gerota's fascia (including contiguous extension into the ipsilateral adrenal gland)
Nx	Regional LNs cannot be assessed
N0	No regional LN metastasis
N1	Metastasis in regional LN
M0	No distant metastasis
M1	Distant metastasis

Table 15.5 TNM (8th edition) classification for prostate cancer

TX	Primary tumour cannot be assessed
T0	No evidence of primary tumour
T1	Clinically inapparent tumour not palpable or visible by imaging
	T1a: Tumour incidental histological finding in 5% or less of tissue resected
	T1b: Tumour incidental histological finding in more than 5% of tissue resected
	T1c: Tumour identified by needle biopsy (e.g. because of elevated prostate-specific antigen level)
T2	Tumour that is palpable and confined within the prostate
	T2a: Tumour involves one-half of one lobe or less
	T2b: Tumour involves more than half of one lobe, but not both lobes
	T2c: Tumour involves both lobes
T3	Tumour extends through the prostatic capsule
	T3a: Extraprostatic extension (unilateral or bilateral) including microscopic bladder neck involvement
	T3b: Tumour invades seminal vesicle(s)
T4	Tumour is fixed or invades adjacent structures other than seminal vesicles: external sphincter, rectum, levator muscles, and/or pelvic wall
Nx	Regional lymph nodes cannot be assessed
N0	No regional lymph node metastasis
N1	Regional lymph node metastasis
Mx	Distant metastasis cannot be assessed
M0	No distant metastasis

(Continued)

Table 15.5 (*Continued*) TNM (8th edition) classification for prostate cancer

M1	Distant metastasis
	M1a: Non-regional lymph node(s)
	M1b: Bone(s)
	M1c: Other site(s)

Table 15.6 TNM (8th edition) classification for testicular cancer

pTX	Primary tumour cannot be assessed
pT0	No evidence of primary tumour (e.g. histological scar in testis)
pTis	Intratubular germ cell neoplasia (testicular intraepithelial neoplasia)
pT1	Tumour limited to testis and epididymis without vascular/lymphatic invasion; tumour may invade tunica albuginea but not tunica vaginalis
pT2	Tumour limited to testis and epididymis with vascular/lymphatic invasion, or tumour extending through tunica albuginea with involvement of tunica vaginalis
pT3	Tumour invades spermatic cord with or without vascular/lymphatic invasion
pT4	Tumour invades scrotum with or without vascular/lymphatic invasion
NX	Regional lymph nodes cannot be assessed
N0	No regional lymph node metastasis
N1	Metastasis with a lymph node mass 2 cm or less in greatest dimension or multiple lymph nodes, none more than 2 cm in greatest dimension
N2	Metastasis with a lymph node mass more than 2 cm but not more than 5 cm in greatest dimension, or multiple lymph nodes, any one mass more than 2 cm but not more than 5 cm in greatest dimension
N3	Metastasis with a lymph node mass more than 5 cm in greatest dimension
MX	Distant metastasis cannot be assessed
M0	No distant metastasis
M1	Distant metastasis
	M1a: Non-regional lymph node(s) or lung
	M1b: Other sites
SX	Serum marker studies not available or not performed
S0	Serum marker study levels within normal limits

	LDH (U/L)	hCG (mIU/mL)	AFP (ng/mL)
S1	$<1.5 \times N$ and	<5,000 and	<1,000
S2	$1.5–10 \times N$ or	5,000–50,000 or	1,000–10,000
S3	$>10 \times N$ or	>50,000 or	>10,000

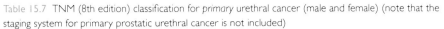

Table 15.7 TNM (8th edition) classification for *primary* urethral cancer (male and female) (note that the staging system for primary prostatic urethral cancer is not included)

Tx	Primary tumour cannot be assessed
Tis	Carcinoma *in situ*
T0	No evidence of primary tumour
Ta	Non-invasive papillary, polypoid or verrucous carcinoma
T1	Tumour invades subepithelial connective tissue
T2	Tumour invades any of the following structures: corpus spongiosum, prostate, peri-urethral muscle
T3	Tumour invades any of the following structures: corpus cavernosum, invasion beyond prostatic capsule, anterior vaginal wall, bladder neck
T4	Tumour invades other adjacent organs (bladder proper, rectum)
Nx	Regional lymph nodes cannot be assessed
N0	No regional lymph-node metastasis
N1	Metastasis in a single lymph node
N2	Metastasis in multiple nodes
Mx	Distant metastasis cannot be assessed
M0	No distant metastasis
M1	Distant metastasis

FURTHER READING

1. Brierley JD et al. *The TNM Classification of Malignant Tumours*, 8th edn. 2017. http://www.uicc.org/resources/tnm/publications-resources

CHAPTER 16
COMMONLY ASKED VIVA QUESTIONS

Contents

ONCOLOGY

1. How would you manage a patient who has a prostate-specific antigen (PSA) of 200 and a positive bone scan with a biopsy proving Gleason 8 adenocarcinoma of the prostate?
2. How would you explain to a GP as to how to start LHRH analogue treatment?
3. When can you give the first luteinizing hormone-releasing hormone (LHRH) injection?
4. How would you manage bone pain in metastatic prostate cancer?
5. What are the 2-week guidelines for referral of suspected malignancy?
6. How would you investigate a 50-year-old male with painless haematuria?
7. How would you investigate a 3 cm mass in the kidney detected on renal ultrasound scan (USS)?
8. How would you manage a newly diagnosed pT1G3 tumour in the bladder?
9. What if the patient with a pT1G3 bladder tumour also has carcinoma *in situ* (CIS)?
10. What is the TNM classification for bladder cancer?
11. Draw the transverse appearance of the prostate as it would appear on transrectal ultrasound scan (TRUSS).
12. Discuss the role of interferon-α in the treatment of renal cell cancer (RCC).
13. What are the complications of radical prostatectomy?
14. What are the complications of radiotherapy for carcinoma of the prostate?
15. What are the risks of ureterolysis?
16. What is the role of finasteride in prostate cancer prevention?
17. How would you investigate a female patient with painless haematuria who is on methotrexate treatment?
18. How do you administer Mitomycin C?
19. Tell me about the Bosniak classification.
20. Describe the technique of TRUSS and prostate biopsy.
21. What are Partin's tables?
22. Tell me about prostate brachytherapy.
23. What happens to PSA levels after radiotherapy treatment?
24. What is the aetiology of carcinoma of the bladder?

25. What is an acceptable glomerular filtration rate (GFR) prior to undergoing chemotherapy?
26. What is accelerated MVAC?
27. How common is cord compression in advanced carcinoma of the prostate?
28. What is the half-life of PSA?
29. What is the significance of a high PSA nadir following LHRH analogue treatment?
30. What chemotherapy can be used in advanced prostate cancer?
31. Tell me about von Hippel–Lindau (VHL).
32. What is the incidence of upper tract transitional cell carcinoma (TCC)? How often would you image the upper tracts in a patient with a history of bladder cancer?
33. How would you manage a T3b RCC? What is the prognosis?
34. A 37-week pregnant woman presents with haematuria. What would be the investigation and treatment?
35. A male patient aged 73 presents with lower urinary tract symptoms (LUTS) and is noted to have a PSA of 140 and an obvious prostate cancer on digital rectal examination (DRE). How would you discuss the findings with the patient? How would you manage this patient?
36. When would you start hormone treatment in the patient in the previous question? Why does a flare response occur? What are the side effects of LHRH analogues? How do you avoid osteoporosis?
37. How many cores should you take on a TRUSS biopsy of the prostate? What is the benefit of increasing the number of cores?
38. What is PSA density, PSA velocity, Free:total PSA?
39. Classify PIN. What is the incidence of CaP and PIN. What would you do if PIN was found on a prostate biopsy?
40. What are the different types of testicular tumour?
41. How would you counsel a patient regarding orchidectomy?
42. How many cycles of chemotherapy are used in seminoma and teratoma?
43. A 40-year-old man has renal mass diagnosed. What are the indications for partial and radical nephrectomy?
44. What are the surgical approaches to the kidney?
45. What are the indications for nephron-sparing surgery?
46. How would you investigate a caval thrombus?
47. A patient presents with a testicular tumour, does it make any difference performing orchidectomy through the scrotum or inguinal region?
48. How would you follow up a patient with a T1b renal cell carcinoma post-operatively?
49. What is the role of neoadjuvant chemotherapy in carcinoma of the bladder?
50. Which investigations would you perform before giving cisplatin therapy?
51. What are the autocrine mechanisms of carcinogenesis?
52. What is the management of a male aged 65 with a PSA of 5?
53. What do you understand by the term *age-related PSA*?
54. How would you counsel a patient for biopsy of the prostate?
55. Discuss the significance of a negative prostate biopsy in a patient with a PSA of 5.
56. What is a tumour suppressor gene?
57. What is the impact on the management of prostate cancer with seminal vesicle involvement?
58. What are the indications for adjuvant treatment post radical prostatectomy?
59. What do you know about anti-angiogenic therapy for cancer and monoclonal antibodies for cancer?
60. What are the British Association of Urological Surgeons (BAUS) guidelines for metastatic prostate cancer?
61. What is the PRO7 trial?
62. What do you know about zoledronic acid? What is the evidence for the use of zoledronic acid and what are the complications?

63. How would you manage adenocarcinoma at the dome of the bladder?
64. What is the management of urachal carcinoma? The margins are positive, what further treatment is required?
65. What do you know about familial prostate cancer? What is the relevance of breast cancer?
66. How does the androgen receptor work?
67. What is the management of keratinizing squamous cell metaplasia? What is the risk of progressing to SCC?
68. What is malakoplakia of the bladder?
69. What is the management of a 6 cm angiomyolipoma?
70. What is the evidence for performing an extended lymphadenectomy for invasive bladder cancer?
71. What is the role of neoadjuvant chemotherapy for invasive bladder cancer?
72. What is an oncogene? How does ras oncogene cause a malignant phenotype?
73. What is a mutation?
74. What are the indications for a partial nephrectomy? How do you perform a partial nephrectomy? What is the warm ischaemia time?
75. What is the management of metastatic renal cancer?
76. What is the literature for adjuvant treatment of renal cancer?
77. What is the management of classical seminoma?
78. What is the toxicity of bleomycin, etoposide and cisplatin (BEP)?
79. What is a tumour suppressor gene?
80. What is the evidence for post-operative intravesical Mitomycin C?
81. What percentage of people with a normal PSA has underlying prostate cancer?
82. What is the pickup rate of prostate biopsy?
83. Tell me about the European screening program for prostate cancer.
84. What are the predisposing conditions for carcinoma of the penis? What are the metastatic sites?

PAEDIATRIC UROLOGY

1. What is the classification of vesico-ureteric reflux (VUR)?
2. What associated abnormalities are found with VUR?
3. How would you manage grade III VUR?
4. How do you measure GFR?
5. How do you do a renogram?
6. Describe how you would perform an orchidopexy.
7. What is the management of an undescended testicle?
8. How do you do a Whitaker test?
9. What are the indications and how would you do a pyeloplasty?
10. How does isotope renography work?
11. What are the phases in a renogram? How long do you wait before scanning?
12. What are the symptoms of pelviureteric junction (PUJ) obstruction? Which renogram would you perform? What are the treatment options?
13. What is the incidence of undescended testes?
14. Describe the Fowler-Stephens procedure.
15. What is the differential diagnosis of the acute scrotum?
16. What is the management of a 2-year-old with cryptorchidism?
17. Describe the descent of the testes.
18. What is the natural history of cryptorchidism?
19. What is the fate of undescended testes?
20. What about bilateral undescended testes?

21. A 3-year-old girl with a first urinary tract infection (UTI) has been treated and completely recovers. When would you organise the DMSA? If photopenic areas are found what would you do?
22. What prophylactic antibiotic would you use in the above case?
23. Define reflux and what classification is used.
24. Draw me the glomerulus. What happens to the GFR when the efferent and afferent arterioles constrict?
25. What is the presentation of ureteroceles? What are the treatment and complications?
26. How do you do a laparoscopic pyeloplasty?
27. What other methods of pyeloplasty do you know?

ANDROLOGY

1. What are the side effects of sildenafil?
2. What are the contraindications for sildenafil?
3. Draw the nitric oxide/cyclic guanosine monophosphate (NO/cGMP) pathway.
4. What are the differences between high- and low-flow priapism?
5. How would you manage a penile fracture which presents within 24 hours?
6. A man wants to undergo a vasectomy. How would you counsel him?
7. What would you do if persistent sperm are seen following a vasectomy?
8. How do you assess a man with erectile dysfunction (ED)? What tests would you ask for?
9. What are the side effects of a PDE-5 inhibitor?
10. What is the incidence of chronic scrotal pain post vasectomy?
11. Tell me about haemospermia.
12. What are the indications of varicocele repair in adolescent males?
13. What is the evidence that varicocele repair improves semen parameters?
14. What are the approaches available for varicocele repair?
15. Who would you scan the upper tracts in when presented with a varicocele?
16. What is the risk of ED in a patient presenting with a fractured penis?
17. How would you treat high-flow priapism?
18. Tell me about Peyronie's disease.
19. Tell me about the testosterone pathway.
20. How is testosterone released from the adrenals?
21. What is testosterone bound to?
22. What happens to testosterone during the day?
23. When should a testosterone assay be performed?
24. How is testosterone converted to dihydrotestosterone (DHT)?
25. What is the rate of infection of a penile prosthesis?
26. What is the risk of priapism for someone using intracavernosal prostaglandin?
27. Classify priapism. What are the investigations and treatment?
28. What precautions would you take in order to minimise the risk of infection when inserting a penile prosthesis?
29. Describe the Lue procedure for the management of Peyronie's disease.
30. Anatomically describe a hydrocele.

STONES AND UTI

1. How would you manage a 1.5 cm lower pole calyx stone?
2. What are the contraindications for extracorporeal shock wave lithotripsy (ESWL)?

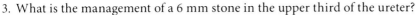

3. What is the management of a 6 mm stone in the upper third of the ureter?
4. Draw an obstructed renogram curve.
5. What is Homsy's sign?
6. What is the incidence of asymptomatic bacteriuria in pregnancy?
7. What is the incidence of pyelonephritis in pregnancy?
8. Which antibiotics are contraindicated in pregnancy?
9. How do you define *urinary tract infection*?
10. Describe the concept of bacterial adherence.
11. Where did the 10^5 CFU definition arise from?
12. What is the epidemiology of urinary tract calculi?
13. What is the composition of stones and their frequency?
14. What is the management of a 3 mm distal ureteric stone?
15. What is the role of α-blockers in ureteric stones?
16. What is the management of first-time stone formers?
17. How would you do a 24 urine analysis in a recurrent stone former?
18. What is the effect of calcium restriction on stone disease?
19. What are the causes of stone formation? How would you treat hypercalcaemia?
20. What is the management of a child with a large distal ureteric stone?
21. What analgesia would you use for ESWL? What sort of machine do you use in your department?
22. How do you locate the stone?
23. Which energy level do you start at?
24. What are the contraindications to performing an intravenous urography (IVU)?
25. What conditions cause calcified cysts in the kidney?
26. What are virulence factors?
27. What is the dosing regime for gentamicin?
28. How does gentamicin work?
29. Describe the various lithotriptors and how they work.
30. What sort of antibiotic is trimethoprim?
31. Define *recurrent UTI*.
32. What are the risk factors for UTI? What investigations would you do?
33. How would urine dipstick help in UTI?
34. What defences against *Escherichia coli* are there?
35. What is the role of *Lactobacillus* in preventing *E. coli* colonisation?
36. What does P-fimbriae attach to?
37. What is the Stamey test?
38. What is the classification of prostatitis?
39. How do you treat prostatitis medically?
40. What are the risks of percutaneous nephrolithotomy (PCNL)?
41. What is the management of post-PCNL bleeding via the nephrostomy?
42. What is the prevalence of UTI before and after starting sexual activity?

FEMALE AND RECONSTRUCTIVE UROLOGY AND BLADDER DYSFUNCTION

1. How would you treat interstitial cystitis?
2. How would you investigate a female with incontinence?
3. How would you manage a 20-year-old female with urgency and frequency?
4. How does tolterodine XL work as extended release?

5. What are the problems associated with ileocystoplasty?
6. How would you manage chronic pelvic pain syndrome?
7. A 55-year-old female with multiple sclerosis is bed bound with a problematic catheter. What is the investigation and management?
8. How do you do a bladder neck closure?
9. What is Ulmstein's integral theory of continence?
10. What is Delancy's hammock theory?
11. What are the complications of tension-free vaginal tape (TVT) and transobturator tape (TOT)?
12. What do you understand by types I and III incontinence?
13. How does BOTOX work in the bladder and what are the risks?
14. What changes occur in the urinary tract during pregnancy?
15. How would you manage loin pain and hydronephrosis in a 35/40 pregnant woman?
16. What is Fowler's syndrome?
17. Draw the neurophysiology of micturition.
18. What are the complications of an ileal conduit?
19. What are the principles of reservoir reconstruction?
20. What is Laplace's law?
21. How do you perform a video cystogram?
22. What are the causes of painful urinary retention in a 25-year-old woman?
23. What are the urodynamic findings in a patient with multiple sclerosis?
24. What are the risk factors for upper tract deterioration in a neurogenic bladder?
25. What is the management of overactive bladder (OAB) in MS?
26. How do you do a Boari flap and Psoas hitch?
27. What are the causes of a urethral stricture?
28. What are the narrowest parts of the urethra?
29. How do you deal with a post-transurethral resection (TUR) bulbar stricture?
30. What is the value of urethrography in stricture disease?
31. What do you understand about interstitial cystitis?
32. How do you diagnose interstitial cystitis?
33. What is a Koch pouch?
34. What is a Mainz 2 pouch?
35. What are the provocative manoeuvres during urodynamics?
36. What is the stop test?
37. What is PSA? What causes PSA elevation?
38. How do you consent for TRUSS and what are the side effects?
39. What is the definition of detrusor instability? What is the medical and surgical treatment?
40. How many times should a patient cough during urodynamic evaluation?
41. Which types of neobladder do you know using small bowel?
42. How does trospium chloride work?
43. What types of BOTOX are there?
44. How many types of detrusor sphincter dyssynergia (DSD) are there?
45. How do you diagnose a urethral diverticulum?
46. Why does a urethral stricture give a flat curve?
47. What is the evidence for intermittent self-catheterisation (ISC) in urethral stricture management?
48. What is the significance of mast cells in a biopsy from a patient with interstitial cystitis?
49. How is interstitial cystitis classified? What are the disadvantages for this classification?
50. How would you do a colposuspension?
51. Which antibiotic prophylaxis would you use in a colposuspension?

52. How would you manage a pelvic haematoma post colposuspension?
53. What are the risks of nephrostomy insertion in a pregnant female?
54. Why do you detubularise the ileum in pouch formation?
55. What end fill pressure on urodynamics would be significant for a neuropath with reduced compliance?
56. What is the Mitrofanoff principle?
57. What are the metabolic consequences of a continent pouch? What happens to serum calcium?
58. What is the risk of UTI in clean intermittent self-catheterisation (CISC)?
59. How common is bacteriuria in patients with an ileal conduit?
60. What is the most common urethral stricture?
61. Where are strictures most commonly located post transurethral resection of the prostate (TURP) and why?
62. What is the calibre of the urethra?
63. Draw a picture of the bulbar urethra and corpus spongiosum.
64. What makes bladder muscle contract?
65. Where is the sacral micturition centre?
66. How do sympathetic fibres get to the bladder?
67. What is the nerve supply and structure of the urethral sphincter?
68. How do the sphincter arrangements differ in females?
69. What sensations can you feel in the bladder?
70. What is DSD? Where is the site of the lesion?
71. Which sensory neurotransmitters are in the bladder?
72. What injuries would you get with an open book pelvic fracture?
73. Explain a urethral distraction defect.
74. Draw a picture of the micturition pathway.
75. Who described the pontine micturition center?
76. Where is the social control of voiding?
77. What happens to micturition with lesions above pons and below the pons?

UROLOGICAL EMERGENCIES

1. How would you take your SHO through insertion of a suprapubic catheter?
2. What are the advantages of a suprapubic catheter over a urethral catheter?
3. You are called to the gynaecology ward to see a patient who is 3 days post-hysterectomy and has clear fluid draining vaginally. What would you do?
4. What would you do with a 12-year-old boy with an acutely painful scrotum?
5. How would you classify acute scrotum diagnosis according to age groups?
6. How would you diagnose idiopathic scrotal oedema?
7. How would you manage a ureteric injury which occurs during aneurysm repair?
8. A patient arrives having been involved in a road traffic accident and presents with haematuria. What is the subsequent management?
9. How would you perform a urethrogram in a patient with a fractured pelvis?
10. What is the management of a patient with pelvic fracture and urethral and bladder trauma?
11. Classify renal trauma.
12. What is shock?
13. What is the relationship between the uterine artery and ureter?
14. What is the definition of systemic inflammatory response syndrome (SIRS)? What is septic shock? What are the clinical features of shock?

TECHNOLOGY IN UROLOGY

1. What types of contrast media do you know?
2. What do we worry about with contrast media?
3. What are the components of a cystoscope?
4. How is a cystoscope constructed?
5. What is the physics behind the Hopkins' lens system?
6. What does 'LASER' stand for?
7. What are the settings for your diathermy machine when performing a TURP?
8. Draw the circuit diagram for diathermy.
9. Show the waveform for diathermy.
10. Tell me about green light laser.
11. What are the advantages and disadvantages of laser?
12. How do you perform sphincter electromyography (EMG)?
13. How would you do a flexible cystoscopy?
14. Which local anaesthetic agent would you use?
15. What angle lens is used in a flexible cystoscope?
16. What is a dual energy x-ray absorptiometry (DEXA) scan?

BENIGN PROSTATIC ENLARGEMENT

1. What is the meaning of F (in terms of catheter size)?
2. What is the role of urodynamics in men?
3. How would you set up a LUTS clinic?
4. How many uroflows would you do in each patient in a LUTS clinic?
5. What do you understand by a frequency-volume chart?
6. How can you improve patient compliance with a frequency-volume chart?
7. Draw a uroflow showing normal male flow and one showing a male with BPH.
8. What are the indications for TURP?
9. How would you manage a diabetic patient undergoing TURP post-operatively?
10. What are the pharmacotherapies used in BPH?
11. How would you manage a patient who has been on combination treatment and presents with retention?
12. How would you design a trial of laser prostate versus standard TURP?
13. What are the complication rates for TURP?
14. What do you know about warfarin?
15. A patient presents with haematuria and is on warfarin and has bleeding secondary to BPH. What would you do?
16. What are the surgical treatments for BPH?
17. What is on the International Prostate Symptom Score (IPSS) sheet?
18. What is the disadvantage of the IPSS?
19. Tell me about the concept of uroselectivity in α-blockers.
20. Tell me about MTOPS. What are your recommendations for combination therapy?
21. How do 5-α-reductase inhibitors work? What is the benefit of dutasteride?
22. Regarding BPH, what are the messages from MTOPS?
23. What is the difference between dutasteride and finasteride?
24. What are the absolute indications for surgery?
25. What is IPSS? How is it used?
26. What are the complications of bladder outflow obstruction?

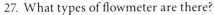

27. What types of flowmeter are there?
28. How do you interpret a flow rate?
29. How do you work out the voided volume on a flow rate?
30. What is the mortality from TURP?
31. Tell me about laser prostatectomy.
32. What is the bladder outflow obstruction index?
33. What irrigation fluid do you use during a TURP?
34. Why use 1.5% glycine and not 3%?
35. Tell me about TUR syndrome.
36. How can you monitor for TUR syndrome during surgery?
37. What are the risk factors for acute urinary retention?
38. What are the treatment options for men with LUTS?
39. Tell me about the BAUS guidelines for LUTS.
40. How do you manage patients with acute urinary retention (AUR)?
41. What is the efficacy of α-blockers prior to undergoing a trial without catheter?
42. What is the significance of a residual volume during AUR?
43. Tell me about chronic retention.
44. What is the physiological basis of post-obstructive diuresis. Distinguish between pathological and physiological diuresis.
45. Draw the zones of the prostate gland.
46. Where does BPH originate?
47. Describe the embryology of the prostate.
48. How would you consent for a TURP?
49. Tell me about the national prostatectomy audit.
50. What is nocturnal polyuria?

INDEX

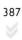

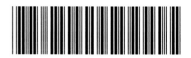